DICTIONARY OF REHABILITATION

Myron G. Eisenberg, Ph.D., is Chief of the Psychology Service at the Department of Veterans Affairs Medical Center in Hampton, Virginia, and is Associate Professor of both Physical Medicine and Rehabilitation and of Psychiatry and Behavioral Sciences at Eastern Virginia Medical School, Norfolk, Virginia. He obtained his doctorate from Northwestern University and received postdoctoral training at the University of Toronto's Clarke Institute. Dr. Eisenberg has published extensively in the area of rehabilitation, holds editorial board positions on several journals, serves as Editor of *Rehabilitation Psychology* and as Editor of the *Key Words* book series for rehabilitation, and is a member of several national task forces charged with investigating various quality-of-life issues of importance to persons with chronic disabling conditions. A Fellow and Past President of the American Psychological Association's Division of Rehabilitation Psychology, he is actively involved in the development of standards that will establish a more effective and consistent basis for evaluating the performance of individual rehabilitation service providers.

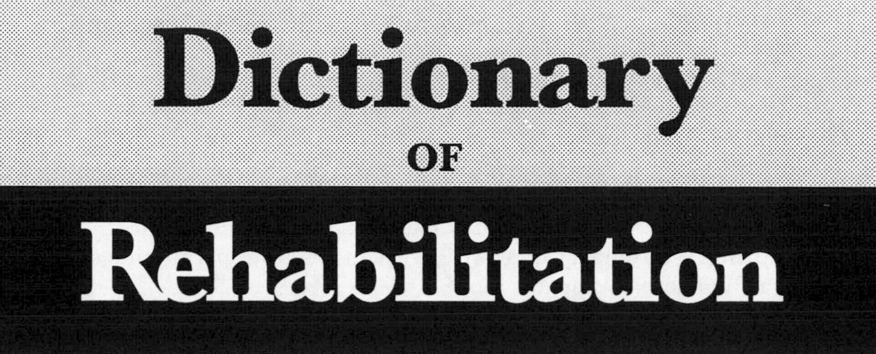

Myron G. Eisenberg, PhD

With Section III prepared by Timothy J. Meline, PhD

SPRINGER PUBLISHING COMPANY

This volume is based on the *Dictionary of Rehabilitation Medicine* by Herman L. Kamenetz, MD, published by the Springer Publishing Company in 1983.

Springer Publishing Company, Inc.
536 Broadway
New York, NY 10012

Cover design by Tom Yabut
Production Editor: Pam Lankas

95 96 97 98 99 / 5 4 3 2 1

Library of Congress Cataloging-in-Publication Data

Dictionary of rehabilitation / M.G. Eisenberg, editor
p. cm.
Includes bibliographical references and index.
ISBN 0-8261-8890-7
1. Medical rehabilitation—Dictionaries. I. Eisenberg, Myron G.
RM930.D455 1955
617'.0'03—dc20 94-48400
CIP

Printed in the United States of America

To my wife, Ellen, and our daughter, Toby

M.G.E.

Contents

Preface

This text, a revision of Kamenetz's *Dictionary of Rehabilitation Medicine* (1983), represents a significant departure from the original book in at least three ways. First, the present text's focus has been enlarged from a primarily medical emphasis to a multidisciplinary perspective. This was done in order to more accurately reflect an expanded definition of the rehabilitation process and to acknowledge the critical role played in this process by allied disciplines. Although the original *Dictionary* did include some terms common to the practice of psychology and social work, it overrepresented the vocabulary specific to the discipline of rehabilitation medicine. By doing so it appeared to emphasize the importance of that field over others. This new multidisciplinary emphasis can be found in the book's changed title.

A second difference between the Kamenetz text and this one is its updating of terminology. This was done to ensure accurate representation of current patterns of language usage.

The third way by which the present text differs from the original *Dictionary* is through its inclusion of two new sections. The first describes selected organizations and research centers and institutions that deal with rehabilitation-related issues. The second section, authored by Timothy Meline, is a comprehensive list of health care abbreviations and symbols commonly used in rehabilitation settings. The reader is referred to "Scope and Arrangement" for additional information about the text's organization and structure.

The rapid expansion and accumulation of knowledge required in the health sciences, coupled with a decrease in the time available to acquire this knowledge, has created the need for a new dictionary of terminology that helps the reader to quickly and easily assimilate this information. The present text is the only book currently available that presents a compilation of terms that comprise the core of information commonly used in describing and explaining the rehabilitation process. The *Dictionary of Rehabilitation* was developed to meet a need by presenting a brief and "to the point" explanation of the distinctive language of the rehabilitation practitioner. For extended discussions of certain critical words and terms, the reader is referred to other texts, including *Key Words in Psychosocial Rehabilitation* (Springer Publishing Company, 1994) and *Key Words in Physical Rehabilitation* (Springer Publishing Company, 1995).

The more than 3,500-word vocabulary and 2,400 abbreviations and symbols included in the *Dictionary of Rehabilitation* were selected with the intended audience of students of the rehabilitation process in mind. An attempt to avoid arbitrary inclusions and exclusions was made by conducting an extensive review of the current professional literature and through consultation with other rehabilitation specialists. To reflect contemporary developments, terms that were only recently introduced but are gaining wide acceptance have been included. A limited number of obsolete terms were retained for historical perspective.

Special attention has been given to the vocabulary used in the definition. Each definition was developed to be as simply, clearly, and concisely worded as possible. Efforts were made not to begin the definition with a broad conceptual statement, and whenever possible, the use of words that would require additional reference has been avoided. Finally, the section describing rehabilitation organizations, research centers, and institutions and the list of commonly used abbreviations were included in the *Dictionary* to further increase the reader's access to the rehabilitation process, its sometimes unique language, and its literature.

Scope and Arrangement

The *Dictionary of Rehabilitation* is divided into three sections. Section I, Vocabulary, comprises the bulk of the text and includes a core vocabulary specific to the practice of rehabilitation. Definitions were designed to encourage appropriate use of terminology commonly used in rehabilitation settings. Definitions were developed to be current and concise.

Section II of the *Dictionary*, Rehabilitation Organizations, was prepared to offer convenient access to selected programs of the nation's most important rehabilitation organizations. This section is organized in the following manner.

1. *National and International Associations.* Contained under this heading are selected medical societies, professional and voluntary associations, advocacy groups, and other not-for-profit organizations that provide rehabilitation services on a national or international level. Information supplied for each entry includes address, telephone number, name of director, staff, membership, programs and purposes, and publications. Arrangement within this heading is alphabetical by name.
2. *Research Centers and Institutes.* Organizations represented under this heading are university-related research centers and independent nonprofit research institutes that are engaged in rehabilitation-related research on a continuing basis.

Section III, Health Care Abbreviations and Symbols, was developed by Timothy J. Meline and contains abbreviations and symbols commonly used today in rehabilitation settings. The

Latin origins of many abbreviations are provided for the user's information. In addition, many Spanish abbreviations are included in this comprehensive collection. Abbreviations are arranged alphabetically, and symbols are found at the end of the section.

Abbreviations Used in This Dictionary

ca.	circa, about
cf.	compare
e.g.	for example
etc.	et cetera
i.e.	that is
UK	United Kingdom
US, USA	United States of America
q.v.	which see; see this term

Abbreviations of units are found among the entries. Greek letters are listed under their English equivalents:

μ	(mu) see *m*
ψ	(omega) see *o*

SECTION I

VOCABULARY

A

A

1. In electricity: ampere(s).
2. In measurements of length: Ångström unit(s) or angstrom(s).
3. In the description of an orthotic or prosthetic joint, referring to its motion: assist.

Å Symbol for Ångstrom unit(s) or angstrom(s).

a-, an- Prefix denoting without, lacking, or away from.

abasia Inability to walk due to impaired motor coordination.

abducens Term used with the names of muscles or nerves that abduct a part.

abduct To move away from the midline. A limb, hand, or foot is abducted from the midline of the body; a digit is abducted from the midline of the hand (third digit) or the midline of the foot (second digit). Antonym: **adduct**.

abduction

1. Act of moving a limb, a hand, or a foot away from the midline of the body, or of moving a digit away from the midline of the hand (third digit) or the foot (second digit).
2. Result of such a motion: position away from the respective midline.

Antonym: **adduction**.

ablution Action of sponging or pouring water (or other liquid) over the body or part of it. As a therapeutic measure its duration may vary from a few seconds to a few minutes.

abnormalization Ascribing supernatural powers to explain observed behavior or accomplishments as, for example, believing that people who are blind must have a "sixth sense" allowing them to perform functions believed to be impossible without sight.

abrachia Absence of arms.

accelerometer Instrument for measuring the rate of change of velocity (acceleration or deceleration) of an object. Used in kinesiologic work.

acceptance of disability A phenomenological, subjective experience in which a person with a disability develops a personally meaningful view of life following a disability. The experience is considered a process, and emphasis is given to the subjective interpretation by the person with the disability.

accessibility symbol Symbolizing a person in a wheelchair, this stick figure indicates places that allow access by individuals in wheelchairs, on crutches, or otherwise disabled. Examples of such places are reserved parking space wide enough for complete opening of car door, ramp with an incline not greater than 8.3% (1 cm rise in 12 cm), door at least 80 cm wide, toilet with grab bar, low-placed telephone. Also used to identify the vehicle of a person with a disability; some states in the US have adopted the symbol to mark license plates of automobiles. Designed by Susanne Koefoed of Denmark as a project of the Scandinavian Design Students Organization and adopted internationally in 1969 by the eleventh World Congress on the Rehabilitation of the Disabled.

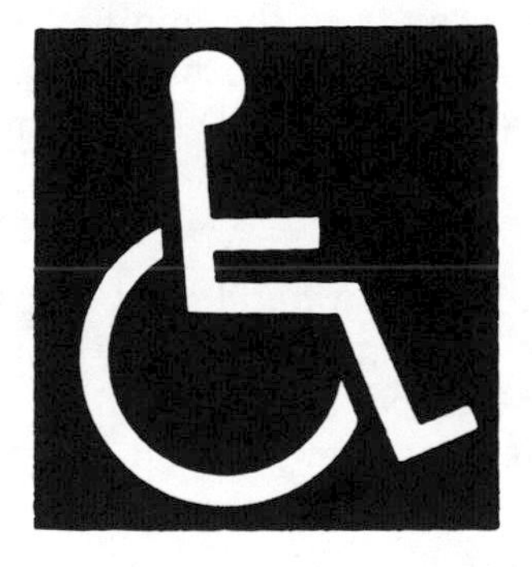

accommodation The act of accommodating, the state or process of being accommodated, and a process of mutual adaptation between persons or groups that supplies a need, want, or convenience. Within rehabilitation, the term is closely related to the principle of normalization, a concept introduced by Nirje (1969).

acroagnosis Absence of sensory recognition of a limb.

acroanesthesia Lack of sensation in the extremities.

acrometagenesis Congenital deformity of the extremities.

acromyotonia Rigidity of the hands or feet, resulting in spasmodic deformity.

actin A muscle protein that, together with myosin, is responsible for muscular contraction.

actinic Pertaining to radiation, and more specifically to radiation with chemical effects, i.e., in the ultraviolet portion of the electromagnetic spectrum.

actinotherapy Treatment by actinic radiation. Term specifically applied to ultraviolet radiation.

active-assisted (or active-assistive) exercise See under **exercise**.

activities of daily living (ADL) The range of common activities in which performance is required for personal self-maintenance and independent community residence.

- **Physical ADL.** The most basic personal care tasks, such as eating and bathing.
- **Instrumental ADL.** Complex activities needed for independent living, such as homemaking skills.

activities-of-daily-living test (ADLT) An assessment of a patient's level of performing activities of daily living. A great variety of tests is in use. See also the following entries: **Barthel index, Donaldson scale, Katz index, Kenny self-care score, pulses profile**.

activity limitation A measure of disability defined as long-term reduction in activity resulting from chronic disease or impairment.

activity program Program of various directed activities, most often used in long-term institutions. It aims at maintaining and developing the physical and mental potentials of patients or residents and at enhancing their interactions with others.

activity therapy Therapeutic use of any of a great variety of activities, such as physical, diversional, and social ones. Usually administered to mental or older patients in institutions.

acupressure Pressure applied by the fingertip or a pointed object to a small area of the body. This area is usually one of many points known in acupuncture.

acupuncture A traditional form of Chinese medicine that involves puncturing the skin with fine needles at strategic points for a desired therapeutic effect.

acute brain syndrome Sudden, often reversible impairment of brain function, secondary to other conditions, such as drug ingestion or systemic metabolic disorders; manifested by faulty perception and interpretation, usually with delirium.

-ad Suffix denoting direction toward.

adaptation A condition that meets two criteria: (a) the individual meets the demands of the environment, and (b) the individual experiences a sense of general well-being in relation to the environment. The term has also been defined as an intrapsychic evaluation of general life quality that is operationalized through such concepts as morale, life satisfaction, and happiness.

adapted housing Housing specially adapted for people with disabilities. It provides maneuverability and easy reach of doors, electric switches, cupboards, stove, and other utilities for persons in wheelchairs, on crutches, or with visual or auditory deficiencies.

adapted physical education Medically oriented physical education, comparable to corrective therapy (q.v.) but mostly adapted to the special needs, in schools or colleges, of subjects with or without physical disabilities.

adaptive capacity

1. The ability to change structural, physiologic, or behavioral characteristics to suit a new or changed environment.
2. The ability to maintain performance in the face of altered circumstances.

adaptive equipment A generic term for a wide range of items that aid persons with disabilities in their everyday life by improving function and compensating for physical, sensory, or cognitive limitations.

adaptive seating A term that encompasses the many devices designed to improve sitting balance or to relieve pressure on the bony prominences of a nonambulatory person.

adduct To move toward the midline. A limb, hand, or foot is adducted to the midline of the body; a digit is adducted to the midline of the hand (third digit) or the midline of the foot (second digit).

Antonym: **abduct**.

adduction

1. Act of moving a limb, a hand, or a foot toward the midline of the body, or of moving a digit toward the midline of the hand (third digit) or the foot (second digit).
2. Result of such a motion: position close to the respective midline.

Antonym: **abduction**.

adductor A structure, such as a muscle, that draws a part toward an axis of the body.

adhesion The union of two surfaces.

adjustable leg, adjustable limb See **adjustable prosthesis**, under **prosthesis**.

adjustment (to disability)

1. To bring into balance or achieve homeostasis after a disruption.
2. The process of establishing an identity that provides meaning and quality to life.

aerobic work, sport, exercise See under **exercise**.

aero-Kromayer lamp See under **Kromayer**.

affusion The pouring of water from a hose, a pitcher, a pail, or any other receptacle upon the body or a part of the body.

ageism A process of systematic stereotyping and discriminating against people because they are old.

agnosia A failure to recognize familiar objects despite intact vision, hearing, sensation, and language functions.

agonist A muscle in a state of contraction opposing the action of another muscle, its antagonist, which at the same time relaxes.

agraphia Loss of the power to communicate ideas in writing, due to a cerebral lesion.

aid

1. The help given by a person.
2. Any of various objects that help a person with a disability in a given activity. For examples, see following entries.

• **ambulation (ambulatory, or gait) aid.** Walking aid (q.v.).

• **hearing aid.** Any of various types of mechanical or electric devices carried in or close to the outer ear in order to improve hearing. For details about types, see **hearing aid**, under **hearing**.

• **low-vision aid.** Any device that helps persons with low vision to make better use of their residual eyesight. There is a great variety of optical, mechanical, electric, and electronic low-vision aids. Examples: magnifiers, special lights, strong reading glasses, handheld and eyeglass telescopes, video-magnifiers (closed-circuit television monitors adapted for reading).

• **mobility aid for the blind.** One of several devices that help a blind person to move about. Also called travel aid. Examples: long cane, laser cane, various sensoring devices. See also **ultrasonic mobility aid**.

• **mobility aid used in locomotor deficiencies.**

1. A walking aid (q.v.).
2. A wheelchair, movable lifter, or other vehicle for persons with disabilities.

• **self-help aid.** Any of various objects that make it possible or easier for a person with a physical disability to perform certain activities such as eating, washing, dressing, writing, picking up an object, using a telephone, without help by another person. Examples: button hook, long-handle brush or shoe-horn, combination knife and fork, typing stick, etc.

• **sensory aid.** Any device worn or held by the user to improve a sensory deficiency, usually visual or auditory. Examples: a hearing aid, magnifying glass, eyeglasses.

• **travel aid.** See **mobility aid for the blind**.

• **ultrasonic mobility aid.** A sensoring device for the blind. It emits a high-frequency, inaudible vibration, similar to radar, that strikes objects in the user's path and is reflected to a pair of earphones. The signals warn of objects that cannot be detected by the long cane.

• **walking aid.** Any object used to make walking easier or safer. Canes, crutches, and walkers are most often referred to, but walking belts and orthoses of the lower limb may be included.

aide A nonlicensed helper who has received appropriate on-the-job training in certain routine duties under the supervision of a licensed worker.

Air-Boot Proprietary name for an air split used as a temporary lower-limb prosthesis. A pneumatic prosthesis.

air conduction The conduction of sound waves carried as far as the inner ear.

airline gymnastics or exercise See **air travel exercises**, under **exercise**.

akinesia, akinesis Loss, absence, or poverty of motion.

akinetic Adjective referring to akinesia.

Alexander technique A system for developing one's kinesthetic sense and awareness of posture and everyday movements. It comprises the inhibition of faulty postural habits and aims at conscious control of body and mind. Developed (after a personal experience of the importance of the neck muscles) at the turn of the century by the Australian elocutionist F. Matthias Alexander (1869–1955), who published the method in articles and books between 1907 and 1941. Together with his brother, Albert R. Alexander (1874–1947), he taught it in London and the USA.

alexia A form of aphasia in which brain damage causes inability to grasp the meaning of written or printed words; also called visual aphasia and word blindness.

algesthesia Perception of pain.

alienation State of a muscle that after paralysis due to an acute condition has objectively improved but has not regained its ability to contract properly upon volition. Observed after a long period of inactivity, in poliomyelitis and similar disorders.

Allen exercises See **Buerger-Allen exercises**, under **exercise**.

Allison headrest Headrest used in the prone position, consisting of an individually made support of clear plastic with a cutout for eyes, nose, and mouth and of a soft resilient padding. Described in 1965 by John D. Allison, physical therapist in Minneapolis.

almoner A social worker in the UK.

alphabet board See under **board**.

alternating-pressure bed, mattress, pad See under **mattress**.

ambidextrous, ambidexter Able to use either hand about equally well.

ambiguity Uncertainty or lack of clarity in situations, roles, and behaviors, a term typically used by rehabilitation professionals when there is unclear communication and role assignment.

ambivalence-induced behavioral amplification A theory introduced by Paul Katz (1981), which maintains that attitudes toward certain groups in society, such as persons with physical disabilities, older adults, racial and ethnic minority groups, and persons with mental disabilities, tend to be ambivalent rather than simply positive or negative.

ambulator Walker (q.v.).

American sign language Language by signs, used by most deaf persons in the USA. It is a visual language expressed through positions and movements of the hands, expressions of the face, and positions of the body. Fingerspelling is usually included. Abbreviated: Ameslan or ASL.

American standard sign language See **American sign language**.

Americans with Disabilities Act of 1990 An act signed into law on July 27, 1990, that guarantees the rights of persons with disabilities to be free of discrimination by private employers, private health service providers, or private facilities with public access.

Amer-Ind Abbreviation for American Indian signs.

Ameslan Abbreviation for American sign language.

ammeter Instrument to measure amperage, i.e., the intensity of strength of an electric current. Also called amperemeter.

ammotherapy Treatment by sandbaths. Also called psammotherapy. From the Greek *ammos* or *psammos* (sand).

ampere (A) Unit of intensity of electric current. A current of one volt through a resistance of one ohm produces an intensity of one ampere. (See also **Ohm's law**.) Named after André-Marie Ampere (1775–1836), French physicist.

amperemeter Ammeter.

amphiarthrosis A joint or articulation that allows only slight motion, for example, between the bodies of the vertebrae.

amputee A person with one or more amputated limbs.

anaerobic work, sport, exercise See under **exercise**.

analgesia Absence of sensibility to pain.

analgesic

1. Relieving pain.

2. A medication that relieves pain without affecting consciousness; the most commonly used analgesic is aspirin.

analgia The condition of being without pain.

anarthria Loss of the ability to articulate properly.

anatomic position See under **position**.

anatripsis Obsolete term, of Greek origin, meaning therapeutic friction, massage.

anelectrode Anode.

anelectrotonus See **electrotonus**.

angstrom, Ångström unit (A, Å) A unit of length, equal to 10^{-10}m. Used for the measurement of electromagnetic radiations, blood cells, etc., the angstrom is now being officially supplanted by the nanometer, which is 10 times larger. Named after Anders Jonas Ångström (1814–1874), Swedish physicist.

anion Negative ion, i.e., ion with a negative electric charge, therefore migrating toward the positive electrode, the anode. Examples of anions: acids and acid radicals, Cl^-, I^-, SO_4^{2-}.

ankle cuff Usually weighted with lead, it is used for strengthening exercises of the lower limb, less often to steady the lower limb in walking.

ankle disk Circular board, about 35 cm in diameter, screwed in its center to a half sphere of wood, on which it is balanced. The patient stands on the board, attempting to keep it horizontal—a balancing exercise activating joints and muscles of feet and ankles.

anklet A soft orthosis of leather, textile, or similar material, embracing the ankle so as to support or protect it in cases of weakness, instability, or pain, notably after injury.

ankylosis Abnormal immobility and fixation of a joint.

anode The positive electrode or positive pole of an electric source. Thus called because it attracts anions.

anomia Inability to name or to recall the names of objects.

anosognosia A term, coined by Babinski, that applies to a condition in some patients with left hemiparesis or hemiplegia who do not recognize their left extremities as their own or who do not recognize the disabilities in those extremities.

antagonist Contraction of anti-agonist: a muscle opposing another muscle called the agonist.

antalgic Contraction of anti-algic, i.e., against pain, and referring to a gait, limp, or posture that tends to avoid pain in a certain area.

anteroposterior Relating to both the front and back.

anticipatory grief The process of being confronted with impending loss and initiating the grieving process before the event actually occurs.

anti-embolism stocking An elastic stocking that, by its elasticity and resulting relatively tight fit, compresses superficial varicose veins, thus assumed to improve venous circulation. It exists in various lengths, reaching to the knee, the thigh, or the waist.

antigravity muscle A muscle that normally, in the erect body, helps to support or lift a body segment against gravity. Examples: elbow flexors, knee extensors.

antispasmodic An agent that prevents or relieves involuntary muscular contractions.

anuresis Total retention of urine in the bladder; failure to urinate.

anxiety A feeling of uneasiness, distress, or dread concerning some impending or anticipated ill.

• **state anxiety.** Transitory, situationally specific anxiety.

• **trait anxiety.** A relatively stable characteristic persisting across situations and over time.

aphasia An impairment in the ability to interpret and formulate language symbols as a result of brain damage.

• **Broca's aphasia.** A type of aphasia characterized by effortful and halting speech and reduced grammar.

• **conduction aphasia.** Selective loss of the ability to repeat.

• **global aphasia.** A type of aphasia characterized by severe deficits in all language processes, including speech production, auditory comprehension, and writing.

• **transcortical motor aphasia.** A rare syndrome of aphasia characterized by the preserved ability to repeat fluently to a degree that would not be expected from observing spontaneous speech.

• **Wenicke's aphasia.** Aphasia characterized by fluent speech with paraphasic errors (sounds in words substituted for one another) and impaired auditory comprehension, reading, and writing.

apollo cover Canopy placed over a bed in order to provide a sufficient level of temperature, thus allowing the patient, usually with extensive burns, to remain unclothed. Made of transparent acrylic plastic with electrically conductive metal, the device was developed in the 1960s and also became known as omtru, or optimum metabolic temperature regulator unit.

appraisals The cognitive process through which individuals evaluate their physical, social, and psychological environments as well as events around them. These appraisals are of importance to the rehabilitation process because research indicates that certain types of appraisals are associated with adaptive coping responses. For instance, a person who was recently disabled and who views the event in terms of loss will likely cope differently than if he/she had viewed the event as a challenge to be overcome.

apraxia The inability to perform purposeful learned motor acts in the absence of paresis, sensory loss, lack of coordination or comprehension, or attentional deficits.

• **ideomotor apraxia.** The inability to imitate gestures.

• **constructional apraxia.** An impairment in the ability to perform activities in which parts are put together to form a single entity.

• **dressing apraxia.** An impairment in the ability to align the clothes to one's body in order to dress oneself.

APRL Abbreviation for Army Prosthetics Research Laboratory, established after World War II in Washington, D.C., where prosthetic hands, hooks, and other parts were developed; subsequently renamed Army Medical Biomechanical Research Laboratory (AMBRL). Some of the items were later manufactured privately by Sierra Engineering Company in Sierra Madre, California, and became known under their proprietary name, notably the Sierra hand and hook.

• **APRL hand.** Prosthetic hand of the voluntary-closing type developed at the Army Prosthetic Research Laboratory (APRL).

• **APRL hook.** Terminal device of an upper-limb prosthesis with voluntary closing, developed at the Army Prosthetic Research Laboratory (APRL). The hook fingers are lyre-shaped, made of aluminum and lined with neoprene.

arc, electric Flame caused by the electric current that bridges the gap between two conductors. The resulting heat is so intense that vapor is produced from the substance of the conductors. See **carbon arc lamp**, under **lamp**.

architectural barriers Structural obstacles barring access by the physically handicapped to a place, building, installation, or vehicle. Examples: electric switches, door knobs, elevator buttons, drinking fountains, and telephones out of reach of a person sitting in a wheelchair; doors too narrow or washrooms too small to accommodate a wheelchair; unramped curbs and steps without ramps or elevators; visual signals imperceptible to blind persons, not combined with an audible tone; or audible signals imperceptible to deaf persons.

Arica gymnastics See under **exercise**.

arm

1. The part of the upper limb between shoulder joint and elbow joint. Term less correctly used for the entire limb.
2. The part of a chair that supports the forearm.

• **Boston arm.** Above-elbow prosthesis activated by minute electric signals given off by muscles in the arm stump. Developed in the 1960s by Melvin J. Glimcher, orthopedic surgeon at Massachusetts General Hospital, and Robert W. Mann, engineer at Massachusetts Institute of Technology, Boston.

• **desk arm.** A wheelchair with an armrest that is not of full length, thus allowing a closer approach to a table, desk, or workbench.

• **domestic arm or armrest.** British term for desk arm.

• **fixed arm.** The arm of a chair, usually of a wheelchair, that cannot be removed.

• **Heidelberg arm.** A pneumatic prosthesis with hand for amputations at any level of the upper limb, powered by carbon dioxide gas and providing a great variety of functions. It was created about 1951 at the University Clinic in Heidelberg, Germany.

• **Hendon arm.** Upper-limb prosthesis for children, powered by carbon dioxide gas. Developed at the West Hendon Hospital, England, about 1966.

• **Hepp-Kuhn arm.** Munster prosthesis. See under **prosthesis**.

• **retractable arm.** Wheelchair arm that can be retracted for a closer approach to a table, desk, etc. Most often it is only the upper part of the arm, i.e., the armrest itself, that is retractable.

• **Russian arm.** A myoelectric prosthesis (see under **prosthesis**) for the upper limb. Developed by the Russians and exhibited at the Brussels World's Fair in 1958.

• **training arm.** An artificial upper limb used as a training device by therapists. Applied to their own normal limb it provides a valuable experience for teaching amputees the use of such a prosthesis. Also called simulated arm prosthesis.

arm pedaling The turning by the hands of a pair of levers similar to the pedals of a bicycle.

armrest The upper part of the arm of a chair, on which the forearm rests. For various types of armrests, notably of wheelchairs, see under **arm**.

armtray Support for the forearm and hand, usually attached to the arm of a wheelchair. It is most often used by the hemiplegic patient with a flaccid shoulder or forearm.

Arsonval, arsonvalism, arsonvalization See under **d'Arsonval**.

arthralgia Pain in a joint.

arthrectomy Removal of a joint.

arthrodesis Surgical fixation of a joint.

arthrogryposis Permanent or persistent flexure of a joint.

arthrometer Device to measure angles or range of motion at joints. Also called goniometer.

arthropathy Any disease of the joints.

Arthur Point Scale of Performance See under **test**.

artificial larynx An electronic device resembling a telephone receiver or a flashlight, used after loss of one's larynx or its function. It is held against the throat or cheek and emits a buzzing sound that is modulated into understandable speech by the action of the articulatory muscles. Also called electrolarynx.

artificial muscle Device used for the replacement of a paralyzed muscle (in an orthosis) or absent muscle (in a prosthesis). There are essentially two types.

1. Usually a nylon mesh in the shape of a small sausage that enlarges, hence shortens (like a contracting muscle), upon being

filled by carbon dioxide gas from a reservoir of liquefied CO_2. The patient operates the appliance by a simple motion of another body part, thus activating a pneumatic valve. A cable attached to the "muscle" pulls the part of the orthosis or prosthesis to be moved. The device was invented about 1956 by Joseph L. McKibben, physicist at Los Alamos Scientific Laboratory, New Mexico. Called also McKibben muscle or pneumatic muscle.

2. Another device, powered by electric current, performs a similar function by pulling a cable.

art therapy The therapeutic use of art in its various forms, such as drawing, painting, sculpturing, crafts, music, dance, drama, and creative writing, executed by the patient. Most often practiced with groups of psychiatric patients.

asasmolytic Antispasmodic; a drug that reduces spasm.

Asclepiades Greek physician (124–56 B.C.) from Bithynia, Asia Minor, called by some the "Hippocrates of Chronic Disease," by others the "Father of Geriatrics," by others again the "Father of Physical Medicine." He advocated massage, bathing, and exercise.

assistance The amount of help needed from one person to perform any part of a functional activity and/or cognitive assistance to perform gross motor actions in response to directions.

• **maximal assistance.** The need for 75% or more assistance from one person to perform physical or cognitive activities.

• **moderate assistance.** The need for 50%–75% assistance from one person to perform physical activities or constant cognitive assistance to sustain/complete simple, repetitive activities safely.

• **minimal assistance.** A need for 25%–50% assistance from one person for physical activities and/or periodic cognitive assistance to perform functional activities safely.

astasia Inability to stand, due to incoordination or hysteria.

astasia-abasia Inability to stand or to walk, due to incoordination or hysteria.

asthenia Loss of strength; weakness.

ataxia Motor incoordination due to a deficit in the cerebellar or proprioceptive system.

ataxic Pertaining to ataxia.

athetoid Pertaining to athetosis.

athetosis Distortions of volition producing motions that have been described as writhing, twisting, or wormlike.

atonic Lacking normal tone or strength.

atrophy A wasting, progressive degeneration and loss of function of any part of the body.

attitude ambivalence A concept that holds that members of groups perceived as having marginal status in a society, such as persons with disabilities, tend to be stigmatized and perceived by others as both deviant and disadvantaged.

Attitudes Toward Disabled Persons Scale A scale developed by Yuker and Block, 1986, that measures attitudes toward persons with disabilities.

attitudinal barrier Attitude of an individual or society toward persons with disabilities that imposes an unjustified limit to the latters' achievements or potentials. Term created by analogy with architectural barriers (q.v.).

attribution A social psychological process through which individuals come to believe that certain events, actions, or characteristics are linked to the behavior of self or others.

A.U. Ångström unit. See **angstrom**.

audiogram A chart plotted from the results of hearing tests with the audiometer.

audiologist A specialist in audiology, particularly in the rehabilitation of persons with hearing impairment. Usually not a physician. A physician who practices audiology is most often an otologist.

audiology The field of hearing, particularly of rehabilitation of individuals with impaired hearing. Term popularized in 1945 by the US otologist Norton Canfield and the speech pathologist Raymond Carhart.

audiometer An instrument to test the acuity of hearing. The result of the audiometric test is the audiogram.

audiometrist One who performs audiometric tests. See **audiometry**.

audiometry The testing and measuring of the acuity of hearing. See also **pure-tone test** and **speech reception test**, under **test**.

auditory training Education of the hard-of-hearing to improve their ability to understand spoken language by better use of residual hearing, together with other cues related to the person speaking, the circumstances, and the environment.

augmentative communication Any approach designed to support, embrace, or augment the communication of individuals who are not independent verbal communicators in all situations.

autocondensation couch Table with large autocondensation pads for general diathermy.

autocondensation pad Large metal plate electrode enclosed in a thin cover of insulating material. Two of these pads may be used for diathermy therapy.

autogenic training See **Schultz autogenic training**.

automatism

1. Involuntary or automatic action.
2. A condition in which activity is carried out by the patient without his conscious knowledge, often inappropriate to circumstances.

autonomic dysreflexia An extreme elevation of blood pressure, resulting in headache, slowing of the pulse, flushing and sweating of the face, and nasal congestion.

avoidance learning A phenomenon described by Stoyva (1981) that typically occurs in response to actual or perceived aversive events whereby the individual develops a specific set of responses to reduce the likelihood of coming into contact with the aversive stimulus or event.

B

B = F(P,O,E) A formula used to describe the balance among variables that determine health status, wherein behavior (B), or health, is seen as a function of the interaction of psychosocial (P), biological-organic (O), and environmental (E) influences.

back

- **flat back.** Back in which the curves are less marked than normally.
- **hollow back.** Back in which the lordosis extends to part or the total of the thoracic segment.
- **poker back.** Straight back with no or very little mobility, such as in rheumatoid spondylitis.
- **sway back.** Back with exaggerated lumbar lordosis.

back knee Lay term for **genu recurvatum** (q.v.).

bahnungstherapie German term meaning therapy by grooving a path. It refers to repetitive motions that may be passive in the beginning because of insufficient volitional control. It is assumed that, thanks to the repetition and with the appropriate guidance by the therapist and effort by the patient, the motion becomes more or less voluntary, and lost coordination is partly regained. This is the principle of Frenkel exercises (see under **exercise**). The term was introduced in 1902 by the Berlin physician Paul Lazarus, who applied the procedure to hemiplegia.

baker Jargon for heat cradle (q.v.).

balance beam Gymnastics apparatus consisting of a wooden beam, 5 m long and 10 cm wide. The type used in women's competitions is raised 120 cm from the floor; others, for balancing exercises, are usually lower.

Balance Theory of Expectations A theory developed by Heider (1958), which contends that pain and suffering are subjectively equated with punishment or trial by ordeal, while the expectation of relief is subjectively equivalent to purification and exoneration.

Balkan frame See under **frame**.

Balmoral (balmoral) shoe See under **shoe**.

balneary A place for bathing. From the Latin *balnearium*.

balneology The study of therapeutic baths and bathing. It includes balneotherapy.

balneotherapy Treatment by baths.

band

• **pelvic band.** The metal part of the pelvic belt of a prosthesis or orthosis. In a lower-limb appliance it gives support to its hip joint, connecting the belt with the thigh section of the device. In a lower-limb prosthesis the band is about one-third of the length of the entire belt.

• **Silesian band.** Silesian bandage. See under **bandage**.

bandage

• **Esmarch bandage.** Elastic bandage wound around a limb in such a way as to squeeze blood out of its superficial vessels. The limb in an elevated position is bandaged from its extremity toward its root. Suggested by the German surgeon Friedrich von Esmarch (1823–1908).

• **Scultetus bandage.** A many-tail bandage. A bandage with many tails or strips. Each strip is held in place by the following one. It is used as abdominal bandage. Named after the German surgeon Johann Schultes, latinized Scultetus, (1595–1645).

• **Silesian bandage or band.** Light belt, usually of webbing, attached to a lower-limb prosthesis as a means of suspension. Origin of term obscure.

bandy leg Bowleg, *genu varum*. See under **genu**.

bar, bars

• **C bar.** A component of a hand orthosis, in the shape of a C, placed between the second metacarpal bone and the opposed thumb to maintain the webspace.

• **chinning bar.** A horizontal bar, usually of steel and about 3 cm in diameter, used as an apparatus for gymnastics. One of the fundamental exercises consists in flexing the forearms while being suspended at the bar by the hands, so as to raise the chin to the level of the bar, i.e., to chin oneself; hence its name.

• **comma bar.** A metatarsal bar applied to the outsole of a shoe, just posterior to the metatarsal heads. Shaped like a comma, its larger end is thicker than the rest and is most often turned laterally, in order to pronate the anterior part of the foot. Called also Hauser bar, after Emil D. W. Hauser (1897–1981), Chicago orthopedic surgeon, who proposed it in 1939.

• **Denver bar.** See under **Denver**.

• **grab bar.** A sturdy bar, solidly fixed, usually to the floor or the wall, providing a hold and stability to a person for standing up, sitting down, or otherwise moving.

• **Hauser bar.** See **comma bar**.

• **lumbrical (or lumbricales) bar.** A flat bar in a hand orthosis, placed across the dorsal aspect of the proximal phalanges ii to V, preventing their extension.

• **metatarsal bar.** A strip of leather or comparable material applied to the outsole of a shoe across the metatarsal bones. Used to relieve pressure on the metatarsal heads.

• **parallel bars.**

1. An apparatus for gymnastics. The bars are usually at the level of the elbows or shoulders or even higher.
2. An apparatus used in physical or corrective therapy to facilitate a patient's walking after an injury or disease. The bars are at a comfortable height and distance from each other, to give support to the hands of the individual walking between them.

• **stall bars.** Gymnasium device made of wood, comparable to a ladder, usually fixed to the wall, with rungs about 1 m long and between 10 and 15 cm apart.

• **standing bar.** A horizontal bar at a convenient level for a standing person (e.g., the level of the chest) to support the hands while standing. Used by patients with insufficient stability to maintain a standing position. Similar to a grab bar.

barbell The object used in weight lifting, to be held in both hands. It consists either of an iron bar having at each end a sphere like a cannon ball, thus resembling the much smaller dumbbell (q.v.), or of a steel bar with removable disks of various weights. The latter type allows progressive addition of disks, up to hundreds of kilograms. While a barbell is normally lifted while standing, paraplegics practice weight lifting from the supine position.

barrel A bolster (q.v.) of the larger type.

barrier-free Refers to an environment that is accessible to the handicapped. Whether barriers such as stairs and narrow doors exist or not, there are means that allow wheelchair users and other individuals with physical disabilities access to the facility in question. Such means are appropriate parking places, ramps, elevators, wide doors, grab bars in toilets, low water fountains and telephones, etc. See also **access, accessibility**.

Barthel index A scale that permits measurement of one's activities-of-daily-living skill level. These activities include feeding, continence, transferring (moving in and out of bed or chair), attending to self at the toilet, dressing, and bathing. Each scale is subdivided to provide detailed analysis of skill in each activity. For example, feeding is subdivided into drinking from a cup and feeding from a dish, and four specific types of transfers are described.

Baruch, Simon New York physician (1840–1921). A pioneer in hydrotherapy, he introduced this branch of medicine to the USA and was the first teacher of physical medicine at Columbia University College of Physicians and Surgeons.

• **Baruch law.** A therapeutic rule, according to which a bath at skin temperature is sedative, whereas, if the water temperature is warmer or colder, it is stimulating. Proposed by S. Baruch.

• **Baruch table.** A table for hydrotherapy. Developed by S. Baruch.

bath

1. Immersion of the body or part of it in water, vapor, air, or other gas or fluid for hygienic or medical purposes.
2. Substance in which such immersion takes place.
3. Receptacle used for such immersion.

• **brine bath.** A bath in water rich in salt, such as sea water.

• **bubble bath.** A bath in a liquid containing or enriched by air or other gas.

• **cabinet bath.** Heat cabinet bath (q.v.).

• **carbon dioxide bath.**

1. Bath in water rich in carbon dioxide gas. Used in cardiovascular diseases. See also **Nauheim bath**.
2. Carbon dioxide gas bath. The patient sits or lies inside a tightly closed cabinet filled with carbon dioxide gas, with head and neck outside the enclosure.

• **chalk bath.** Bath in water to which chalk has ben added. Already known in ancient Rome, where chalk was used in the form of marble dust, it was reintroduced in the mid-1930s at the hospital of Bergen on the island of Rügen in the Baltic Sea, under its German name *kreidebad.*

• **Charcot bath.** Sponging with cold water of a patient standing in ankle-deep hot water. Suggested for patients with arterial disorders by Jean-Martin Charcot (1825–1893), Paris neurologist.

• **contrast bath.** A bath, most frequently for the hands or feet, in which there is alternation between cold and hot water. Temperature ranges are 5° to 15°C and 37° to 47°C, respectively.

• **electrostatic bath.** Treatment by static electricity. The patient sits on an insulated stool and is connected with an electrostatic machine.

• **faradic bath.** Bath in water charged with faradic current (see under **current**).

• **Finnish bath.** Sauna bath (q.v.). So called because it probably originated in Finland, where the exposure to heat is often accompanied by flogging with leafy branches.

• **Finsen bath.** General ultraviolet irradiation. See also entries under **Finsen**.

• **footbath.** A bath of one or both feet.

• **four-cell bath.** See **Schnee bath**.

• **galvanic bath.** Bath in water charged with galvanic current (see under **current**).

• **half bath.** Bath in which only the lower limbs and pelvis are immersed.

• **heat cabinet bath.** Bath of hot dry air in a heat cabinet (q.v.).

• **hip bath.** Sitzbath (q.v.).

• **hydroelectric bath.** A bath in water exposed to a direct current (hydrogalvanic bath; see next entry) or a low-frequency alternating current (see also **Schnee bath**).

• **hydrogalvanic bath.** Bath in water charged with direct current of very low voltage. Formerly used in the treatment of certain rheumatologic and neurologic conditions.

• **light bath.** Exposure of the body or part of it to the heat of electric light bulbs, either under a heat cradle, in a heat box, or in a heat cabinet. The term rarely refers to exposure to ultraviolet irradiation.

• **light cabinet bath.**
1. Bath of hot dry air in a heat cabinet (q.v.).
2. Total irradiation in an ultraviolet cabinet (q.v.).

• **Nauheim bath.** A bath in water rich in carbon dioxide gas, as, e.g., water in Saratoga Springs, New York. Named for Bad Nauheim, a German spa.

• **needle bath.** Projection of a filament of water against the body.

• **paraffin bath.** Application of paraffin at a temperature of about 52°C, either by brushing it on the skin or by dipping the area repeatedly into it. Also called wax bath (British term). See also **paraffin**.

• **peat bath.** A bath in peat (q.v.), which may be mixed with water.

• **sauna bath.** Bath in the hot dry air of a sauna, a specifically built room, with occasional production of steam, and followed by a cold plunge or other cold application to the entire body.

• **Schnee bath.** A hydroelectric bath in which four small insulated buckets are used, one for each hand and foot, the patient being seated. Each of the four receptacles contains a weak saline solution and a metal plate connected by a wire to the source of a low-frequency current. Devised at the end of the nineteenth century by Schnee in Carlsbad (Karlovy Vary), Czechoslovakia. Called also four-cell bath.

• **sitzbath.**
1. A bath in which only the pelvis is immersed, the lower limbs being kept outside. From the German noun *sitz*, seat.
2. A tub for such a bath.

• **sponge bath.** Washing of the body or part of it by using a wet sponge.

• **Stanger bath.** Hydrogalvanic bath (q.v.), to the water of which tannic acid is added. Suggested about 1900 by J. Stanger, a tanner in Ulm, Germany, and electrically improved in the early twentieth century by his son, engineer Heinrich Stanger.

• **sweat bath.** A bath of various kinds (hot air, hot water, vapor, etc.) to induce sweating.

• **Turkish bath.** A progressive hot-air bath taken in two or three rooms of increasing levels of temperature, followed first by a hot and thereafter a cold shower.

• **wax bath.** British term for paraffin bath.

• **whirlpool bath.** Bath in which the water is agitated and air injected by a powered device, the agitator.

bath chair, bathchair See under **chair**.

bath lift A device, usually hydraulic and operated by hand, to lift a patient in and out of the bathtub.

Batrow (or batronic) stimulator Proprietary name of an electric stimulator with a current of high voltage, small amperage, extremely short duration (7 μs) and damped oscillations.

baunscheidtism A method of producing counterirritation by scarification, i.e., cutting the skin with an instrument containing several small blades. A chemical irritant such as mustard or croton oil is then rubbed into the skin. Named after the German wheelwright and inventor Karl Baunscheidt (1809–1873).

BC bone conduction (q.v.).

beach ball A large air-filled plastic ball, up to 1 m in diameter or larger. It is used in exercises, whereby it may be held between the hands, the feet, or the knees; it is also tossed or pushed between members of a group. A child may also lie prone or sit on it, for stimulation of righting and other reflexes, for balancing and other exercises.

beam walking Balancing exercise consisting in walking on a beam of any width or length, placed on the floor or raised to a certain height.

beating A maneuver of massage, essentially percussion with the ulnar border of the hand and the little finger or the flat side of the fist.

Beck Depression Inventory A scale that measures depressive symptomatology.

bed

• **air bed.** A bed with an air-filled mattress.

• **air-fluidized bed.** A bed whose mattress consists of small ceramic beads, about 0.1 mm in diameter but in such number (hundreds of millions) as to form a layer of about 30 cm. They are suspended by a stream of warm air and covered by a polyester sheet on which the patient floats. Used for the treatment and prevention of decubitus ulcers.

• **Arnott bed.** A water bed devised by Neil Arnott (1788–1874), Scottish physician, and used in the treatment of bedsores.

• **CircOlectric bed.** Proprietary name of a bed in which the mattress can be turned around its transverse axis together with the patient. It can be operated electrically by the patient or by an attendant. Developed in 1960 by Michigan orthopedic surgeon Homer H. Stryker (1894–1980).

• **Emerson rocking bed.** A bed that rocks back and forth by electric power, providing mechanical assistance to the diaphragm of a patient with respiratory paralysis. Developed in 1953 by John H. Emerson Co., Cambridge, Massachusetts.

• **fluid bed.** Water bed.

• **Foster bed.** See **Foster frame**, under **frame**.

• **fracture bed.** A bed with an overhead frame and attachments for traction, suspension, and other procedures; used primarily in the treatment of patients with fractures. A board under the mattress prevents its sagging and consequent displacement of a fractured spine or limb.

• **Gatch bed.** A bed in which the support of the mattress is made of three parts that can be operated separately, permitting various positions of the trunk, thighs, and legs. Introduced in 1909 by Willis Dew Gatch (1879–1961), US surgeon.

• **Guthrie-Smith bed.** See under **Guthrie-Smith**.

• **high-low bed.** A bed the mattress of which can be lowered and raised, either mechanically (by the hand or the foot) or electrically. Some electrically operated beds may be controlled by the bed occupant.

• **hydrostatic bed.** Water bed.

• **oscillating bed.** A bed that oscillates either around its transverse axis, i.e., a rocking bed (q.v.), or around its longitudinal axis, i.e., a rolling bed (q.v., 2nd definition).

• **ripple bed.** See **alternating-pressure mattress**, under **mattress**.

• **rocking bed.** A bed that oscillates around its transverse axis. See **Sanders oscillating bed** and **Emerson rocking bed**.

• **rolling bed.**
1. A bed on rollers or wheels.
2. A bed that oscillates slowly around its longitudinal axis, completing one side-to-side motion in four minutes or more. Designed to prevent prolonged pressure on any area of the bedfast patient.

• **Royalaire bed.** Proprietary name of an air-fluidized bed (q.v.). Developed originally in the uk in the late 1960s.

• **Sanders oscillating bed.** Rocking bed that moves slowly around a transverse axis through an arc of 60°; gravity thus aids in the draining and filling of the vessels of the lower limbs and in the respiratory motions of the diaphragm. Proposed in 1936 for the treatment of cardiovascular and peripheral vascular diseases by Kansas City, Kansas, physician Clarence Elmer Sanders (1885–1949).

• **Stryker bed.** See **Stryker frame**, under **frame**.

• **turning bed.** One of several types of beds in which the patient can be turned together with the mattress.

• **water bed.** A bed with a water-filled mattress of rubber or similar material. It is used for the treatment or prevention of decubitus ulcers or for relaxation.

bed activities Locomotion in bed, such as turning from the supine position to one side and the other, to the prone position and return, rising to the sitting position in or at the edge of the bed. The term may also comprise activities such as adjusting the bed covers, operating a bell or a light switch, using the telephone, etc.

bedboard See **fracture board**, under **board**.

bed positioning See **positioning**.

behavior modification
1. A treatment modality that emphasizes the social–environmental causation of human behavior.
2. Viewing ineffective or maladaptive behavior as learned and thus amenable to change by altering the environmental contingencies controlling the behavior. Techniques employed usually focus on specific, observable symptoms or behaviors as targets for change.

behavioral analysis Identification of problematic behaviors and factors responsible for behavior change through objective observations and quantitative recordings, which is typically expressed in an A-B-C format, in which antecedents (A) and consequences (C) of the behavior (B) are noted, as well as the behavior itself.

behavioral medicine A field of study that focuses on reducing risk factors for serious illness and premature death that are lifestyle and behavioral in nature.

behaviorism A school of psychologic theory concerned with the observable, tangible, and objective facts of behavior, rather than with subjective phenomena such as thoughts, emotions, or impulses.

belt

• **breathing belt.** A strap of webbing or similar material, about 5 to 8 cm wide, slung around the lower ribs and crossing in front. The patient, by pulling at one or both ends, applies pressure on one or both sides, assisting expiration or providing resistance to inspiration in the respective area of the lungs.

• **emphysema belt.** A canvas belt with a suprapubic pad that, with the help of elastic springs, compresses the abdomen, thus pushing the diaphragm slightly higher and facilitating expiration. Suggested for patients with pulmonary emphysema. Called also Gordon-Barach belt, after the physicians Burgess L. Gordon (1892–), who devised it in 1934, and Alvan L. Barach (1895–1977), who modified it in 1950.

• **Gordon-Barach belt.** See **emphysema belt** (preceding entry).

• **pelvic belt.** A belt that encircles the pelvis and is attached to a lower-limb prosthesis or brace.

• **Silesian belt.** Silesian bandage. See under **bandage**.

• **transfer belt.** Leather or webbing strap held by the therapist or a helper around the patient's waist (or at the axillary level in children) to prevent or control a fall during walking and transfer activities. Also called walking belt.

• **vibratory belt.** A large strap fixed at both ends, usually to a wall, and slung around the hips or waist of a standing person. An electromotor produces vibrations that are transmitted to the involved area for purposes of massage, allegedly to reduce weight.

• **walking belt.** Transfer belt.

bench press A resistance exercise performed while astride a padded bench, the trunk usually in the supine position (supine press), less often in the upright position (sitting press). It consists in lifting a weight over a pulley by extending (pressing) the upper limbs upward over the head (shoulder press) or forward (chest press) or, with the feet in a more elevated position, by extending the lower limbs (leg press).

Bender test See **Bender gestalt test**, under **test**.

bibliotherapy The therapeutic use of reading. Reading as directed by health professionals for the purpose of helping patients in their programs of recovery or rehabilitation.

biceps curl Flexion of one or both forearms against resistance, which may be a weight either held in the hand (dumbbell) or attached to a pulley.

bicycle ergometer An apparatus measuring energy expended during the operation of a stationary bicycle.

binder Flexible orthosis in the shape of a belt, to be applied around the chest (rib binder), the lower segment of the trunk (abdominal binder), the thigh, or another body part.

• **Scultetus binder.** See **Scultetus bandage**, under **bandage**.

Binet test See under **test**.

bioenergetics System that combines psychotherapy with muscular manipulation and physical exercises, including specific body positions and respiratory training. Based originally on the psychoanalytic method (character analysis) of Wilhelm Reich (1897–1957), it purports to free the body's energy by releasing muscular tension considered to be the cause of various dysfunctions. Developed in the 1950s by US psychiatrist Alexander Lowen (1910–1983).

bioengineering Biomedical engineering; the application of engineering principles to solve biomedical problems, e.g., design and construction of devices, using suitable materials, for implantation within the body or of life-supporting apparatus for external use.

biofeedback Method of monitoring the function of a physiologic system in an individual and returning—i.e., feeding back—to him the information obtained. An instrument with sensitive detectors is used to reveal otherwise unperceived responses. In biofeedback therapy the patient is informed by the instrument of the level of control he has achieved over a muscle or single muscle fiber, amplitude of motion, tonus, posture, amount of weightbearing, relaxation, or even involuntary functions, such as heart rate, blood pressure, or brainwaves. It is used to intensify and expand the awareness of such biologic processes and hence to influence them.

• **alpha wave biofeedback.** Biofeedback centered on alpha waves, a slow rhythmic form of brain waves. Developed in the late

1960s after a report that alpha waves were associated with a relaxed and creative state of mind.

• **electromyographic biofeedback.** Technique of teaching control over the level of relaxation or the contraction of individual muscles or even single muscle fibers by the use of an electromyograph, which detects and demonstrates the muscular activity, feeding this information back to the user by visual information (on an oscilloscopic screen) and audible information (on a loudspeaker).

biogenics A method of self-education by means of exercises in relaxation, focusing of attention, and spiritual attunement, taking elements of techniques from Emile Coué, J. H. Schultz, Carl G. Jung, Edmund Jacobson, Gestalt psychology, Roberto Assagioli, and others. Developed in the 1970s by US neurosurgeon C. Norman Shealy.

biomedical engineering The field and study of engineering in the service of biomedical sciences, including rehabilitation.

biothesiometer An instrument for measuring the threshold of vibratory perception in a subject.

bipolar stimulation Stimulation by two electrodes placed at a short distance from each other on the same nerve or muscle, usually at the two ends of the muscle. Cf. **monopolar stimulation**.

Blindengarten German for "Garden for the Blind," which is part of a public park (Wertheimstein Park) in Vienna, Austria. At the garden entrance is an embossed map with legends in braille. Stone paths and rails guide blind visitors to odoriferous plants, to tame animals that can be touched, to a sculpture that captures and projects sounds, and to a twelve-tone acoustic fountain in which water plays on brass cymbals. See also **garden for the blind**.

blindness The legal definition of blindness in the USA, as amended in 1967, is a central visual acuity of 20/200 or less in the better eye with use of a corrective lens or a reduction of the visual field to 20° or less.

blind training Training of the blind in the use of a cane, other assistive devices, or a dog when walking; in braille reading and writing; in typing; and in many other activities of daily living. This might include prevocational and vocational training.

Bliss symbols, Blissymbols A collection of symbols in a system of communication for nonvocal persons, such as the deaf, aphasic, and mentally retarded. The symbols, which are very elementary line drawings, can be combined to form more complex meanings and sentences, independent of any spoken or written language. Developed by Austrian-born Charles K. Bliss, who published it in 1949 in his book *Semantography*. Instructors are taught the system at the Blissymbolics Institute in Toronto, Canada. Later, raised-surface Blissymbols were developed for use by blind, nonspeaking persons.

blow bottles A pair of bottles containing water that is blown from one to the other through an interconnecting tube. Used for the practice of expiration against resistance. Developed in 1918 by US physician Conreid Rex Harken (1884–1975).

Blucher (blucher) shoe See under **shoe**.

Blythemobile Combination wheelchair-stretcher for self-propulsion. It allows its user to keep the knees extended while being supine or sitting. Developed in the 1960s at Blythedale Children's Hospital, Valhalla, N.Y.

board

• **alphabet board.** A board used by a person who cannot speak but can compose words or sentences by pointing to the letters of the alphabet on the board. Numbers and certain often-used words such as eat, water, toilet, tired, cold, may be included in full. See also **communication board**.

• **balance board.** A board mounted on an unstable support under its center, used for the evaluation and education or reeducation of the sense of balance. The subject may either sit or stand on the board. It may be rectangular, square, or round, and of various sizes. The support may also be of different dimensions and shapes, providing for a seesaw motion or, if it is a hemisphere resting on its pole, for mobility in all directions. Called also rocker, rocking, or seesaw board, or vestibular board because of the role played by the vestibule of the ear in the maintenance of balance.

• **bedboard.** See **fracture board**.

• **bridge board.** Transfer board.

• **communication board.** A board divided into a certain number of small fields displaying words, phrases, or pictures. Used by persons who cannot speak or write but can express simple messages and thoughts by pointing to these fields. In case of associated quadriplegia where only the head can move, a flashlight or a stick attached to the forehead or a stick held in the mouth may serve as a pointer. See also **alphabet board**.

• **crawl board.** See **prone scooter**.

• **exercise board.** A board of wood or synthetic material with a smooth surface to facilitate the gliding of a limb or other part of the body placed on it for exercises. In order to further decrease friction of the moving part, talc may be used (see **powder board**) or a skate may be attached to the moving limb (see **skate board**).

• **finger board.** A device for exercises of the hand and its digits.

• **footboard.** A board, usually plywood, placed vertically at the foot end of the bed in order to keep the bedclothes off the feet, thereby giving the latter more freedom and decreasing the danger of pressure and plantarflexion deformity.

• **fracture board.** A board, usually plywood, placed under the mattress of a bed in order to overcome its sagging and to provide a better horizontal position for its user. So named because of its indication for patients with fractures of thoracic or lumbar vertebrae. Also used in low back pain and other conditions.

• **hip board.** An exercise board (q.v.) in the form of a half disk with a central cutout, used for exercises of the lower limb.

• **inclined board.** Slant board.

• **lapboard.** A board of wood, plastic, or other rigid material, placed on the arms of a wheelchair or other chair with arms, thus providing a table surface for its occupant.

• **picture board.** See **communication board**.

• **powder board.** Exercise board on which talc or a similar powder is spread to diminish friction of the moving part.

• **prone board.** A board on which the patient, usually a child, is placed or strapped in the prone position. It can remain horizontal or, if provided with a footboard, be raised at its head end to a vertical or intermediate position. It allows its user to perform activities in various positions. Called also standing board.

• **rocker (or rocking) board.** Balance board.

• **scooting board.** See **prone scooter**.

• **seatboard.** A board applied to the seat of the common type of collapsible wheelchair to overcome the sag.

• **seesaw board.** Balance board.

• **skate board.** Board on which part of the body, supported by a skate, moves with little friction, either for exercise or to counteract a tendency to contracture deformity. For example, a hip or knee flexion contracture is counteracted in supine position with a skate under the heel. See also **skate**.

• **slant board.** A board placed in an inclined position; used for bronchial drainage or certain exercises.

• **sliding board.** Transfer board

• **spelling board.** Alphabet board.

• **standing board.**

1. Prone board (q.v.).
2. A board used like a tilt table. With the patient strapped on it in the supine position, it is raised and attached by hooks to a bed frame or a wall bar, thus providing the patient with a more or less upright position.

• **testing board.** A wooden board with an assortment of objects of various shapes and sizes (square blocks, disks, dowels, screws, bolts, wingnuts, keys, etc.), to be handled by a patient. It serves to assess dexterity, e.g., in the use of an orthosis or prosthesis of the upper limb, and to develop skill, hand-eye coordination, etc.

• **transfer board.** A board aiding in the transfer of a patient by spanning the space between bed and wheelchair, wheelchair and car, etc. It measures about 30 by 75 cm and is made of wood or rigid plastic. Its surface is smooth for easy sliding. It may also have one or two hooks so that it can be attached to the wheelchair. Called also sliding board or bridge board.

• **turtle board.** See **prone scooter**.

• **vestibular board.** See **balance board**.

Bobath method of exercise A system of therapeutic exercise for patients with lesions of the central nervous system, notably children with cerebral palsy and adults with hemiplegia. The treatment, which is strictly individual, progresses from the horizontal position (including rolling over) to sitting, kneeling, and standing. By manipulation and precise guidance of the patient's head, trunk, and limb motions, the therapist suppresses undesirable reflexes and abnormal postural reactions, concentrating on certain "key points of control." These reflex-inhibiting movement patterns and controlled postures facilitate active automatic and voluntary movements, which are further elicited or facilitated by proprioceptive and tactile stimuli (e.g., tapping). First published in 1948 by London physical therapist Berta Bobath and in 1950 by her husband, neurologist Karel Bobath, the method is often called the Bobaths method.

Bobath Test Chart of Motor Ability A chart for the evaluation of a child's postures, their degrees of abnormality, and the child's ability to control them. Refers to Bobath method (see preceding entry).

Bock knee See under **knee**.

body building A program of physical training aiming at the development of a hypertrophic general musculature, yet avoiding the preponderance of any one muscle or group of muscles.

body ego technique A system of physical reeducation for individuals with disturbances of body image and identity. Developed initially from teaching children modern dance, it evolved into a predominantly nonverbal method that is applied to psychiatric patients of all ages.

body image theory The application of psychoanalytic or psychoanalytically derived principles to explain the development of the concept of and set of attitudes toward oneself as a bodily entity.

Böhler exerciser A device for exercising the knee extensors. A cylinder-shaped bolster is placed in the popliteal space of the recumbent patient, and the exercise consists in raising the leg to full extension. The height of the bolster can be adjusted, as it is fixed between two notched uprights of a support. Sandbags of various weights are placed over the dorsum of the foot to add resistance. Devised by Vienna orthopedic surgeon Lorenz Böhler (1885–1973).

bolster A cushion or pillow in cylinder form, made of foam rubber or similar material, between 30 and 60 cm in diameter and between 60 and 120 cm in length. When used for testing of reflexes and for balance exercises, the subjects sit on it astride or sideways; for other exercises, for relaxation or stretching, they may lie prone or supine. A child may be placed on it in the prone position in order to stimulate creeping movements. There are also air-filled bolsters of the same shape and sizes or larger. Both types are also called spot trainers or, if of the larger dimensions, barrels.

bone conduction The conduction of sound waves by the bones of the skull.

bootee

1. A knitted shoe for infants.
2. A short and light boot or overboot for women or children.

boot therapy Treatment aimed at the prevention of postoperative thrombophlebitis by using a pair of plastic boots intermittently inflated to a pressure sufficient to empty the veins yet without interfering with the arterial blood flow.

boot weight A weight attached to a weight boot (q.v.) to be lifted in resistance exercises of the leg or the entire lower limb. The amount to be lifted is obtained by selecting the appropriate size and number of the weight plates.

Boston Diagnostic Aphasia Examination A standardized test commonly used to evaluate language disturbances in adults that evaluates auditory comprehension, oral expression, understanding of written language, and writing.

Boston naming test See under **test**.

bowleg A lower limb with lateral convexity. See **genu varum**.

box toe A spacious toe (q.v.) of a shoe with more or less rigid walls, designed to provide comfort and protection to the toes of the foot.

brace

1. The noun: an orthosis (q.v.), a term with which it is often used interchangeably, as it is with other terms: splint, collar, corset, etc.
2. The verb: to provide with a brace, to support, to make more rigid.

• **caliper brace.** An orthosis for the lower limb, whose two upright bars articulate with the shoe at the level of its sole or do not articulate at all.

• **cast brace.** Articulated cast. When applied to fractures of the femur, the cast of the thigh and the cash of the leg are connected by an incorporated metal knee joint. It combines the advantages of partial immobilization, mobility, and early ambulation.

• **chairback brace.** See **Knight brace**.

• **coil-spring brace.** A brace with a single or double coil spring hinge. The coil is usually made of stainless steel spring wire. By far the most frequent example is the coil-spring ankle brace with a double coil around a steel axis placed at the level of the sole. Designed to support the foot in dorsiflexion, it is particularly useful in flaccid footdrop.

• **Dropfoot brace.** Brace that holds a foot with insufficient voluntary dorsiflexion in a neutral or near-neutral position.

• **Hessing brace.** One of a great variety of braces with steel skeleton and molded leather encasing a body part. Named after Friedrich von Hessing (1838–1918), German orthopedic surgeon and bracemaker, who used the same construction.

• **Klenzak brace.** A brace with a Klenzak joint, usually a double-bar ankle brace used for footdrop: the spring assist provides dorsiflexion of the ankle. For Klenzak joint, see under **joint**.

• **knee brace.** A support for the knee, extending from about mid-thigh to about mid-leg. It may be with or without a joint; in the former case there is also a lock for the joint.

• **Knight brace.** A thoracolumbosacral orthosis. It comprises two lateral and two posterior uprights and a full-front abdominal flexible support. Called also chairback brace. Devised in 1874 by Maryland physician James C. Knight (1810–1887).

• **Knight–Taylor brace.** A thoracolumbosacral orthosis that combines the chairback brace according to Knight (see preceding entry) with features of the Taylor brace (q.v.), including shoulder straps. It restricts in particular flexion and extension of the spine in the thoracolumbar area.

• **long leg brace.** Knee-ankle-foot orthosis, i.e., extending from the thigh (usually close to the inguinal area) to the foot.

• **Milwaukee brace.** See **Milwaukee corset**, under **corset**.

• **PA brace.** Abbreviation for Pull-and-Adjust brace, an orthosis for footdrop. So named by its manufacturer to indicate the manner of its adjustment for each individual patient.

• **short leg brace.** Ankle-foot orthosis, i.e., an orthosis extending from below the knee to the foot.

• **standing brace.** Standing orthosis. See under **orthosis**.

• **stirrup brace.** An orthosis for the lower limb, whose two upright bars articulate at the level of the ankle with a stirrup-like shoe attachment.

• **Taylor brace.** Thoracolumbar orthosis with pelvic band, full-front abdominal support, paraspinal uprights, and shoulder straps. It restricts in particular flexion of the thoracic and lumbar vertebrae. Devised in 1863 by New York orthopedic surgeon Charles Fayette Taylor (1827–1899).

• **Thomas brace.** See **Thomas splint**, under **Thomas**.

• **tractive brace.** A brace for the stretching of tight structures with the help of turnbuckles or other means.

• **Williams back brace.** Thoracolumbosacral orthosis keeping the spine in a slightly flexed position. Constructed on the three-point-pressure principle, it comprises a low front part with abdominal pad and two posterior transverse bars, one at the lower thoracic level, the other over the buttocks. Thus it allows flexion but restricts other motions, especially extension. Developed by Paul C. Williams (1900–1978), Dallas orthopedic surgeon.

brachial Relating to the arm.

brachiotomy Incision into or amputation of an arm.

brachium The arm, especially above the elbow.

bradykinesia Slowness of motion.

Braille, Louis Blind French teacher of blind persons (1809–1852).

• **braille alphabet, system, or symbols.** The alphabet in which each letter is represented by a different arrangement of between one and six raised dots that can be felt by one finger. Created in 1829 by Louis Braille and introduced in the USA in 1860. It can also be written with the aid of a metal slate or typed with a braille typewriter.

Braillophone Device that combines the telephone with the braille system of raised symbols. It enables individuals who are both blind and deaf to use the telephone. The spoken message is typed out on a keyboard and printed in braille symbols embossed on a narrow ticker tape. Developed in the early 1970s by the Siemens Company in Germany.

breath control Mode of operating an apparatus, most often a wheelchair, by a patient with quadriplegia: the forward, backward, and turning motions and the stop are controlled by various types of breathing, i.e., soft or intense inspiration or expiration. The system, which may be part of a larger one (see **environmental control system**), is also called sip-and-puff control, referring to the inspiration (sip) and expiration (puff) of a small amount of air used to operate it. Some units may be activated by the user's voice (voice control).

bridge board Transfer board. See under **board**.

bronchospirometer Instrument to determine oxygen intake and carbon dioxide output of the lung.

Brown–Sequard syndrome Damage of a lateral half of the spinal cord, causing motor and sensory disturbances below the level of the lesion, i.e., motor paralysis and loss of joint position sense and vibration sense on the same side of the body and loss of pain and temperature sensation on the opposite side.

Brunnstrom method of exercise An exercise method for patients with lesions of the central nervous system, primarily hemiplegics. It uses reflexes, associated reactions, and mass synergies and stimulates the patient to intense participation in order to achieve the desired movements. The treatment, strictly individual, combines techniques of proprioceptive and exteroceptive stimulation, central facilitation, and inhibition. Proprioceptive stimulation includes stretching of selected muscles; exteroceptive stimulation comprises stroking, rubbing, and tapping. Resistance is often applied. The method was developed about 1951 by Signe Brunnstrom, Swedish physical therapist, who practiced in the USA between 1928 and 1974.

buck, vaulting buck A thickly padded, leather-covered, firm, heavy bolster about 60 cm long and 35 cm wide, with a wooden core and standing on four heavy, adjustable legs. Used mostly for vaulting. Is comparable to the vaulting horse (see **horse**).

bucket Pelvic socket of a lower-limb prosthesis.

Buck extension or traction Traction of the extended lower limb of a recumbent patient by means of a weight over a pulley. The rope of the pulley is attached to the limb by a bandage. Used in fractures of a long bone of the limb. Technique devised by Gurdon Buck (1807–1877), New York surgeon.

Buerger exercises, Buerger-Allen exercises See under **exercise**.

Bunnell block A flat block of wood, between 1 and 2 cm thick, with rounded edges, held in the hand to exercise stiffened joints. Recommended by San Francisco hand surgeon Sterling Bunnell (1882–1957).

burnout The state of emotional and physical fatigue experienced by individuals who have incurred excessive psychological demands in their roles of helping other people.

butterfly Gluteal attachment to or extension of the pelvic band of a back or lower-limb orthosis. shaped like the lower half of a disk, it is designed to push the buttock forward in order to correct hip flexion. If bilateral, it vaguely resembles a butterfly in shape (butterfly pads). In a back brace the pelvic band may have a double downward curve (butterfly pelvic band).

C

C

1. Symbol for Celsius.
2. Symbol for electric capacitance.

c

1. Symbol for cycle(s).
2. Symbol for the prefix centi-.

cable In diathermy, an applicator in the form of a coil that covers an area or encircles a limb or part of it. See also **inductance cable**.

Cage questionnaire A measure of alcohol use.

Cal, cal Abbreviations for large calorie (Cal) and small calorie (cal). See **calorie**.

Calcutta technique Refers to the addition of a ventilator to therapeutic irradiation by infrared rays. The draft produced upon the irradiated area of the skin prevents the accumulation of sweat and thus allows a higher temperature and a deeper penetration of the tissues. Suggestion published in 1960 by R. Harris and S. K. Sarkar, after observations made in Calcutta, whence the name of the technique.

California Psychological Inventory (CPI) A 480-item inventory that evaluates the "normal" personality.

caliper British term for splint or brace, notably a limb brace with two uprights. Also called caliper splint.

• **walking caliper.** A caliper for the lower limb, whose uprights fit into a channel at the level of the shoe heel. See also **caliper brace**, under **brace**.

calipers (plural) A pair of compasses whose legs are formed so as to measure the thickness of a body part (e.g., a skinfold, measured by skinfold calipers) or the width of an opening.

calisthenics Calisthenic exercises. See under **exercise**.

calorie (cal) A unit of heat, also called small calorie or gram calorie. It is the amount of heat required to raise the temperature of 1 ml of water by 1°C. The unit used in the study of human metabolism is the large calorie or kilocalorie, abbreviated Cal, kcal, or kg-cal, which is equal to 1,000 calories.

cane A walking aid, make of wood or metal, to be held in one hand. It is used to add to stability while walking or to take some of the weight off one foot. Called also walking cane or walking stick.

• **broad-based cane.** Cane with three or four tips providing a relatively wide base of support. Examples: three- or four-point cane, three- or four-legged cane.

• **C cane.** Regular cane, i.e., a cane of the most frequently used type, with curved, C-shaped handle.

• **crab cane.** Cane with three or more tips.

• **crook-handle cane, crook-top cane.** C cane (q.v.).

• **English cane.** Forearm crutch. See under **crutch**.

• **four-legged cane.** A cane with four relatively long tips.

• **four-point cane.** A cane with four tips.

• **glider cane.** Four-legged cane, the two inner legs of which have wheel tips so as to glide on the floor when the outer tips are raised by tilting the cane. Also called cane glider.

• **Hoover cane.** Cane for blind persons. See **long cane**.

• **hospital cane.** Standard wooden cane. Called also regular cane or C cane (q.v.).

• **laser cane.** A long cane for blind persons, containing three lasers. Held in front of the body, it sends out light beams, warning by auditory and tactile signals when its user is approaching a stairway, a curb, or other obstacle. Developed in the 1960s.

• **long cane.** A guidance device for blind persons. It is a light and thin cane, longer than a walking cane, reaching from the ground vertically to about the level of the base of the neck of its user, with a crook (C-shaped) top. It is held like a pencil obliquely in front of the body. (See also **cane travel of the blind**.) Developed during World War II by Richard E. Hoover (before he became a physician and later an ophthalmologist) and associates at US Army General Hospital, Valley Forge, Pennsylvania. Hence also called Hoover cane.

• **offset cane.** Cane in which about one-third of the upper part of the stem is offset so that the handle is placed vertically above the lower part.

• **quad cane.** Colloquialism for quadripod, four-point, or four-legged cane.

• **quadripod cane.** Four-point or four-legged cane.

• **regular cane.** Cane with curved handle, the most common type of cane.

• **single-point cane.** A cane so named to emphasize that it does not have more than the usual single tip, as opposed to tripod and other canes.

• **T cane.** A cane whose top resembles the letter T, the handle being at a right angle to the shift.

• **three-legged cane.** A cane with three relatively long tips.

• **three-point cane, tripod cane.** A cane with three tips.

• **T-top cane.** T cane (q.v.).

• **typhlocane.** Cane for blind persons. After the Greek adjective *typhlos*, blind. Refers usually to the so-called long cane (q.v.) rather than the white cane.

• **white cane.** A cane used by a blind person. Its white color has become traditional to inform others of its user's disability. Usually held vertically, it cannot be used to probe very far in advance of the body during walking because it is much shorter than the so-called long cane (q.v.) by which it is being more and more supplanted.

cane glider Glider cane. See under **cane**.

cane travel of the blind Walking of a blind person with the use of a cane, particularly out of doors. There are essentially two techniques of using the so-called long cane (q.v.) by a blind person. In the *cross-body technique* the cane is held like a pencil, obliquely in front of the body. If it is held in the right hand, without being moved its tip points to the floor in front of the left foot, thus more or less shielding the body. In the *rhythm*, or *touch, technique* the cane is held like a pointer, the index finger lying on it, and is swung from side to side at every step. When the left foot moves forward, the cane moves to the right, its tip lightly touching the ground so as to probe the area before the right foot advances, and so forth. There are some variations of this touch method.

capacitance (or capacity), electric (c) The ability to store an electric charge. Its unit is the farad.

CAPP Child Amputee Prosthetics Project (University of California, Los Angeles), in operation since 1954, where various protheses or parts of prostheses for the upper or the lower limb and other devices were developed, among which are the following.

• **CAPP cart.** Electric cart designed to provide mobility for children with quadruple amputations or other severe limb deficiencies.

• **CAPP terminal device.** Terminal device of an upper-limb prosthesis. Without being a prosthetic hand or hook, it is a voluntary-opening device. It is made of plastic with a soft palmar surface.

capuchin monkey helper Capuchin monkey from Central America, trained as helper for physically disabled individuals in feeding, opening doors, fetching small objects, turning lights and other electric equipment on and off, and doing other chores. The method of training was developed in the mid-1970s by Mary Joan Willard, psychologist, at Tufts–New England Medical Center, Boston.

carbon dioxide snow A substance consisting of compressed, or solid, carbon dioxide, also known as dry ice, having a temperature of −79°C. It is used to treat acne, angiomas, skin tuberculosis, etc. It was introduced in 1905 for such treatment by William A. Pusey (1865–1940), US dermatologist. **Carbon dioxide slush** is a mixture of carbon dioxide snow with acetic acid and precipitated sulfur, used for the same purpose.

cardiac rehabilitation An interdisciplinary, goal-oriented rehabilitation program designed to restore patients with cardiac disease to their optimal medical, physical, psychological, emotional, social, vocational, and economic status.

career assessment inventory An instrument that measures the degree to which one's interests match those in various occupations with modest educational requirements.

caregiver burden Negative consequences of caring for individuals who have chronic disability, typically occurring when demands of care exceed the caregiver's coping resources.

• **objective burden.** Observable changes in the personality and behavior of the person receiving care, as well as environmental changes for the caregiver, such as financial strain, changes in routine, changes in living conditions, and changes in social activities.

• **subjective burden.** The caregiver's negative reaction resulting from the presence of objective burden.

carpal tunnel syndrome A complex of symptoms caused by any condition that compresses the median nerve in the carpal tunnel of the wrist; marked by pain and numbness in the area of the hand innervated by the median nerve.

case management Coordination and integration of services and other resources designed to enhance the functioning of a client or group of clients.

cast A rigid casing, usually made of bandages impregnated with plaster of Paris, applied to or around a body part in order to support it.

• **walking cast.** A cast for the leg or the entire limb with a heel or similar support incorporated in the sole, for walking.

casterchair See under **chair**.

castercommode A casterchair with a removable seat over a removable bedpan.

casterwalker A walker, the four legs of which are fitted with casters.

cataplasm A pack, usually a hot pack, containing a substance other than water. Also called poultice.

cataplexy A sudden and temporary loss of muscle tone and of postural reflexes, causing limpness of the body or a part, usually triggered by an emotional surge, such as sudden elation, anger, etc.

catapult seat A seat that tilts forward, thus helping its occupant to stand up. It can be powered either mechanically or electrically.

catelectrotonus See **electrotonus**.

cathode The negative electrode or negative pole of an electric source. Thus called because it attracts cations.

cation Positive ion, i.e., ion with a positive electric charge, therefore wandering to the negative electrode, the cathode. Examples of cations: metals such as Cu^{+}, Ca^{2+}, Mg^{2+}, bases, and alkaloids.

cauda equina syndrome Dull pain and anesthesia of the buttocks, genitalia, and/or thigh, with impaired bladder and bowel function; caused by compression of the spinal roots.

C bar A component of a hand orthosis in the shape of a C, placed between the second metacarpal bone and the opposed thumb to maintain the webspace.

Celsius (C) Temperature scale, in which the boiling point of water is one hundred degrees (100°C) and the ice point is zero degrees (0°C). Invented in 1742 by Anders Celsius (1701–1744), Swedish astronomer.

centi- (c) Prefix meaning one hundredth of a measure (10^{-2}).

centigrade One grade of a centesimal system. The temperature scale that is abbreviated C, together with its degrees, are correctly called Celsius, not centigrade.

chair See also under **wheelchair**.

• **Bath chair.** Known throughout the nineteenth century as a vehicle for outdoor use, developed in Bath, the English spa, it usually had three wheels and a hood and was pulled or pushed by an attendant. After many changes it was supplanted by a handier vehicle for indoor and outdoor use, which adopted its name modified as bathchair. See next entry, first definition.

• **bathchair.**

1. A term used mostly in the UK for the large pushchair of old standing.
2. A metal chair, either stationary or on casters, used in a shower; a shower chair.

• **casterchair.** A chair on casters. Its user pulls it forward or pushes it backward by applying the feet against the floor or the hands against the wall or a piece of furniture. Rarely, the occupant uses a pair of canes in the manner of ski poles, punting the chair. Also called swivel chair, glide-about chair, roll-about chair.

• **commode chair.** A chair with a removable seat over a removable bedpan. If on casters, such a chair may be called a castercommode.

• **geriatric chair.** A combination of rolling armchair and tabletop. Also called table chair.

• **glide-about chair.** See **casterchair**.

• **growing chair.** Chair constructed in such a way that its dimensions can be modified, accommodating a child during several years of growing.

• **lift-seat chair.** A chair with a lift (or catapult) seat. See **catapult seat**.

• **pushchair.** A wheeled chair that is not fitted with handrims or another device for self-propulsion but is designed to be pushed by an attendant. It might still be possible for the user to "walk" the chair, i.e., using his or her feet against the ground, or to punt it along with a pair of canes.

• **relaxation chair.** One of several types of chairs most frequently used by children or adults with cerebral palsy and similar conditions in which spasticity and hyperreflexic muscles interfere with quiet sitting. Usually constructed so as to support large parts of the user's body in a position of flexion of the neck, trunk, hips, and knees, a posture conducive to relaxation in many patients.

• **roll-about chair, swivel chair.** See **casterchair**.

• **table chair.** See **geriatric chair**.

• **walking chair.** A walker with a seat, usually a foldaway seat.

chairback brace, corset, or orthosis See **Knight brace**, under **brace**.

chair dancing Wheelchair dancing.

chairlift See **stairlift**.

chair–table combination See **geriatric chair**, under **chair**.

chalybeate Containing iron, such as the waters of certain spas.

Chandler collar A felt collar, usually covered with stockinette.

charley horse Postexertional myalgia, i.e., muscle pain and stiffness after physical activities, particularly of prolonged and arduous nature.

chest physical therapy See under **physical therapy**.

chest press See under **bench press**.

chest weights Weights of various amounts to be raised and lowered, usually along a wall (in that case, also called wall pulleys). Most frequently moved by the upper limbs for the strengthening of muscles attached to the chest. They can also be used for many other muscle groups.

chimney, standing chimney Stand-in table. See under **table**.

chin control System of activating an apparatus used by a person with absent or completely paralyzed upper limbs: the chin mobilizes a multidirectional switch. It is often used for the control of a wheelchair.

Chinese fingertrap See **fingertrap**.

chinning (oneself) To pull oneself up while being suspended by the hands, to a position in which the chin is above the level of the hands. See also **chinning bar**, under **bar**.

chiropodist, chiropody See **podiatrist** and **podiatry**.

chiropractic A system of treatment consisting essentially in manipulations of the vertebral column, originally based on the assumption that minor displacements of the vertebrae are the cause of most diseases. Founded by Canadian-born Daniel David Palmer (1845–1913), who in 1898 opened the first school of this method in Davenport, Iowa.

chiropractor One who practices chiropractic.

chorea Any of a group of disorders characterized by a brief, rapid, involuntary movement of the limbs, face, trunk, and head; flailing or jerky motions of segments of extremities.

choreiform movements Flailing or jerky motions of the limbs, abnormal postures of the head, and facial grimaces that occur during attempts at voluntary movement or generalized activity or in response to emotional stimulation because of impaired capacity for inhibition.

choreo-athetoid Combination of choreiform and athetoid.

chronaximeter Apparatus for the measurement of rheobase and chronaxy, also used for treatment by electric stimulation. The earlier apparatus with condenser discharges has been replaced by electronic generators of two types:

1. Voltage-stabilized (constant voltage) stimulator of low output impedance (500 Ω or less), giving the rheobase in volts. Little used in USA.
2. Current-stabilized (constant current) stimulator of high output impedance (100,00 Ω or more), giving the rheobase in milliamperes. Commonly used in USA.

chronaximetry Measurement of chronaxy.

chronaxy The minimum time required for an electric stimulus at an intensity double that of the rheobase to provoke the contraction of a muscle. Also spelled **chronaxia** and **chronaxie**, the latter corresponding to the French term proposed in 1909 by Louis Lapicque (1866–1952), French physiologist.

chukka, chukka boot, chukka shoe See under **shoe**.

cine-, cinesi- See **kine-, kinesi-**.

circuit training

1. A program of physical fitness training that consists in jogging or running along a prescribed circuit studded with a number of stations (10, 20, or more). At each station different exercises are performed, e.g., situps, pushups, climbing a ladder, lifting weights, pedaling on a stationary bicycle, performing on a rowing machine. The paths between the stations may be level, descending, or ascending. There is grading and variation, depending upon the aim of the program and the level of the subject's fitness. See also **Parcours**.
2. Use of a multiexercise apparatus (see **universal gymnastic machine**) by moving from one station to another to perform various exercises.
3. A program of a variety of exercises for the overall preparation of an athlete for a competition.

circumduction

1. Circular motion of a body part.
2. Circumduction gait. See under **gait**.

circumductor A small wheel with a handle. It is turned by the circumduction of the wrist while the forearm is strapped to a troughlike support so as to avoid all motion proximal to the wrist.

clapping A massage maneuver, essentially a type of percussion by the hand kept either flat or slightly hollowed. It is often used on the chest for the dislodging of bronchial secretions, particularly in combination with postural drainage.

clasp, (posterior clasp, shoe clasp) A clip or clasp that is attached to a single posterior bar of an ankle-foot orthosis and held in place by being clipped to the upper border of the shoe. Used together with the orthosis to stabilize the ankle and prevent plantar flexion, it allows easy change of the orthosis from one shoe to another. Developed by the Veterans Administration Prosthetics Center, it is also called VAPC posterior clasp.

claudication Limbing.

• **intermittent claudication.** A condition marked by cramplike pains and weakness of legs induced by walking and by the disappearance of all discomfort when at rest; caused by sclerosis with narrowing of the arteries of the legs.

clawfoot A disabling deformity of the foot in which the longitudinal arch is extremely high, the toes are clawed, and the forefoot is dropped.

Clias method of exercise See under **exercise**.

climatology The science of climates.

climatotherapy The therapeutic use of climate.

climbing activities See **elevation activities**.

clonic perseveration Active, unconscious repetition of a motion that has first been performed as a passive motion by the examiner or on his order by the patient. Cf. **tonic perseveration**.

coaptation The fitting together of parts, such as the ends of a broken bone.

cognition

1. The intellectual process by which knowledge is acquired as opposed to emotional processes.
2. The product of this process; also called comprehension, judgment, perception.

cogwheel resistance, rigidity, or phenomenon Stepwise resistance felt by the examiner on passive motion, as, e.g., on passive elbow flexion and extension in a patient with parkinsonism.

coil A type of applicator in shortwave diathermy. See also **inductance cable or coil**.

coil field heating One type of electromagnetic-field heating.

cold quartz ultraviolet lamp See under **lamp**.

cold spray See **spray-and-stretch therapy**.

cold therapy The local application of cold for therapeutic purposes, including the treatment of muscle spasm and spasticity, mechanical trauma, burns, pain relief, and arthritides.

ColPaC Proprietary name of a pack for cold applications. See under **Hydrocollator**.

COMET Acronym for Child-Operated Mobile Electric Transport, an indoor vehicle for children without lower limbs. Developed in 1970 at the Chailey Heritage Craft School and Hospital, Chailey, Lewes, Sussex, England.

Communicative Abilities in Daily Living Test (CADL) See under **test**.

compensated work therapy Incentive therapy.

compensatory education Motor education of a child who, because of motor, sensory, or mental deficiencies, has never learned to perform certain physical activities. Term sometimes used as a synonym of habilitation (q.v.).

compensatory model A theory hypothesizing that persons with physical disabilities are likely to emphasize positive attributes over which they have some control to compensate for perceived deficits.

Comprehensive Assessment and Referral Evaluation (CARE) instrument An instrument designed to measure the functioning of elderly community residents in two cultures, the United States and Great Britain.

Comprehensive Occupational Assessment and Training System (COATS) A work evaluation and training system for vocational rehabilitation.

Comprehensive Outpatient Rehabilitation Facility (CORF) A facility that is recognized as a provider of comprehensive outpatient rehabilitation services under the Medicare Act and, as such, eligible for reimbursement for services provided to Part B Medicare beneficiaries.

compression device

• **elastic compression device.** Elastic garment for the mild but continuous compression of a smaller or larger part of a limb or even of both lower limbs, including the pelvis, used in the treatment of edema and varicose veins. See also **stump shrinker**.

• **pneumatic compression device.** Inflatable cuff or air bag for a limb or the distal part of a limb. It is submitted to intermittent or continued pressure by the inflation of air and used for the reduction of edema or to prevent orthostatic hypotension.

computer adaptive systems The modification of computer, keyboard, monitor, modem, or other equipment, as well as programs, to accommodate disabled and/or physically challenged individuals to achieve independent usage of the system.

condenser field heating See **electric-field heating**.

condenser pad or plate A device used in shortwave diathermy with electric-field heating.

conductance The capacity for conducting. Electric conductance is the reciprocal of electric resistance.

conduction time The time between the stimulation of a nerve and the response, as measured by a recording device, such as an electromyograph.

conduction velocity The speed, expressed in meters per second, of the propagation of a nerve impulse after stimulation, as recorded with an electromyograph. The normal values average between 40 and 60 m/s.

conductive heat or heating See under **heat, heating**.

confusion pattern, confused motion A type of synkinetic, automatic, or reflex motion, occurring in upper motor neuron lesions as part of a more complex reflex pattern. See also **zero cerebral muscle**.

connective tissue massage See under **massage**.

containment The limiting of the experience of loss to functions that are directly affected by a disability of other types of loss or misfortune.

contingency contract A mutual agreement, frequently in writing, between the treating practitioner and the client, in which the individual agrees to treatment and the targeted behaviors, the reinforcers, and the contingencies are specified.

continuous positive airway pressure (CPAP) A technique of respiratory assistance administered by a respirator, used in particular for infants with hyaline membrane disease.

contraction See also under **exercise**.

- **anisometric contraction.** Contraction of a muscle in which the distance between its origin and its insertion changes. This is usually called isotonic contraction.

• **anodal closing contraction (ACC).** Contraction of muscle at the anode upon closure of the electric circuit. See also **Erb's formula**.

• **anodal opening contraction (AOC).** Contraction of muscle at the anode upon opening of the electric circuit. See also **Erb's formula**.

• **cathodal closing contraction (CCC).** Contraction of muscle at the cathode upon closure of the electric circuit. See also **Erb's formula**.

• **cathodal opening contraction (COC).** Contraction of muscle at the cathode upon opening of the electric circuit. See also **Erb's formula**.

• **closing contraction.** Contraction of muscle due to electric stimulation upon the closing of the circuit. See also **Erb's formula**.

• **concentric contraction.** Usual activity of a muscle, which shortens because of the contraction of its fibers. Strictly speaking it is simply a contraction, but the term is used in opposition to eccentric contraction (see next entry), an expression equally objectionable.

• **eccentric contraction.** Action of a muscle that takes place while its length increases, because the force it develops is smaller than the outside force against which it contracts. Example: the action of the elbow flexors while slowly letting a weight down on the floor. Called also lengthening contraction. In fact it is a contraction of decreasing intensity.

• **galvanotonic contraction.** Prolonged contraction of a muscle produced by galvanic current.

• **idiomuscular contraction.** Contraction of a denervated muscle that is not stimulated by its diseased motor nerve but by direct electric stimulation.

• **isokinetic contraction.** See **isokinetic exercise**, under **exercise**.

• **isometric contraction.** Contraction of a muscle without appreciable change in its length, since there is no joint movement. Also called static contraction. See also **isometric exercise**, under **exercise**.

• **isotonic contraction.** Contraction of a muscle that results in a motion, hence in a change in its length. See also **isotonic exercise**, under **exercise**.

• **lengthening contraction.** Eccentric contraction.

• **opening contraction.** Contraction of a muscle due to electric stimulation upon the opening of the circuit. See also **Erb's formula**.

• **sluggish contraction.** Slow, wormlike contraction, as seen on electric stimulation of a denervated muscle.

• **static contraction.** Isometric contraction.

contracture Shortening of soft tissue that cannot be brought to its normal length. In physiology, this term denotes a prolonged contraction of muscle without propagation of an impulse.

cookie Colloquialism for navicular pad. See under **pad**.

Cook shingle Pressure pad of rectangular shape, for rigid support of the lumbosacral area.

coordination The ability of muscles or groups of muscles to work together to produce controlled movements that are needed for task performance.

• **bilateral integration coordination.** The coordination of both sides of the body during activity (e.g., writing with the right hand while stabilizing the paper with the left).

• **eye-hand coordination.** The use of the visual system to guide movement.

• **fine motor coordination.** The controlled use of small muscle groups.

• **gross motor coordination.** The use of large muscle groups for controlled movements.

coping The cognitive and behavioral efforts to reduce, master, or tolerate stressful situations and the emotional reactions that accompany them.

Cordo insert Socket liner made from stockinette impregnated with a thinner (called Cordo-Bond) and a plasticizer. Developed in 1971 by US Veterans Administration Prosthetics Center, New York.

Cornell Medical Index A measure of physical health, developed by Brodman, that is composed of 195 items categorized into 12 different areas of physical health.

coronary-prone behavior The concept that behavior and emotions might contribute to the development of coronary heart disease.

• **Type A behavior.** Behavior that increases the prevalence of heart attacks, sudden death, and angina, such as impatience, competitiveness, and hostility.

• **Type B behavior.** Behavior that does not contribute to heart attacks, sudden death, and angina.

corrective therapist A physical educator, administering therapeutic exercises, training in locomotion, games, sports, etc., as ordered and supervised by a physician, usually in a US Veterans Administration hospital.

corrective therapy In a general sense, any medical or surgical therapy purports to be corrective. In a more restricted sense, the term refers to medically oriented and medically prescribed exercises and other physical activities for the physically or mentally impaired, administered by corrective therapists (see preceding entry) in Veterans Administration hospitals. **Corrective medical gymnastics** is applied to scoliosis, flatfoot, poor posture, faulty walking or breathing, etc. See also **adapted physical education**.

corselet A small corset.

corset Named after the Latin *corpus*, for "body" (hence the related term "bodice") and originally meaning a garment around the trunk. It refers to an orthosis or orthotic part that encircles the trunk or part of it or a segment of a limb. Examples: thoracic, thoracolumbar, lumbar, lumbosacral, sacroiliac, thigh, knee, calf corsets.

• **Boston corset.** A prefabricated corset, comparable in its design to the Milwaukee corset (q.v.). Developed in Boston in 1974 by John E. Hall, surgeon, and William Miller, orthotist.

• **Hoke corset.** Thoracolumbosacral canvas corset with front opening and multiple stays. Developed about 1930, primarily as a support in scoliosis due to poliomyelitis, by Warm Springs, Georgia, surgeon Michael Hoke (1874–1944). Called also Warm Springs corset.

• **metatarsal corset.** An elastic cuff slipped over the midportion of the foot. It usually incorporates a metatarsal pad (see under **pad**), which can thus be applied and removed as desired. Without the pad, it may be used as a support in splayfoot.

• **Milwaukee corset.** A body brace reaching from the pelvis to the occiput and chin, designed to distract all vertebrae while allowing certain motions of the trunk. Created in 1945 for the treatment of scoliosis by orthopedic surgeon Walter P. Blount and coworkers in Milwaukee, Wisconsin.

• **Warm Springs corset.** Hoke corset.

cosine law See **Lambert's cosine law**.

cosmesis, cosmetic As applied to a prosthesis, these terms refer to its appearance, being as similar as possible in shape, color, surface, and feel to the body part it replaces. As applied to an orthosis or other device, they express its relative unobtrusiveness.

Cosom hockey Sport combining ice hockey and basketball. It originated in Battle Creek, Michigan, in 1962 and was adapted for the physically handicapped in wheelchairs, who played it first in 1967 at the University of Virginia Children's Rehabilitation Center. Named after the manufacturer of the equipment used.

coulomb The unit of electric charge, or quantity of electricity. The coulomb is the quantity of electricity carried in one second by a current of one ampere. Named after Charles Auguste de Coulomb (1736–1806), French physicist.

counter The part of a shoe that is attached to its heel and embraces the heel of the foot. Thus it has a medial and a lateral extension, also called medial and lateral counter.

counterextension Traction applied coincident with, but in a direction opposite to, another traction. Example: in a recumbent patient, traction by a pelvic belt is applied toward the feet, while a thoracic harness applies countertraction toward the head. Thus the lumbar vertebrae are submitted to counterextension.

counterirritation An irritation, therapeutically produced, usually to an area of the skin, in order to relieve an irritation situated in another area.

coupling agent for ultrasound A substance used to ensure close, uninterrupted contact between the soundhead of an ultrasound apparatus and the skin, indispensable to achieving transmission of energy. A simple coupling agent is mineral oil. Special products are marketed. Under water, no further coupling agent is needed.

cow horn A support of the axilla that extends from the dorsal part of a back brace to the anterior part of the chest.

coxa plana (plural coxae planae) A flattening of the femoral head, due to osteochondrosis of the epiphysis. Also called osteochondrosis, Legg-Calvé-Perthes disease, or other names.

coxa valga (plural coxae valgae) Femur in which the angle between neck and body is greater than normal, i.e., greater than about 130°.

coxa vara (plural coxae varae) Femur in which the angle between neck and body is smaller than normal, i.e., smaller than about 120°.

cradle Frame protecting the patient's body or part of it from the contact of the upper bed sheet. See also **heat cradle**.

craunotherapy Crenotherapy.

crawler See **prone scooter**. Cf. also **creeper**.

crawling Mode of locomotion in which chest and abdomen touch the ground (or other surface of support). A child may begin to crawl at the age of seven months. Often called creeping (q.v.).

creative therapy General term, often used in the plural (creative therapies). It includes art, dance, horticulture, music, occupational, and possibly other therapies used in rehabilitation.

creeper A low rolling support for a subject, usually a child, in the quadruped position. Although the term is interchangeably used with crawler, the latter term is preferably used for still lower supports (see **prone scooter**).

• **suspension creeper.** A framelike construction with four legs on rollers. A harness hangs from above, supporting the trunk of the subject, whose hands and knees (or feet) rest on the ground. Used to assist in normal locomotion on all fours.

creeping Mode of locomotion on hands and feet, or hands and knees, seen in children after the age of nine months. No part of the trunk touches the ground, as opposed to crawling (q.v.). However, the terms are often interchangeably used. therefore, in order to underline the fact that the chest, the abdomen, and the thighs do not touch the floor, the term high creeping is sometimes used.

crenotherapy Treatment by mineral waters, notably at the spring itself. From the Greek words for spring and treatment.

crisis theory A conceptual framework that views the onset of disability or illness as a crisis-inducing event.

Crooke's metal Electrode foil: a flexible sheet metal. Consisting mainly of lead, with small amounts of tin, zinc, or other metals, it is easily cut with ordinary scissors and molded over a body part. Named after the John J. Crooke Company in New York and Chicago, which manufactured it early in the twentieth century for Chicago radiologist Émil H. Crubbé (1875–1960), who used it to protect healthy tissues from untoward x-ray effects during radiotherapy. Later, notably in the second quarter of the century, it was also used as material for electrodes in certain therapeutic applications. Also called Grubbé x-ray foil (obsolete), or, in the same or similar composition, sheet lead, lead foil, tinfoil, block tin, and rolled tin.

cross-body method (or technique) of travel See **cane travel of the blind**.

cross-legged Referring to walking, the toes turned in and one foot in front of the other.

crouch, crouching See under **gait** and **position**.

crounotherapy Crenotherapy.

CRUMBS Acronym for continuous, remote, unobtrusive monitoring of biobehavioral systems, a technique of quantitative evaluation of patient performance, used in rehabilitation.

crutch A support for standing and walking, made of wood or metal, extending from the ground to a level between the elbow and the axillary cavity, held by the hand or attached to the upper limb.

• **axillary crutch.** The most common kind of crutch, having a crossbar just below the axilla.

• **California crutch.** Canadian crutch. See next entry.

• **Canadian crutch.** A wooden crutch that is slightly shorter than, but similar to, an axillary crutch. Its upper extremity consists of a leather cuff at or a little above mid-arm level. Suggested term: wooden triceps crutch.

• **crab crutch.** A crutch with three or more tips.

• **Everett crutch.** Aluminum variety of Canadian crutch. Named for Charles E. Everett, a patient at Georgia Warm Springs Foundation, Warm Springs, Georgia, for whom the first crutch of this type was made. Also called Warm Springs crutch. Suggested term: metal triceps crutch.

• **folding crutch.** Single upright metal crutch that can be folded at a joint just above the hand piece for use as a cane or for storage.

• **forearm crutch.** Cane, usually made of aluminum, with hand piece pointing forward at a 90° angle and forearm extension deviating posteriorly at a 15° angle. At its upper end, reaching about two to three fingerbreadths below the elbow, is a hinged open cuff. Also called Lofstrand crutch.

• **full-length crutch.** Axillary crutch.

• **German crutch.** Forearm crutch.

• **Kenny crutch.** Double upright wooden forearm crutch with leather cuff at the upper end. Named after Elizabeth Kenny (1886–1952), Australian nurse known as Sister Kenny.

• **Lofstrand crutch.** Forearm crutch. Named after Adolf Lofstrand, Rockville, Maryland, who developed it about 1944.

• **mat crutch.** Shortened axillary crutch, the lower part of which reaches to the level on which the user sits, i.e., the floor or an exercise mat. Mat crutches are used to prepare paraplegics or bilateral lower-limb amputees for regular crutches.

• **platform crutch, shelf crutch.** Crutch of either the axillary or forearm type, with a horizontal support (the platform or shelf) for the forearm and usually a peg for the hand. Used when for any reason the elbow is kept flexed or the hand is unable to grasp the handle in the usual way.

• **short crutch.** Mat crutch.

• **sling-top (axillary) crutch.** An axillary crutch in which the rigid axillary crosspiece is replaced by a slinglike support, usually made of leather.

• **standard crutch.** Axillary crutch, made of wood.

• **tricepts crutch.** Crutch ending with a cuff at about mid-arm level. It can be made of wood, with a leather cuff, or of aluminum, in which case the cuff is usually covered with leather. The former is also called Canadian crutch; the latter, Warm Springs or Everett crutch.

• **underarm crutch.** Axillary crutch.

• **Warm Springs crutch.** Aluminum variety of Canadian crutch. Named for Georgia Warm Springs Foundation, Warm Springs, Georgia, where it was originally devised. Suggested term: metal triceps crutch.

• **weighted crutch.** Crutch made heavy by lead or other means for easier studying of an uncoordinated upper limb. A good technique is to take a metal crutch and weight its hollow uprights with lead pellets.

crutch paralysis Paralysis due to pressure on the brachial nerves by the axillary piece of a crutch.

crymo-, cryo- Prefixes referring to cold.

Cryogel Proprietary name of cold packs.

cryotherapy Treatment by cold substances, such as ice, ethyl choride, carbon dioxide snow, etc.

cue A signal to begin a specific behavior.

• **physical cue.** A cue that involves touching to prompt the desired physical movement.

• **verbal cue.** A spoken prompt in which the level is variable, ranging from a sound to a complete instruction.

• **visual cue.** Any visible gesture, posture, and/or facial expression that is used to aid in the performance of a task.

cued speech A system of eight hand signals (manual cues) made in four positions close to the mouth, so as to produce a total of 32 combinations supplementing spoken words in order to facilitate lipreading by the deaf, particularly the congenitally deaf. The cues represent phonetic signs. Thus, three different cues help to distinguish between the consonants in **ba, pa,** and **ma**, three syllables spoken with the same lip movement. Developed in 1966 by American physicist R. Orin Cornett (1913–1983), Washington, D.C.

cuff suspension Method of attachment of a below-knee prosthesis, consisting of a strap—called a cuff—that is attached to the socket and is applied to the thigh just above the patella.

curb jumping Negotiating a curb while sitting in a wheelchair.

current, electric The flow or movement of electrons in certain bodies called conductors. The flow of electric current, i.e., electricity, in a circuit is ruled by **Ohm's law** (q.v.).

• **alternating current (AC, ac).** Electric current changing its direction periodically.

• **conduction current.** Current due to movement of electrons from atom to atom. Type of current along metal conductors.

• **constant current, continuous current.** Direct current of steady flow.

• **cutting current.** Electric current used for surgical cutting.

• **d'Arsonval current.** High-frequency current of low voltage. Current of a frequency as high as not to produce muscular contraction but heat. Introduced for therapeutic use by Arsène d'Arsonval (q.v.).

• **diadynamic current.** Sinusoidal current of low frequency (commonly between 50 and 1,000 Hz), with continuous modulation, which, depending upon the variations in frequency, intensity, and duration, has various physiologic effects. Developed in the 1940s by the French physician Pierre M. Bernard; little used in the USA.

• **diathermy current.** High-frequency current that alternates so rapidly that it usually neither stimulates motor nerves nor causes burns.

• **direct current (dc, dc).** Unidirectional current. Electric current that does not change polarity.

• **faradic current.** An alternating, asymmetric current that stimulates muscle through its nerve. It is in effect, however, a direct current abruptly interrupted about 80 to 100 times per second. It is therefore one kind of tetanizing current. Originally it was produced by a faradic coil. This has been replaced by a thermionic grid-glow tube. Developed by Michael Faraday (q.v.).

• **galvanic current.** Direct current of steady flow. Term mostly used in medicine. Same as constant or continuous current. Named after Luigi Galvani (q.v.).

• **high-frequency current.** Alternating current of frequencies above 100,000 Hz, i.e., above frequencies resulting in muscular contraction. The frequencies used in diathermy are over 10,000,000 Hz and are also referred to as ultrahigh frequencies.

• **induced current.** Current generated by induction, i.e., by the presence of another electric current nearby.

• **interference current.** Current resulting from the intersection of two independent circuits in one apparatus. One produces a sinusoidal current of a constant frequency of about 3,000 or 4,000 Hz; the other generates a current of a slightly different and variable frequency, e.g., between 2,900 and 3,100 Hz or between 3,900 and 4,100 Hz, respectively. Developed in 1951 by the Austrian physicist Hans Nemec.

• **low-frequency current.** Current of a frequency between 5 and 3,000 Hz, usually between 50 and 100 Hz, i.e., current capable of stimulating muscle and nerve. It is of low voltage. Also called tetanizing current. See also **low-volt currents** (next entry).

• **low-volt (or low-voltage) currents.** Term embracing constant, faradic, and sinusoidal currents. Also called low-frequency currents, though the constant current has, of course, no frequency.

• **modulated (or modulation) current.** Current whose intensity is cyclically reduced to zero. An example of modulated current is surging current (q.v.).

• **oscillating current.** Alternating current.

• **Oudin current.** A high-frequency current of particularly high voltage, obtained by a special coil of wire, called Oudin resonator. Invented by Paul Oudin (1851–1923), French electrotherapist.

• **progressive current.** Electric current that increases relatively slowly before reaching its maximum intensity.

• **pulsating current.** Electric current that increases and decreases in intensity in a regular fashion.

• **sine wave (or sinusoidal) current.** A type of alternating current increasing and decreasing in intensity with symmetric variation.

• **surgical current.** Electric current used for surgical purposes, either cutting or fulguration.

• **surging current.** Modulated current (AC or DC), whose peak intensity gradually increases and decreases at a rate (called modulation rate) of from once a second to once every ten seconds.

• **Tesla current.** A high-frequency current, comparable to d'Arsonval current but of higher voltage, adjustable by an induction coil. Proposed by Nikola Tesla (1856–1943), Serbian physicist in New York.

• **tetanizing current.** Electric current contracting a muscle to the point of tetanus. This is usually a current with a frequency between 50 and 200 Hz for normal muscles and between 5 and 10 Hz for denervated muscles.

current-stabilized stimulator See **chronaximeter**.

curvature A bending or curving.

Cybex exerciser Proprietary name of an isokinetic device.

cycle As referring to an alternating current, it is the passage from zero through a positive maximum, then back to zero, through a negative maximum and again back to zero. The time required to complete one cycle is a period.

D

dactylology Fingerspelling (q.v.).

Dalcroze Eurhythmics A method of musical education in which the body is called upon to experience and to express musical rhythms. Customarily taught to children in groups, it was developed in the 1890s by the Vienna-born Swiss composer and educator Emile-Jaques Dalcroze (1865–1950).

dance notation A method of recording body movements, in particular those of a dancer, by simple symbols that can be written. A typewriter with such symbols became commercially available in 1973, developed by New York City's Dance Notation Bureau and International Business Machines Corporation. Its ball-shaped typing element carries 88 symbols indicating the body parts, directions, and other details of the movements. See also **movement notation**.

dance therapy Therapeutic system consisting in guiding subjects toward self-expression by dancing or simply performing rhythmic movements of their bodies. Applied most often in groups of individuals with emotional, less often with physical, disturbances. Pioneered in 1940 by Marian Chase.

d'Arsonval, Arsène French physicist and physician (1851–1940).

• **d'Arsonval current.** See under **current**.

• **d'arsonvalism, d'arsonvalization.** The therapeutic use of d'Arsonval currents.

dBA Decibels measured on the "A" scale of soundlevel meters, the most frequently used of the scales A, B, and C, because it most closely reflects the way the human ear hears.

deaf A term with an audiological meaning and, for many, a sociocultural meaning, referring to persons whose hearing loss is of such severity that oral/aural communication in ineffective in most settings.

deaf-mute An individual who can neither hear or speak.

deafmutism Inability to speak due to congenital or early deafness.

deafness Inability to hear, partial or complete.

- **acoustic trauma deafness.** Loss of hearing caused by prolonged exposure to excessive noise.
- **cerebral deafness.** Deafness caused by a lesion in the auditory area of the brain.
- **conductive deafness.** Loss of hearing caused by disease of or injury to the tympanic membrane or ear ossicles.
- **nerve deafness.** Deafness caused by damage to the cochlear division of the vestibulocochlear nerve.
- **sudden deafness.** A sudden loss of hearing, thought to be related to systemic disease, including fat metabolism and hypercoagulation (diseases that block the circulation).
- **toxic deafness.** Loss of hearing caused by certain chemical agents.
- **word deafness.** Acoustic or auditory aphasia; inability to understand the spoken word.

deafness symbol Emblem showing an ear crossed by a diagonal bar denoting impairment. Preferably white on a dark blue background, it may serve to identify a person with impaired hearing (by a lapel pin, carrying card, etc.), television programs either captioned or interpreted for the deaf, access to a teletypewriter (TTY) or other telecommunication device for the deaf (see TDD), etc. Developed by an international team, it was approved in 1979 by the World Federation of the Deaf, in 1980 by the National Association of the Deaf (Usa) and adopted internationally.

Deaf Olympics World athletic games for the deaf, a quadrennial contest organized by the International Games for the Deaf, founded in 1924.

Deaver, George G. New York physiatrist (1890–1973), who coined the expression "activities of daily living." He considered maximum use of the hands and independence in these activities as the primary objectives of rehabilitation. These were followed by independence in locomotion, i.e. either walking and climbing stairs or wheelchair propulsion; maximum ability to hear and speak; and functioning in a manner as close to normal as possible.

• **Deaver method.** Applied in particular to patients with cerebral palsy or other brain injuries resulting in locomotor disabilities, it consists in restricting most movements by extensive bracing, except for one body segment that is left free for motor reeducation. Once an acceptable level of function in that segment has been achieved, the neighboring segment is freed from orthotic restriction and submitted to reeducation, so that progressively less and less bracing is needed.

debilitate To make weak or feeble.

debility The condition of abnormal bodily weakness; lack or loss of strength.

deci (d) Prefix meaning one tenth of a measure (10^{-1}).

decibel (dB) Unit of intensity of sound. It is a proportional unit that indicates a difference of loudness, just noticeable under certain conditions. Examples of decibel levels:

Whispering	30 dB
Normal conversation at 4 m	50 dB
Light auto traffic at 30 m	50 dB
Freeway at 15 m	70 dB
Industrial noise limit	85 dB
Shouting into one's ear	100 dB
Auto horn at 1 m	110 dB
Jet aircraft taking off at 60 m	120 dB

Named after Alexander Graham Bell (1847–1922), inventor of the telephone.

decubitus

1. The act or position of lying down.

2. Incorrectly used for decubitus ulcer, pressure sore, bedsore. The term "decubti" as plural is inadmissible, being grammatically incorrect.

degenerative joint disease (DJD) A chronic disorder marked by degeneration of articular cartilage and hypertrophy of bone, accompanied by pain that appears with activity and subsides with rest; a common form of chronic joint disease in the middle-aged and the elderly; also called osteoarthritis and degenerative or hypertrophic arthritis.

Delorme method of exercise See under **exercise**.

Delsarte system, Delsartism A school of posture, gesture, expression, breathing, speaking, and singing, originally for singers and actors, developed by the Frenchman Francois-Alexandre-Nicolas Delsarte (1811–1871). His method was popularized by his pupils and further developed into a system of calisthenics, with emphasis on breathing, grace, and relaxation, by Genevieve Stebbins in New York, who in 1885 published *The Delsarte System of Expression.*

dementia An impairment of global cognitive function that results in a decrease in the patient's ability to function in the environment.

denervated Refers to an organ or a tissue, especially muscle or skin with interrupted nerve supply.

denervation The state of an organ or a tissue, especially muscle or skin, with interrupted nerve supply.

densitometry Technique for measuring the density of a substance, especially bone.

Denver bar, Denver heel A metatarsal bar. Usually attached to the outsole of the shoe, it is thinner and extends farther posteriorly than the common type. The **internal Denver bar** is inserted between outsole and insole. Used by the English orthopedic surgeon Sir Robert Jones (1858–1933), it was named after the city where it was observed in the late 1930s by a New York orthopedist.

deossification Removal of the mineral elements of bone.

depersonalization The tendency of rehabilitation professionals to detach from feelings of concern for clientele moving toward a regard for clients as impersonal objects. This state usually is present in individuals who have burnout.

Derby (derby) shoe See under **shoe**.

dermohmmeter Instrument that measures electric skin resistance. See next term.

dermohmmetry Measurement of electric resistance of the skin. This is an objective, though not completely reliable, test of involvement of a sensory nerve accompanied by dryness of the skin in the area of its distribution and reflected in an increase of electric skin resistance. It is also used to assess the result of sympathectomies and paravertebral blocks. The electric resistance of a sweating skin might be 100,000 ohms or less. The resistance of denervated skin can reach 60,000,000 ohms and above.

dermometer, dermometry See **dermohmmeter** and **dermohmmetry**.

devaluation A process through which some view persons with disabilities as lacking something of importance, with the result that their worth is devalued and their being held in lower social esteem.

developmental therapy A psychoeducational approach to the treatment and rehabilitation of children with emotional disturbances. The therapist, on the basis of the child's stage of development, plans an appropriate sequence of experiences to help the pupil to progress. The term sometimes refers to physical or occupational therapy of children with cerebral palsy and other locomotor dysfunctions.

developmental stage models Conceptualizations of the adjustment process in which stages are proposed in an attempt to describe characteristic patterns of behavior.

diagnosis The determination of the nature of a disease.

- **clinical diagnosis.** A diagnosis based on the signs and symptoms of a disease.

- **diagnosis by exclusion.** A diagnosis made by excluding all but one of the disease processes, thought to be possible causes of the symptoms being considered.

- **differential diagnosis.** The determination of which of two or more diseases with similar symptoms is the one with which the patient is afflicted; consideration or listing of diseases possibly responsible for a patient's illness, based on information available at the time, e.g., symptoms, signs, physical findings, and laboratory data.

- **laboratory diagnosis.** A diagnosis made by a chemical, microscopic, bacteriologic, or biopsy study of secretions, discharges, blood, or tissue.

• **pathologic diagnosis.**

1. A diagnosis (sometimes a postmortem diagnosis) made from a study of the lesion present.
2. A diagnosis of the pathologic conditions present, determined by a study and comparison of the symptoms.

• **physical diagnosis.** A diagnosis based on information obtained through physical examination of the patient, using the techniques of inspection, palpation, percussion, and auscultation.

• **postmortem diagnosis.** An autopsy; examination of a dead body, usually to determine cause of death.

diagnostician One who is experienced in determining the nature of disease; formerly used to apply to physicians with extensive training and experience in medicine, comparable to internists of today.

diaphysis The shaft of a long bone.

diaphysitis Inflammation of the body or shaft of a long bone.

diathermy Literally meaning "through-heat" or "heating through." Therapeutic heating of a body part by conversion of high-frequency electric current, electromagnetic waves, or sound waves. The term is most frequently used for shortwave diathermy. An international convention, held in 1947 in Atlantic City, outlawed the previously used longwave diathermy and reserved the following wavelengths (with their corresponding frequencies) for medical use:

0.122	4 m	(2 450 MHz)
7.327	86 m	(40.68 MHz)
11.06	m	(27.12 MHz)
22.123	8 m	(13.56 MHz)

• **conventional diathermy.** Longwave diathermy, more specifically of electric current of frequencies between 0.5 and 3 MHz (corresponding wavelengths, 600 and 100 m, respectively). No longer used in medicine.

• **longwave diathermy.** Diathermy of electric current of frequencies between 0.1 and 10 MHz (corresponding wavelengths, 3,000 and 30 m, respectively.) No longer used in medicine.

• **medical diathermy.** Diathermy for nondestructive purposes, as opposed to surgical diathermy.

• **microwave diathermy.** Deep heating by electromagnetic waves of a frequency between 300 and 300,000 MHz (corresponding wavelengths, 1 m and 1 mm, respectively). A commonly used apparatus emits waves of 122 mm at a frequency of 2,450 MHz. Microwave radiations are "beamed" at the patient with a microwave detector.

• **shortwave diathermy.** Diathermy of electric current of frequencies between 10 and 100 MHz (wavelengths between 30 and 3 m, respectively). The usual frequency is about 27 MHz (wavelength, 11 m). The term diathermy most frequently refers to this type.

• **surgical diathermy.** High-frequency current producing heat of sufficient intensity to destroy tissue by coagulation or desiccation.

• **ultrashortwave diathermy.** Shortwave diathermy, more specifically of frequencies between 25 and 100 MHz (corresponding wavelengths between 12 and 3 m, respectively).

• **ultrasonic (or ultrasound) diathermy.** See ultrasound.

Differential Aptitude Test (DAT) See under **test**.

Digitrap Proprietary name for a tubular device for a finger or toe (see fingertrap) at the tip of which a weight is attached to provide traction to the digit.

Disabilities Factor Scales (DFS) A scale developed by Siller, Chipman, Ferguson, and Vann (1967) that measures attitudes toward persons with disabilities.

disability Status of diminished function, based on the anatomic, physiologic, or mental impairment that has reduced the individual's actual or presumed ability to engage in any substantial gainful activity. Depending upon the individual's age, education, work experience, and other personal factors, disability is a status that is legally determined on the basis of a medically evaluated impairment. Cf. **impairment**.

• **developmental disability.** A chronic disability due to a mental or physical impairment present at birth or which is manifested before the person attains the age of 22 years

disabled Refers to the diminished physical or mental ability of an individual (see **disability**). Adjective or noun, singular or plural. Often used interchangeably with handicapped, which is not always correct. Cf. **handicapped**.

disablement, levels of A generic term referring to any experience identified variously by the terms impairment, disability, or handicap.

disarticulation Amputation of a limb by separating the bones at the joint.

discectomy Surgical removal of an intervertebral disk.

disengagement Withdrawal from roles or activities and reduction of activity levels.

disk Any platelike structure; also written disc.

• **articular disk.** A circular fibrocartilaginous pad present in some synovial joints and attached to the joint capsule.

• **dental disk.** A small disk of paper or plastic, coated with cuttlefish bone, emery, garnet, or sand; used in dentistry to cut, smooth, or polish teeth and dental restorations.

• **herniated disk.** Posterior rupture of the inner portion of an intervertebral disk, causing pressure on the nerve roots with resulting pain; occurring most commonly in the lower back; also called slipped, ruptured, or prolapsed disc.

• **ruptured disk.** See **herniated disk.**

• **slipped disk.** See **herniated disk.**

diskectomy The surgical removal, in part or whole, of an intervertebral disk.

disk syndrome Pain in the lower back, radiating to the thigh with occasional loss of ankle and knee reflexes, resulting from compression of spinal nerve roots by an intervertebral disk.

dislocate To shift from the usual or normal position, especially to displace a bone from its socket; to luxate.

dismember To remove a limb.

distal Farthest from a point of reference.

dog guide See **guide dog**.

Doman-Delacato patterning therapy An exercise method for patients, mostly children, with lesions of the central nervous system. An outgrowth of Fay reflex therapy (q.v.), it attempts to duplicate the phylogenetic development of locomotor patterns. Depending on its developmental level, the child may be kept in the prone position or may be stimulated to crawl or to proceed to other motions by repetitive passive motions. Three, four, or five therapists or helpers, working at the same time with one child, guide its head and each limb individually, also using sensory stimuli such as brushing, pinching, heat, and cold. Frequent, though short, sessions every day of the week restrict this therapy mostly to an institution's inpatients. The method, later extended to speech and reading problems, was established in 1954 by Robert J. Doman, physiatrist; Glenn J. Doman, physical therapist; and Carl H. Delacato, educator.

dominant hand The hand of greater skill, usually the one used in writing.

dominant hemisphere The cerebral hemisphere that seems more important than the other in the control of bodily movements such as handwriting. It is contralateral to the dominant hand.

Donaldson scale Scoring system of a patient's activities of daily living, containing self-care and mobility variables used in other scales, notably those in the Barthel index, the Katz index, and the Kenny self-care score (see these entries). A total of 147 individual items are graded from 1 (independent without assistance or devices) to 8 (unable to, or does not, perform) or by 9 (not applicable) or 0 (not evaluated). Developed by nurse Susanne W. Donaldson at the Department of Physical and Rehabilitation Medicine, Tufts University School of Medicine, Boston, and published in 1973.

Doppler test, Doppler ultrasonic transducer See **Doppler ultrasonic test**, under **test**.

dorsal Relating to the back or to the posterior part of an anatomic structure.

dorsiflexion Term applied to the motion of a toe toward the dorsum of the foot or the motion of the foot toward the anterior aspect of the leg. Also called extension. Opposite: **plantarflexion** or **flexion**. The terms dorsiflexion and palmarflexion, applied to the hand and its digits, are not called for. The correct corresponding terms are extension and flexion. The term volarflexion, instead of flexion, is to be completely abandoned.

dorsum The back of the upper or posterior surface.

dose Amount of therapeutic agent.

• **erythema dose.** Dose provoking erythema, e.g., erythema dose of ultraviolet radiation.

• **minimal erythema dose.** Referring to ultraviolet radiation, the smallest dose provoking an erythema under certain conditions in a given person.

dosimetry Measurement of factors that determine the biological response to ultrasound treatments.

douche Shower bath or irrigation of the surface of the body or of a cavity by a stream of water, which may be adjusted to various shapes, sizes, pressures, and temperatures, depending upon the apparatus used.

• **alternate (contrast, or Scotch) douche.** Alternating application of a standing subject of hot and cold water from two hoses held by an operator at a distance of three meters or more.

do yin Technique of massage of Asian origin.

drip sheet A wet sheet, wrung out and wrapped around the patient.

drive rim (of a wheelchair) Handrim.

driver training As referring to physically disabled persons, it consists in teaching the driving of a motor vehicle usually fitted with special equipment selected according to the physical impairment of the individual. Eg., foot controls may be replaced by hand controls, and other adaptations may be included.

dropfoot A foot that dangles when the leg is lifted, because of weakness or paralysis of the dorsiflexors of the ankle; or a foot in a position of plantarflexion that cannot be overcome.

drop-off at end of stance phase See **drop-off gait**, second definition, under **gait**.

drum A type of applicator in shortwave diathermy. See also **inductance cable** or **coil**.

Du Bois-Reymond law Law expressed in 1848 by Emil Heinrich Du Bois-Reymond (1818–1896), German physiologist, as follows: "It is the variation of current density and not the absolute value of current density at any given moment, that acts as a stimulus to a muscle or motor nerve."

Duchinne-Aran disease Progressive muscular atrophy.

dumbbell A device for exercise, usually made of iron and consisting of two spheres or disks connected by a rod just long enough to be held in one hand. Its weight is usually between 0.5 and 5 kg.

Dutchman A beveled piece of leather inserted between layers of the sole or heel of a shoe. It is usually a lateral sole wedge under the fifth metatarsal bone.

durable medical equipment (DME) Equipment that (a) can withstand repeated use, (b) is primarily and customarily used to serve a medical purpose, (c) generally is not useful to a person in the absence of illness or injury, and (d) is appropriate for use in the home.

dynamometer An instrument for measuring the force of contraction of a muscle or group of muscles.

- **squeeze dynamometer.** An instrument for measuring the intensity of squeeze of a fist.

dysarthria Disordered speech movements characterized by a defect in articulation.

dysbasia Difficulty in walking, especially that due to incoordination or hysteria.

dysgnosia Any disorder of the intellect.

dysgraphia Difficulty in writing, usually due to ataxia, tremor, or motor neurosis.

dyskinesia Impairment of coordinated motion.

dyskinetic Refers to dyskinesia.

dyslalia Impairment of speech due to defective speech organs.

dyslexia Impaired ability to learn to read.

dyslogia Impairment of the thought processes and of speech.

dysmegalopsia A disordered visual perception of the size of objects; called micropsia when objects seem smaller; macropsia, when larger.

dysmetria Impairment of sense of distance in muscular action.

dysphagia Difficulty in swallowing; also called aphagia.

dysphonia Difficulty or pain in speaking.

dysplastic Relating to or marked by abnormality of development.

dysstasia Difficulty in standing.

dyssynergia Disturbance of muscular coordination.

dystonia Spontaneous motion through a very limited range with a high degree of persistent tone during attempted voluntary activity.

E

early ambulation The therapeutic principle of having the patient out of bed and walking as early as possible. Developed in the first half of the twentieth century and strongly advocated by Daniel Leithauser in his book *Early Ambulation*, 1946, it was increasingly applied after childbirth, all types of surgery, myocardial infarction, fractures of the lower limbs, and many other medical and surgical conditions.

early postsurgical fitting Method of prosthetic replacement of a lower limb, similar to immediate postsurgical fitting (q.v.), with a cast applied to the stump at surgery, but weight bearing and ambulation initiated only about 10 to 30 days later.

ectomorph In the somatotype, an individual exhibiting linear and fragile features; a person with a lean and slightly muscular body.

educational therapy Therapy applied by teaching various subjects of basic knowledge, general education, writing, typing, other office activities, etc.

effleurage French for stroking, one of the fundamental maneuvers of massage. Also called stroking.

effluve An electric discharge accompanied by a purplish-blue flame given off by certain electrodes used for high-frequency currents of low amperage. Examples of such electrodes are wirebrush electrode and glass-condenser electrode (q.v.).

electric-field heating Shortwave diathermy using air-spaced plates, condenser pads, or single or double cuffs. Cf. **electromagnetic-field heating**.

electric silence Absence of visible or audible manifestations in the electromyogram.

electric skin resistance test See **dermohmmetry**.

electric stimulation

• **continuous electric stimulation.** Electric stimulation by an electrode either firmly attached to the skin or implanted, for use over hours or longer, monitored by the patient himself after appropriate instruction.

• **functional electric stimulation.** Electric stimulation triggered by a predetermined motion of the patient. It is aimed at increasing the range of active motion. After one or more initial treatment sessions, the electrode, powered by a battery, may be applied for hours or days.

electric stimulation tests See under **test**.

electroaerosol Aerosol whose particles are electrically charged. Its base is usually the mineral water of a spa, used for inhalation, often for a group of patients in a special room saturated with the aerosol.

electrode An object that, as part of an electric circuit, is in proximity to or in immediate contact with the body, receiving or emitting an electric current.

• **active electrode.** In electric stimulation, it is the electrode of smaller size (hence greater concentration of current), as compared with the dispersive electrode. In electromyography, it is the exploring electrode.

• **air-spaced electrode.** An electrode used in shortwave diathermy.

• **Bierman electrode.** Intravaginal diathermy electrode with a thermometer inserted into it. Described in 1936 by William Bierman (1893–1973), New York physiatrist.

• **cable disk electrode.** An electrode used in shortwave diathermy.

• **condenser pad electrode.** An electrode used in shortwave diathermy.

• **contoured electrode.** Hinged electrode (q.v.).

• **cuff electrode.** A flexible electrode in form of a cuff, used single or paired in shortwave diathermy.

• **dispersive electrode.** The electrode of larger size, as compared with the active electrode.

• **exploring electrode.** The active electrode exploring the electric activity of an organ or stimulating a muscle or a nerve for a diagnostic purpose.

• **glass-condenser electrode.** Closed glass tube with partial vacuum, used for high-frequency currents of low amperage.

• **hedgehog electrode.** Wirebrush electrode (q.v.).

• **hinged electrode.** A shortwave-diathermy electrode consisting of one fixed middle part and two lateral wings hinged to it, so as to be better molded over a body part. Called also molded electrode.

• **indifferent electrode.** Dispersive electrode (q.v.) or reference electrode (q.v.).

• **molded electrode.**

1. Hinged electrode for diathermy (q.v.).
2. Electrode cut out of metal foil or wire screen and molded according to need.

• **needle electrode.** An electrode in the shape of a needle to be inserted into tissues for exploration or stimulation. Commonly used in electromyography.

• **pancake electrode.** Shortwave-diathermy coil wound into a flat spiral and enclosed in a flat, round box evoking the shape of a pancake.

• **reference electrode.** The electrode that is used in association with the exploring electrode, as in electromyography.

• **ring electrode.** A metal ring applied around a finger to stimulate a sensory nerve in nerve conduction studies.

• **silent electrode.** Dispersive electrode.

• **skin (or surface) electrode.** Any of a great variety of electrodes of various shapes and sizes, applied to the surface of the body for stimulation, exploration, or dispersion.

• **wirebrush electrode.** An electrode used with Oudin's resonator for the production of high-frequency effluves.

electrodermal response Galvanic skin response (see under **Galvani**).

electrodermatography, electrodermography The measuring and mapping of the electric resistance of the skin. The result is an **electrodermatogram** or **electrodermogram**. See also **dermohmmetry**.

electrodiagnosis Diagnostic procedures by means of electricity (see **electric stimulation tests**, under **test**). In a wider sense it includes diagnostic electromyography but rarely electrocardiography, electroencephalography, and other comparable diagnostic procedures.

electroencephalography The recording of brain waves (which reveal the electric activity of the brain) by means of electrodes usually applied to the scalp.

electrogoniometer Electromechanical device that reads the angle of its two mechanical arms and delivers an electric signal proportional to that angle. It may be used for the measurement of positions and amplitudes of movements in a joint.

electrolarynx A device designed to introduce vibratory sound either directly into the oral cavity through a catheter or indirectly through the neck tissue so as to permit articulation of audible, intelligible words. See also **artificial larynx**.

electrolysis The decomposition of a chemical compound by an electric current. This phenomenon is used, among other things, to remove hair.

electromagnetic-field heating Shortwave diathermy with an inductance cable. Cf. **electric-field heating**.

electromagnetic radiation See under **radiation**.

electromotive force (EMF, emf, E) The force that makes the current flow, i.e., the difference of potential between two points of an electric circuit. It is expressed in volts and is equal to the electric power (in watts) divided by the intensity (in amperes):

$$E = \quad P$$
$$E = \underline{\qquad\quad}$$
$$E = \quad I$$

electromyogram The tracing of the electric potentials registered by an electromyograph.

electromyograph Apparatus that amplifies the electric potentials of muscle tissue for visual and aural display. Its use has been extended to the study of nerve function by the incorporation of a stimulating device.

electromyography The detection of electric potentials by an electromyograph. Primarily used for the study of muscle (myography), the procedure has been extended to the study of other phenomena, conduction of motor and sensory nerves in particular.

electroneurography Recording and measurement of the action potentials and conduction velocities of motor and sensory nerves. Used as a synonym of nerve conduction test (see under **test**).

electroneuromyography General term that includes nerve conduction measurements, electromyography, and classical electrodiagnosis (chronaximetry).

electroneurostimulation Electric stimulation with skin or implanted electrodes. It is used in the treatment of pain of various or unknown origin, of weakness of either a single muscle or a group of muscles, of involuntary motion of various types, and of disturbances of the urinary bladder.

electrophrenic respiration Breathing by electric stimulation of the phrenic nerve at the posterior border of the sternocleidomastoid muscle. Known in the nineteenth century, the method was modernized in 1948 by physician-physiologist Stanley J. Sarnoff and coworkers at Harvard University and in 1969 by surgeon William W. L. Glenn and co-workers at Yale University.

electropuncture Electric stimulation of a nerve or muscle by the application of a current to a needle implanted in the muscle. A therapy first used in 1825 by Sarlandière in France.

electrostatic-field heating See **electric-field heating**.

electrotherapy Literally: treatment by electricity. It refers primarily to electric stimulation and iontophoresis. In a larger sense it includes diathermy, ultrasound, infrared and ultraviolet radiation, and other electrically produced forms of treatment.

electrotonus Modification in the degree of irritability of a nerve during the passage of a galvanic current, which depends upon the position of the electrode. There is an increase in irritability near the cathode (catelectrotunus) and a decrease near the anode (anelectrotonus).

elevation activities Walking up and down stairs, curbs, inclines, and bus steps. It might also include standing up from floor, chair, etc. Also called climbing activities.

elgon Electrogoniometer (q.v.), in which a potentiometer is used as protractor. Term formed by contraction of "electrogoniometer."

Elliott, Charles Robert American gynecologist (1879–1937), who in 1931 published the treatment referred to in the following entries.

• **Elliott apparatus.** Hot-water rubber bag, in which water circulates. It was originally devised only for intravaginal thermotherapy. Later, bags of various shapes for various regions were made. See next two terms.

• **Elliott treatment.** Intravaginal heating by an Elliott apparatus placed in the vaginal cavity. The temperature of the circulating water is usually kept between 50° and 54°C, the pressure at 150 g/cm^2.

• **Elliott treatment regulator.** Device for heating and circulating water of controlled temperature and pressure through one of various Elliott rubber applicators (see **Elliott apparatus**) to be placed in cavities (vagina, rectum, colonic stoma, urethra, nose, mouth), over the eyes, or other regions.

emanatorium An inhalation room in which radon is inhaled for therapeutic purposes.

emanotherapy Inhalation of air charged with natural radioactive elements, usually radon.

empowerment

1. Psychosocial intervention strategies that enhance feelings of self-efficacy, increase the sense of personal control, and instill skills and capabilities essential for self-direction and community participation.
2. A process in which people with disabilities organize to provide mutual support in the struggle for independence and the right to live normal lives in the mainstream of society.

endomorph A person having a body build characterized by prominence of the abdomen and other parts.

endoprosthesis An artificial internal body part for surgical implantation.

environmental control system A system that comprises a control unit and various devices activated or regulated from it, such as heater, air conditioning, lamps, bells, telephone, radio, television set, etc., to be used from a bed or a wheelchair. For the physically handicapped, usually quadriplegics, the switch or switches are arranged for easy reach by the hand, shoulder, chin, cheek, lips, or other functional body part. A great variety of such systems exists, ranging from simple to very complicated.

epilepsy A chronic neurologic disease, marked by sudden alterations in consciousness and frequently by conversions.

• **activated epilepsy.** Seizures induced by drugs or electric shock for the purpose of observation.

• **generalized epilepsy.** A seizure marked by loss of consciousness and spasms of the trunk and extremities, followed by generalized clinic jerking; also called grand mal or major epilepsy.

• **laryngeal epilepsy.** Attacks precipitated by violent coughing.

• **major epilepsy.** See **generalized epilepsy.**

• **musicogenic epilepsy.** Reflex epilepsy characterized by seizures precipitated by listening to a certain type of music.

• **petit mal epilepsy.** A brief or mild seizure, lasting from 5 to 20 seconds, characterized by a sudden cessation of activity and blank stare.

• **psychomotor epilepsy.** A disorder in which the seizure activity originates in or involves the temporal lobe, producing altered, bizarre activity and behavior; also called temporal lobe epilepsy.

• **temporal lobe epilepsy.** See **psychomotor epilepsy.**

Erb, Wilhelm Heinrich German physician (1840–1921), after whom the following are named.

• **Erb's formula.** Formula, now disregarded, relative to electrodiagnosis. Normally, CCC > ACC > AOC > COC: cathodal closing contraction (i.e., contraction of muscle at the cathode upon closure of electric circuit) is larger than anodal closing contraction, which is larger than anodal opening contraction, which is larger than cathodal opening contraction. Because of the German origin of the formula, cathodal is sometimes written with K and abbreviated accordingly. Also called polar formula.

• **Erb's point.** A point where part of the brachial plexus can be stimulated through the intact skin: at the posterior border of the sternocleidomastoid muscle, 2 to 3 cm above the clavicle, at the level of the transverse process of the sixth cervical vertebra.

• **Erb's sign or phenomenon.** Increased electric excitability of muscles and nerves in tetany.

erg A unit of energy equal to the force capable of moving a weight of one gram a distance of one centimeter.

ergogram A graphic recording made by an ergograph.

ergograph An instrument for the recording of movements, e.g., the amplitude and rate of flexion and extension of a body segment.

ergometer An instrument for measuring the work performed by muscular activity.

• **bicycle ergometer.** Instrument for measuring and recording work on a stationary bicycle.

ergometry The measuring of work performed by muscular activity.

ergonomics The field of knowledge of human work in its anatomic, physiologic, and psychologic aspects, as well as its laws of mechanics and efficiency.

ergotherapy Literally: treatment by work. Rarely used in English, it is the term (with slight modifications) for occupational therapy in some other languages, e.g., French, Italian, Dutch.

ERV Expiratory reserve volume. See **lung volumes and capacities**.

esophageal speech The speech an individual may be able to produce after laryngectomy. Air swallowed into the esophagus is belched back up to form words.

ESR Electric skin resistance. See **dermohmmetry**.

esthesiometer An instrument for the examination of the sense of touch.

ethyl chloride A cooling liquid, CH_3CH_2Cl, used to anesthetize the skin. An agent of cryotherapy, used as a spray.

Eurhythmics, Eurhythmy A system of rhythmic movements of the upper limbs, with small movements of head and trunk; performed while walking in dancelike fashion to the accompaniment of spoken words, usually the poetry of Goethe. Named by the term that was also used for Dalcroze Eurhythmics (q.v.), the system was created by the Austrian philosopher and educator Rudolf Steiner (1861–1925), founder of anthroposophy.

eversion tread See **inversion-eversion tread**.

exceptional child In general, this term is used for both gifted children and those with disabilities. Both might require and receive special education (q.v.). Among those with disabilities there may be persons who are deaf, blind, mentally retarded, and those with other physical, psychologic, and educational disabilities. The term "exceptional" is sometimes extended to the parents of exceptional children.

exercise(s) A muscular activity for purposes of sport, hygiene, or therapy. The term, used in singular or plural and, at times, for emphasis, augmented by the adjective "therapeutic," is often equivalent to physical exercise, remedial exercise, medical gymnastics, or corrective therapy.
See also under **contraction**.

• **active exercise.** Exercise performed by the patient without assistance.

• **active-assisted (or active-assistive) exercise.** Exercise performed partially by the patient and aided by the therapist or another individual, by another body part of the patient, or by pulleys or other mechanical devices.

• **aerobic exercise or sport.** An exercise or sport performed while breathing more or less continuously. Examples: walking, running, dancing, swimming. See also **anaerobic exercise**.

• **air travel exercises.** Simple exercises, consisting mostly in small motions or isometric contractions (alternately tensing and relaxing muscle groups) to be performed in the sitting position while traveling by air. See also **fitness in the air**.

• **Alexander exercises.**

1. A system of exercises developing body awareness by perceiving the contact of the body with the ground and with various objects and by recognizing areas of tension. The aim is to achieve a state of ideal tonicity, i.e., eutonia, a term also given to this system, which is based on two other methods, the rhythmic system of Dalcroze and the schooling of Mensendieck. It was developed about 1929 by Gerda Alexander in Copenhagen.
2. Another system of developing body awareness, devised by F. Matthias Alexander; see **Alexander technique**.

• **Allen exercises.** See **Buerger-Allen exercises**.

• **anaerobic exercise or sport.** A sport of exercise that requires short and sudden bursts of energy during which the breath may be held: there might be no need or a reduced need to breathe until the completion of the exercise. Energy is released in spite of limited oxygen intake. Examples: high jump, 100-m dash. Anaerobic training develops the athlete's capacity to sustain an oxygen debt. See also **aerobic exercise.**

• **analytic exercise.** An exercise based on the analysis of a deficient movement. The movement being decomposed into its component parts, each of them is relearned individually and then recombined with the others. Term proposed by Herman L. Kamenetz.

• **Arica gymnastics or exercises.** System of physical and mental exercises that includes meditation, chanting mantras, and dancing. Founded in 1971 by the Bolivian Oscar Ichazo, Arica means "open door" in Quechua, the language of Bolivian Indians.

• **ataxia exercise.** Exercise used for improving balance and gait in ataxia of either spinal or cerebellar origin. See **foot placement exercises** and **Frenkel exercises**.

• **auto-assisted exercise.** See **self-assisted exercise**.

• **automatic exercise or motion.** A motion performed reflexively by a muscle paralyzed by a central lesion. Such a motion can be elicited by applying appropriate resistance to another muscle and is at times used as an exercise.

• **baby exercises or gymnastics.** Exercises for infants. Starting with passive motion, the therapist or the mother stimulates the child to increasing participation. See also **Neumann-neurode exercises**.

• **barrel exercise.** Exercise, usually for balancing, performed on a large bolster, or barrel (see **bolster**).

• **beach ball exercise.** Exercise with a beach ball (q.v.) to be held between the hands, the feet, the knees, etc., or to be tossed to a partner.

• **Billig exercise.** An exercise for dysmenorrhea, counteracting tendency to lordosis and stretching tight fasciae around the pelvis. Published in 1943 by Los Angeles orthopedic surgeon Harvey E. Billig, Jr.

• **blow bottles exercise.** An exercise of expiration against resistance. See **blow bottles**.

• **Bobath exercises or method.** See under **Bobath**.

• **bodily exercise.** Physical exercise.

• **brief maximal exercise.** Exercise in which the maximal load is lifted 1, 2, or 3 times and held for about 5 or 6 seconds. It is performed during 1, 2, or 3 sessions daily. Different techniques show variations in these data based on findings by T. Hettinger and E. A. Müller in Germany, published in 1953.

• **Brunnstrom exercises or method.** See under **Brunnstrom**.

• **Buerger exercises.** A system of exercises for arterial insufficiency of lower limbs, consisting in their elevation, followed by dependency of the legs, and finally their horizontal position for rest. Published in 1924 by Leo Buerger (1879–1943), New York physician. See also next entry.

• **Buerger–Allen exercises.** Buerger exercises (see preceding entry) augmented by active exercises of the feet. These consist in flexion, extension, and circumduction of the ankles and are done during the phase of dependency of the legs, as suggested in 1931 by Arthur W. Allen (1887–1958), American surgeon.

• **calisthenic exercise.** One of a great variety of exercises or simple gymnastics performed without apparatus to maintain or improve posture, harmony of motion, agility, and other attributes of physical fitness. The adjective is derived from the Greek words for beauty and strength. Also known as calisthenics.

• **candle exercise.** Exercise of expiration consisting in blowing out a candle placed at a gradually increased distance.

• **Cawthorne exercises.** Exercises for vertigo and Meniére's disease. They consist in changing from the standing to the sitting position; in walking up and down a slope and up and down steps. each activity is performed first with open, then with closed eyes. Suggested by British physician Terence Cawthorne.

• **Chandler exercises.** Pendulum and circular motions of the upper limb in the prone position, such as performed on a Chandler table (see under **table**).

• **circuit exercise.** See **circuit training**.

• **Clayton exercises.** A small series of simple calisthenic exercises described and named in 1924 by London physician E. Bellis Clayton.

• **Clias exercises or method.** A system of basic, rather rigid exercises, mainly for the young. It was developed by Phokion Heinrich Clias (1780–1854), a Swiss born in Boston, who in 1816 founded in Bern the first *turnverein* (gymnastic association). He published his system in Paris in 1819.

• **Codman exercises.** Shoulder mobilization exercises, recommended notably after repair of the rotator cuff. With the trunk in a forward bent (stooped) position, the upper limb hangs limp and can be moved like a pendulum or in circles by slight motions of the trunk, without contraction of any shoulder muscle. Also called pendulum exercises and stooping exercises. Published in 1934 by Boston surgeon Ernest Amory Codman (1869–1940).

• **Colby exercise.** See **conditioned exercise** (next entry).

• **conditioned exercise or motion.** An exercise taught a child while a specific rhyme is spoken or sung. First it is performed as a passive motion; then the therapist gradually decreases the intensity of guidance as the child, conditioned by the song, takes over and the exercise becomes an active one. Method reportedly initiated by physical therapist Jennie M. Colby (1859–1918), who used it in 1883 for children with cerebral palsy.

• **conditioning exercise.** An exercise aimed at improving a subject's physical condition.

• **convalescence exercise.** Reconditioning exercise aimed at hastening recovery after sickness, injury, or surgical intervention.

• **coordination exercise.** An exercise for improving coordination, such as Frenkel exercises (q.v.).

• **corrective exercise.** An exercise aimed at reducing or eliminating a faulty posture, movement, or breathing; a deformity, muscular weakness, or lack of speed, of coordination, of endurance, or of joint range.

• **crawling exercise.** Exercise performed in the prone position, for reciprocal motion, mobilization, stretching, or strengthening and to prepare for walking on all fours. The term is also used for exercise in the quadruped position (see **creeping exercise**).

• **creeping exercise.** Exercise executed in the quadruped position: on hands and knees. It is used as a passage from crawling to standing, for mobilization of the spine, and for the treatment of spinal deviations. See also **Klapp exercises**.

• **Cureton exercises.** A system of physical education aiming at general physical fitness. Developed by Thomas Kirk Cureton (1901–1976), physical educator at the University of Illinois.

• **DeLorme exercises.** A system of progressive resistance exercises, usually called PRE, in which the loads to be lifted increase progressively during one session as well as during the course of treatment. It was published in 1945 by Boston orthopedic surgeon Thomas L. DeLorme. In 1948 he revised his technique and adopted the term progressive resistance exercise (pre). For other modifications see **regressive resistance exercises**.

• **Delsarte exercises.** See under **Delsarte system**.

• **Doman–Delacato exercises or method.** See under **Doman–Delacato**.

• **Doorframe exercise.** Exercise consisting of moving the hand up along a doorframe to increase the ranges of the upper limb, the shoulder in particular.

• **doorstop exercise.** An exercise to strengthen the muscles of the sole of the foot. The patient, sitting on a chair, places the metatarsal arches of his or her feet over two rubber doorstops and forcibly curls the toes down. Suggested by Chicago orthopedic surgeon Philip Lewin.

• **dynamic exercise.** Exercise in which there is joint motion. So named in order to emphasize this fact, as opposed to static exercise. Also called isotonic exercise.

• **EDF exercise.** Exercise of extension, derotation, and (lateral) flexion of the spine for the treatment of scoliosis, as advocated by Cotrel, who also used the underlying principle in the application of a plaster jacket (see under **EDF**).

• **Fay exercises or method.** See **Fay reflex therapy**.

• **Feldenkrais exercises.** A system that aims at developing body awareness and improving posture and movement. It comprises a great number of physical exercises combined with conscious attention to breathing, to the contact of the body with floor or chair, and to the spatial relationship between moving body parts. Typically, an exercise is performed 25 times and is followed by self-observation. Usually taught in groups, the method was developed by Israeli physicist Moshe Feldenkrais (1904–1979) and published by him in 1972 under the name of "Awareness through Movement." It is also combined with individual sessions of manipulation called "functional integration." The system is remindful of the Alexander technique (q.v.), of the Gindler method (q.v.), and of structural integration (q.v.).

• **foot placement exercises.** Exercises usually executed while standing or walking in any direction. They aim at improving balance and gait. The feet are placed on footprints painted on the floor, on other floor markings, or between the rungs of a foot placement ladder (q.v.). Such exercises are typical of Frenkel exercises (q.v.).

• **Free exercise.** Any exercise that is executed without apparatus and is neither assisted nor resisted in any way other than by gravity.

• **Frenkel exercises or method.** Walking reeducation and other exercises aiming at precision of movement in conditions of incoordination. Proposed as a treatment of tabetic ataxia and published in 1885 by the Swiss neurologist Heinrich S. Frenkel (1860 [Warsaw]–1931 [Berlin]). Practicing in Heiden, Switzerland, he became known as Frenkel-Heiden. See also **Frenkel tracks**.

• **Golub exercise.** An exercise for dysmenorrhea. Standing with abducted lower limbs, the trunk is turned to the side and bent forward. Recommended by Rumanian-born Philadelphia gynecologist Leib J. Golub and co-workers; published in 1957.

• **Gurdjieff exercises.** A system of rhythmic exercises developed in the early 1920s in Paris by philosopher Georg Ivanovich Gurdjeff (1877 [Alexandropol, Armenia]–1949 [Paris]). These exercises, which he called sacred dances or simply movements, were taught in groups as part of a method of self-development of Eastern, notably Sufi, influence.

• **Guthrie–Smith exercises.** See under **Guthrie–Smith**.

• **Guts Muths exercises.** See under **Guts Muths**.

• **gymnasium exercises.** Exercises using various apparatus customarily found in a gymnasium, such as stall bars, pulleys, bicycle, rowing machine, etc.

• **Hébert exercises or method.** See **Hébert system**.

• **interval exercises.**

1. Program of exercises for physical fitness, usually practiced by groups of employees during their working hours at certain intervals (exercise break). Thought to improve the physical condition of the workers and the efficiency in their work and to decrease the number of occupational accidents.
2. Physical training for maintenance of performance between periods of intensive preparation for athletic competition and professional sports.

• **invisible exercises.** Set of exercises described in a book of this title, published in 1922 by Gerald Stanley Lee (1862–1944), an ordained minister. The exercises include "drills" for sitting, standing, walking, lying down, etc. and are based on the system of F. Matthias Alexander (see **Alexander technique**), although without acknowledgment.

• **isokinetic exercise.** An exercise executed with an apparatus that opposes a resistance that varies with the effort of the subject while the motion is kept at a constant, predetermined speed.

• **isometric exercise.** Exercise in which the muscles act against a nonmoving resistance. Their extremities being fixed, they remain isometric, i.e., "of the same length," and, as opposed to isotonic exercise, their contraction does not result in motion. Examples: holding a limb horizontal without support, pushing against a wall. Also called static exercise. Cf. next entry.

• **isotonic exercise.** Exercise in which there is joint motion, as opposed to isometric exercise. In spite of the term "isotonic" (meaning "of equal, or constant, tension"), the tension of the muscle does not necessarily remain the same throughout its contraction. Therefore often called dynamic exercise. Cf. preceding entry.

• **Jahn exercises.** See **Jahn, Friedrich Ludwig**.

• **Kabat exercise.** See **Kabat method of exercise**.

• **Kegel exercise.** Contracting of the muscles of the pelvic floor, monitored by an intravaginal dynamometer, called perineometer, the dial of which is held in the patient's hand for easy reading. Method used in certain conditions of weakness of the perineal muscles. Published in 1948 by Arnold H. Kegel (1894–1972), American obstetrician and gynecologist.

• **kinetic exercise.** Exercise in which there is joint motion. Also called isotonic or dynamic exercise.

• **Klapp exercises.** A system of exercises performed in the quadruped position for weakness of the trunk and deformities of the vertebral column. Created by Rudolph Klapp (1873–1949), German orthopedic surgeon, who published this method of creeping exercises in 1907.

• **Knott exercises or method.** See **Knott method of exercise**.

• **mat activities or exercises.** Various exercises practiced on a mat for comfort and as a protection against injuries. Lower-limb amputees and others unable to stand may perform them in a horizontal or sitting position. Certain sports and acrobatics are also executed on mats.

• **maternity exercises.** See **prenatal exercises**.

• **Mensendieck exercises.** System of physical education consisting of a small number of global movements, each of which requires conscious participation of the entire body in a harmonious coordination of contractions, relaxation, and respiration. Created specifically for women by Bess M. Mensendieck (1861[?]–1957), US physician (M.D., Zurich), who in 1906 published *Körperkultur der Frau* ("Bodily Culture for Women").

• **Mosher exercises.** Four exercises for dysmenorrhea: (1) hooklying: breathing; (2) standing: rising on toes; (3) standing: deep knee bending; (4) hooklying: knees on chest. Advocated in 1914 by California physician Clelia D. Mosher (1863–1940).

• **muscle setting exercise.** Exercise consisting of tension or contraction of a muscle or muscle group, whereby the joint does not show any motion. The muscle may already be in a position of relative shortening. A typical example is the contraction of the quadriceps femoris, with the limb in a cast and the knee in full extension. Also called static exercise. Comparable to isometric exercise but usually less strenuous and may be performed without extrinsic resistance.

• **Neumann-Neurode exercises.** A system of exercises for infants starting at the age of four months. Advocated in 1920 under the name *Säuglingsgymnastik* (baby gymnastics) by the German physical educator Detleff Neumann-Neurode (1879–1945).

• **Ober exercise.** Exercise that stretches a tight fascia lata, as advocated by Frank Roberts Ober (1881–1960), Boston orthopedic surgeon.

• **ocular exercise.** Exercise of the eye muscles aiming at correct accommodation and coordination of the eyes, notably in deficiencies of binocular vision. Called also orthopedic exercise.

• **on-the-job exercise.** See **interval exercise**, first definition.

• **orthoexercise.** See **orthotherapy**.

• **orthoptic exercise.** Ocular exercise.

• **Oxford exercises.** See **regressive resistance exercises**.

• **passive exercise.** Movement executed by the therapist or other individual, another body part of the patient, or a mechanical device.

• **passive vascular exercises.** Treatment for peripheral vascular insufficiency by rhythmic mechanical compression, as achieved by a variety of pneumatic apparatuses. The term was particularly propagated by the Cincinnati surgeon Louis G. Herrmann, who in 1936 published a book under this title.

• **pendulum exercise.** Any exercise in which the forearm, the upper limb, the leg, or the lower limb is swung like a pendulum. If it refers to the upper limb, which is almost always the case, it is also called Codman exercise (q.v.).

• **physical exercise.** So called to emphasize a rather intensive use of muscles and joints.

• **postpartum exercise.** One of several exercises aimed at supporting and hastening the return to normal, particularly of the abdominal wall, after pregnancy.

• **postural exercise.** Exercise for the improvement of posture (lying, sitting, standing, walking). It may be concentrated on a particular body part, such as the feet.

• **prenatal exercises.** Physical part of a method of physical and psychologic preparation during pregnancy, comprising exercises in which breathing and relaxation are emphasized. It is aimed at facilitating the period of delivery and decreasing pain and discomfort as well as the need for anesthetics. Published in 1933 under the name of natural childbirth by the British obstetrician Grantley Dick Read (1890–1959) and other physicians. See also **Lamaze method**.

• **press exercise.** One of various resistance exercises executed on a bench. See **bench press**.

• **progressive assistive exercise.** Modified technique of progressive resistance exercise (see next entry), used when the muscle power is insufficient to perform the motion against gravity. Assistance is given by the elimination of gravity (use of suspension, powder board, or pulleys with counterweights). The amount of assistance is then gradually decreased.

• **progressive resistance exercises.** Resistance exercises of increasing loads. The term, particularly if abbreviated, PRE, refers usually to a system described by Delorme. See **Delorme exercises**.

• **pulley exercise.** Exercise with pulleys either for strengthening, by lifting a weight, or for mobilization, by lifting part of one's own body.

• **range-of-motion exercise.** Motion through the full ranges of a point. It refers usually to a passive motion and is therefore more correctly so called.

• **RCAF exercises.** See **Royal Canadian Air Force exercises**.

• **reciprocal exercise.** Refers usually to a crosswise combination, i.e., the right upper together with the left lower limb, alternating with the two other limbs.

• **reconditioning exercises.** Exercises destined to help a person to recover the strength lost as a result of disease, injury, or decreased activity. Also used in sports.

• **Regen exercise.** Exercise that consists in squatting, emphasizing the convexity of the lumbar area. Also called squat exercise. Advocated in the 1930s by Eugene M. Regen (1900–), Tennessee orthopedic surgeon, published in a film by the Veterans Administration and further developed by Paul C. Williams (see **Williams exercises**).

• **regressive resistance (or resistive) exercises.** A method of progressive resistance exercises in which, while the maximal load is periodically increased, the daily session starts with this maximal load to be lifted. The load then "regresses" after each 10 repetitions by steps amounting to 10% (Oxford technique, named for United Oxford Hospitals in England, from which it was published in 1951 by A. N. Zinovieff) or to 25% (as published in 1953 by R. E. Mcgovern and H. B. Luscombe).

• **resistance (or resistive) exercise.** Exercise against the resistance of the therapist or other individual, another body part of the patient, a weight, or a fixed object.

• **Rood exercise.** See **Rood method of exercise**.

• **Royal Canadian Air Force exercises.** A program of exercises for physical fitness, developed in the late 1940s by the Royal Canadian Air Force. The plan for men, called 5bx (for five basic exercises), is composed of daily sessions of 11 minutes. The plan for women, called xbx (for ten basic exercises), is set for 12-minute sessions. Each plan is arranged to provide several levels of increasing difficulty (six for men, four for women) by modifications of the basic exercises and increases in the number of repetitions, while the duration of the individual sessions remains the same.

• **Schott exercise.** Slow movement against resistance by the therapist. It is part of a therapeutic system for patients with heart disease suggested by the Schott brothers (see **Schott system**).

• **self-assisted (or self-assistive) exercise.** Exercise or stretching, performed by the patient with the aid of another body part, either directly or with the help of pulleys or other mechanical devices. Such self-assisted exercise can therefore be of the active-assisted or the passive type.

• **setting exercise.** Muscle setting exercises.

• **setting-up exercises.** Very simple exercises done at the beginning of an exercise session. They are destined to warm up the muscles, to mobilize them, and to prepare them for the exercises that follow.

• **skating exercise.** Exercise of a weak limb which, supported by a roller skate, ball-bearing board, or similar device, moves on a smooth horizontal surface with little friction.

• **squat (or squatting) exercise.** Exercise consisting in assuming the squatting position, which favors the convexity of the lumbar area. See also **Regen exercise** and **Williams exercises**.

• **static exercise.** Exercise in which muscular effort does not result in any joint motion. Called also isometric or muscle-setting exercise. The term static exercise is used in opposition to dynamic exercise.

• **stick (or broomstick) exercise.** Exercise executed with a wand, broomstick, or cane, usually held in both hands (two-handed stick exercise). One of its indications is to stimulate and facilitate the activity and mobility of an affected upper limb by the more active motions of the unaffected limb.

• **stooping exercise.** Codman exercise.

• **stretching exercise.** Stretching or passive motion aiming at overcoming tightness, hence increasing joint range.

• **stump exercise.** Exercise of the muscles of an amputation stump and the neighboring regions.

• **suspension exercise.** Exercise with elimination of gravity by suspending the body or part of it with springs. See also **Guthrie-Smith exercises**, under **Guthrie-Smith**.

• **sustained exercise.** Static or so-called isometric exercise.

• **Swedish exercises.** System of exercises, originally of military nature, with emphasis on posture, the entire body, including the moving segments, being kept rigid. Developed by the Swedish fencing master Per Henrik Ling (1776–1839), who in 1813 founded the Central Institute of Gymnastics in Stockholm. Thereafter, the medical aspect of the exercises, to which massage was added, developed, and the system became known as Swedish gymnastics and massage.

• **t'ai-chi ch'uan exercise.** See under **t'ai-chi ch'uan**.

• **therapeutic exercise.** See definition of **exercise** (main entry).

• **treadmill exercise.** Exercise consisting in walking on a treadmill. See also **treadmill exercise test**, under **test**.

• **vocal exercise.** Exercise aiming at the correct use and strengthening of the voice in conjunction with that of the respiratory apparatus.

• **Voss exercises or method.** See **Knott method of exercise**, under **Knott**.

• **wand exercise.** Exercise performed with a wand, i.e., a cane, stick, or broom handle. See **stick exercise**.

• **weight-and-pulley exercise.** Exercise using an adjustable weight-and-pulley arrangement for strengthening or mobility.

• **weightless exercises.** Suspension exercises. See under **Guthrie-Smith**.

• **Williams (flexion) exercises.** Exercises to enhance lumbar flexion, avoid lumbar extension, and strengthen the abdominal and gluteal musculature. Systematized in 1937 by Paul C. Williams (1900–1978), Dallas orthopedic surgeon.

• **yoga exercises.** See under **yoga**.

• **Zander exercises.** See under **Zander**.

• **Zinovieff exercises.** See **regressive resistance exercises**.

exercise board See under **board**.

exercise break Period of interruption during working hours (analogous to coffee break) for the purpose of exercise counteracting the relative immobility of certain occupations and promoting physical fitness. See **interval exercises**, first definition, under **exercise**.

exercise glove Glove with hooks at the fingertips for the attachment of weights. Used for strengthening exercises of the digits and the forearm. Cf. **holding glove**.

exercise test or testing See under **test**.

expectation discrepancy A discrepancy between the expectations held by an observer who encounters a person with a disability and the actual observations of the person and his or her characteristics, statements, or behaviors.

expiratory reserve volume (ERV) See **lung volumes and capacities**.

extended care The medical care of patients beyond the acute phase or, in certain cases, beyond the intermediate phase, or their conditions.

exteroceptive Refers to sensory nerves and sensations stimulated by immediate outside influences such as cold, heat, stroking, brushing, light pressure.

extremity End of a pointed structure such as the nose, the clavicle, a digit. The term is frequently, but incorrectly, used instead of limb.

extrinsic muscle Muscle that originates outside the part in which it functions. The extrinsic muscles of the hand originate in the forearm; those of the foot come from the leg. Opposite of intrinsic muscle (q.v.).

eye-switch Device operated by the movements of the eyes, reacting differently to the white and the colored portions of the eyes. Developed by the National Aeronautics and Space Administration, it can be utilized by quadriplegic individuals to propel themselves in wheelchairs and to operate a call board, a typewriter, or other apparatus.

F

F

1. In manual muscle testing: Fair (q.v.).
2. In thermometry: Fahrenheit.
3. In electricity: farad(s) (see under **Faraday**).
4. In the description of an orthotic or prosthetic joint, referring to its motion: free.

facilitation Literally: action of making easier. In neurology, a process or condition that favors the occurrence of a given phenomenon. Opposite of inhibition.

• **neuromuscular facilitation.** Maneuvers and exercises producing or enhancing muscular contraction or relaxation.

• **proprioceptive neuromuscular facilitation (PNF).** Therapeutic maneuvers and exercises utilizing reflex patterns, proprioceptive stimuli, and other facilitatory mechanisms to produce or enhance muscular contraction or relaxation. See **Bobath, Brunnstrom, Fay, Kabat, Knott, Phelps, Rood**.

facilitation technique One of various procedures of facilitating a certain movement of therapeutic exercise or daily living by making use of reflexes and other neurologic phenomena. By extension, the term "facilitation" may include inhibition procedures of antagonists. See also preceding entry.

facultative Relating to a mental faculty.

Fahrenheit (F) Temperature scale in which the boiling point of water is 212 degrees (212°F) and the ice point is 32 degrees (32°F). Invented by the Prussian physicist Daniel Fahrenheit (1686–1736), this scale is now being universally abandoned in favor of the Celsius scale.

Fair A grade in manual muscle testing, given to a muscle or a group of muscles that can lift the corresponding segment through its full range against gravity.

fango Mud of volcanic origin. Used for packs or baths.

fangotherapy Therapeutic application of fango as packs or baths.

far Refers to the position of ultraviolet or infrared radiations in relation to the visible segment of the electromagnetic spectrum. Far ultraviolet rays are of shorter wavelengths; far infrared rays are of longer wavelengths. Opposite of near. See table of **electromagnetic radiation**, under **radiation**.

Faraday, Michael English chemist and physicist (1791–1867), who in 1831 discovered electromagnetic induction.

• **farad (F).** The unit of electric capacitance.

• **Faraday cage.** Copper-screened room or cage inside a room completely enclosing an electric instrument in order to shield it from any outside electric interference. Named after Faraday, it was later used for electromyography.

• **faradic bath.** See under **bath**.

• **faradic current.** See under **current**.

• **faradism, faradization.** The therapeutic use of faradic current (see under **current**).

Fartlek Method of athletic training in which physical performance is combined with the enjoyment of the surroundings. Mostly referring to cross-country long-distance running, it is practiced in beautiful terrain whose diversity invites variations in up- and downhill jogging, sprinting, striding, and running at various places. So called from the Swedish for "speed play" since the late 1940s, when it was popularized by the Swedish Olympic coach Gosta Holmer.

fasciculation Involuntary twitching of a group of muscle fibers. Thus called because thought to correspond to a muscle bundle (fascicle). See next entry.

fasciculation potential Electric potential, detectable by electromyography, of a group of muscle fibers. It corresponds to the involuntary contraction of a motor unit. See preceding entry.

fatigability Condition of becoming easily tired.

fatigue
1. Feeling of tiredness that may result from sustained physical activity, medication, organic disease, or certain states of mind.
2. Reduction or inability of a muscle to respond to stimulation.

Fay reflex therapy An exercise method for patients with neuromuscular disorders, based on the phylogenetic and ontogenetic development of primitive locomotor patterns that pass through the stages of amphibian and reptilian forms of life. By the use of postures (positioning of the body), passive motions, selected normal and pathologic reflexes, and automatic responses, the patient progresses from crawling and creeping to standing and walking. Although most often applied to children with cerebral palsy, the same sequence is used in the treatment of adults. Continued practice of patterns with frequent repetitions is presumed to lead spontaneously to the next, more advanced type of movement. Developed in the 1940s and published in 1954 by Temple S. Fay (1895–1963), Philadelphia neurosurgeon.

feedback, electromyographic See under **biofeedback**.

feeder Mobile arm support (q.v.).

• **ball-bearing feeder.** Balanced forearm orthosis. See under **orthosis**.

• **friction feeder.** A mobile arm support (q.v.) with built-in friction in order to slow involuntary or grossly incoordinated motions of an upper limb, e.g., in certain types of cerebral palsy.

• **link (or linkage) feeder.** Balanced forearm orthosis. See under **orthosis**.

• **suspension feeder.** A mobile arm support (q.v.) suspended from an overhead bar.

feeding tray Lapboard. See under **board**.

FEF Forced expiratory flow. See **forced expiratory volume**.

Feldenkrais method See under **exercise**.

festination See **festinating gait**, under **gait**.

fever bag Large bag, similar to a sleeping bag, used formerly for treatment by artificial fever.

fever cabinet Large box of metal or other material for artificial fever therapy. The patient, sitting or lying inside the cabinet while keeping the head outside bathes in humid air whose temperature is between 40° and 55°C. The relative humidity is kept above 80%. Formerly used in the treatment of gonorrhea and other infectious diseases. See also **heat cabinet**.

fever therapy Artificially induced fever, most often by means of hot air or diathermy, usually for the treatment of syphilis or gonorrhea. Was practiced in the first half of the twentieth century.

fibrillation Involuntary twitching of single muscle fibers due to denervation in lower motor neuron lesions. See next entry.

fibrillation potential Electric potential of a denervated muscle fiber, as demonstrated electromyographically. See preceding entry.

finger board See under **board**.

finger ladder See **shoulder ladder**.

finger reading The reading of braille symbols by using a finger. See under **Braille**.

fingerspelling A conventional system of communication for the deaf in which the letters of the alphabet are expressed by various positions of either one or both hands and their digits. A single-handed alphabet is used in the USA and most European countries. The prevalent system in the UK is two-handed. A deaf-blind person can use a similar system, in which the letters are spelled into the palm.

fingertrap A tubular device of textile or similar material, applied to a finger or toe like the finger of a glove. It is woven diagonally so that it narrows when it is elongated by traction. Used for distracting a digital joint or the fragments of a fractured phalanx.

Finsen, Niels Ryberg Danish physician, founder of modern phototherapy (1860–1904). In 1893 he introduced the short-flame carbon arc lamp for the local treatment of lupus vulgaris and demonstrated the value of actinic radiations. Nobel Prize for medicine in 1903.

• **Finsen bath.** General ultraviolet irradiation.

• **Finsen lamp.** Carbon-arc lamp operating at 50 V and 50 A, emitting concentrated ultraviolet rays and cooled by circulating water.

• **Finsen therapy or method.** Treatment by concentrated ultraviolet rays; usually referring to the treatment of lupus vulgaris.

• **finsen unit or finsen.** Proposed unit of erythemal flux density or intensity of irradiation. It is equal to one unit of erythemal flux per square centimeter of surface irradiated. Named in honor of Niels Ryberg Finsen.

Fitness in the Air (or Chair) A program of simple exercises for air travelers. Developed for Lufthansa Airlines by the German Sports Federation and published in 1976. See also **air travel exercises**, under **exercise**.

fitness, physical State of physical condition with good mobility, muscle strength, coordination, endurance, and readiness to move.

Fitz Gerald method or treatment See **zone therapy**.

5BX Abbreviation for five basic exercises. See **Royal Canadian Air Force exercises**, under **exercise**.

fixation The process of making stationary.

- **external fixation.** The holding together of a broken bone by means of a plaster cast encircling the injured part or a plaster splint until successful healing occurs.

- **internal fixation.** The use of devices such as metallic pins, screws, wires, or plates, applied directly to the bony fragments, to hold them in apposition and alignment.

flaccid Low in tonus; hypotonic.

flaccidity A low degree of tonus; hypotonia.

flagellation

1. A maneuver of massage consisting in whipping the skin with the fingers.
2. Flogging, usually with leafy branches, as used in a Finnish steambath. See **Finnish bath**, under **bath**.

flexor hinge hand Flexor hinge orthosis. See under **orthosis**.

floor loom See under **loom**.

fluidotherapy A type of dry heat treatment for a hand or foot. The extremity to be treated is introduced into a box under a plastic transparent cover; a stream of warm air, in which small particles of corncob are suspended, maintains a temperature of about 50°C. Developed in the 1970s.

Fluori-Methane Proprietary name of a cooling spray consisting of a combination of two chlorofluoromethanes. Used in spray-and-stretch therapy (q.v.).

fomentation The external application of a hot, moist substance or object. Also the substance or object thus applied. Today this is usually a hot, moist pack. Term also used synonymously with cataplasm and poultice.

foot

• **Greissinger foot.** Proprietary name of a prosthetic foot with ankle motion in all directions, including rotation. Developed in the 1950s and 1960s by German prosthetist Georg Greissinger (1903–1972), who had originally devised it in cooperation with Otto Bock at the latter's manufactory. Hence also known as Bock-Greissinger foot.

• **SACH foot.** Prosthetic foot with, as indicated by the acronym, a solid ankle and cushion heel. It is composed of a hardwood keel and a cushion heel of multiple laminations of neoprene and sponge rubber. Thus, the lost mobility of the ankle joint is replaced by the softness of the heel, which provides some mobility in all directions. Ankle and foot are combined into one component firmly attached to the prosthetic leg by a carriage bolt. Developed in 1955 at University of California, Berkeley.

• **SAFE foot.** Prosthetic foot with, as indicated by the acronym, stationary attachment and flexible endoskeleton. It has a flexible keel and is bolted to the leg of the prosthesis. Developed in 1980 by orthotist John W. Campbell and prosthetist-orthotist Charles W. Child.

footboard See under **board**.

footdrop Paralysis or weakness of the dorsiflexor muscles of the foot and ankle causing the foot to fall and the toes to drag on the ground during walking; also called toe drop.

foot eversion (or inversion) tread See **inversion-eversion tread**.

foot placement ladder A ladder-shaped device placed on the floor for exercises of coordination and, depending on the elevation of the rungs, of mobility of the lower limbs.

footprint slipper sock A slipper made of stretchable polyurethane containing fragile microcapsules. Upon pressure, the capsules break, spilling a dye that colors the slipper more or less heavily, according to the amount of pressure. To make a footprint, the slipper sock is worn either by itself or inside the shoe for a test of about 15 steps. Developed in 1967 by surgeon Paul W. Brand, occupational therapist James D. Ebner, and co-workers at US Public Health Service Hospital, Carville, Louisiana.

foot slap Gait deviation of a person with a lower-limb prosthesis in which the foot, instead of coming down to the floor smoothly, lands flat and briskly with a loud slap.

forced expiration A procedure used to remove bronchial secretion.

forced expiratory volume (FEV) The maximum volume of air exhaled (after deep inspiration) during a specified time in seconds as indicated by a number in subscript, e.g., FEV_2.

forced vital capacity (FVC) The vital capacity (see **lung volumes and capacities**) reached with expiration as forceful as possible.

foulage A maneuver of massage consisting in pressing and kneading the tissues in large movements.

four-poster collar, brace, orthosis An orthosis designed to support the neck and greatly reduce its motions. It has four adjustable uprights (posts): two in front, connecting a chin support with a sternal plate, and two in the back, connecting an occipital support with a thoracic plate.

fracture The breaking of a bone or cartilage.

• **articular fracture.** A fracture involving the joint surface of a bone.

• **avulsion fracture.** A breaking off of a small portion of bone at the site of attachment of a tendon or ligament.

• **basal skull fracture.** A fracture occurring at the base of the skull.

• **blow-out fracture.** A fracture of the floor of the orbit caused by a blow to the eye.

• **closed fracture.** A simple fracture, one in which the skin is not broken.

• **comminuted fracture.** A fracture in which the bone is splintered into several pieces.

• **compound fracture.** See **open fracture.**

• **depressed fracture.** A fracture with inward displacement of the skull.

• **fatigue fracture.** See **March fracture**

• **impacted fracture.** One in which one fragment is embedded in the substance of the other and fixed in that position.

• **incomplete fracture.** One in which the line of fracture does not include the whole bone.

• **linear fracture.** A fracture that runs parallel with the long axis of the bone.

• **march fracture.** Fracture of a metatarsal shaft caused by stress associated with prolonged weight bearing, as in walking or marching for a long period of time; seen most commonly in army recruits during basic training.

• **oblique fracture.** One that runs obliquely to the axis of the bone.

• **open fracture.** A fracture that is accompanied by an open wound through which the broken bone may protrude; formerly known as a compound fracture.

• **strain fracture.** The breaking off by sudden force of a piece of bone attached to a tendon or ligament.

• **stress fracture.** One occurring at the site of a muscle attachment and caused by sudden, violent force.

• **supracondylar fracture.** A fracture in the distal end of the humerus.

• **transcervical fracture.** A fracture through the neck of the femur.

• **transverse fracture.** One in which the break line runs perpendicular with the axis of the bone.

fragrance garden See **garden for the blind**.

frame

• **Balkan frame.** Metal construction above a bed, to which it is attached, providing for the suspension of a limb (e.g., after fracture), for the attachment of a pulley for exercise, or of a trapeze to facilitate the patient's moving about. It was reportedly used for the first time in a Dutch ambulance during the Balkan wars between 1908 and 1913.

• **Bradford frame.** Rectangular frame made of gas pipe, covered with heavy canvas. Devised in 1890 by Boston orthopedic surgeon Edward H. Bradford (1848–1926). In a subsequent modification the canvas consisted of an upper and lower half, both movable, so that the patient could use a bedpan without changing position.

• **Foster frame or bed.** Proprietary name of a turning bed permitting easy change of a patient's position. Similar to the Stryker frame (see next entry).

• **Stryker frame or bed.** Proprietary name of a frame with a mattress that can be turned around its longitudinal axis, together with the patient. A second mattress is applied above the patient before turning, providing for the change from the supine to the prone position. Developed in 1939 by Homer H. Stryker (1894–1980), Michigan orthopedic surgeon.

• **walking frame.** Walker, walkerette. Term mostly used in the UK.

• **Whitman frame.** A variant of the Bradford frame but with curved sides.

franklinism, franklinization The therapeutic use of static electricity. Named after Benjamin Franklin (1706–1790), who had used it. See also **static machine**.

FRC Functional residual capacity. See **lung volumes and capacities**.

Frejka pillow splint or abduction pillow A small pillow, made of cotton twill or similar material. Placed between the thighs of an infant and held in place by shoulder straps, it keeps the lower limbs abducted and flexed while allowing them to move. Used in congenital dislocation of the hip joints. Demonstrated in the USA in 1947 by Bedrich Frejka, orthopedic surgeon in Brünn, Czechoslovakia.

Frenkel tracks Footprints or other marks painted on the floor. Suggested by Heinrich S. Frenkel as a guide in the walking reeducation of patients with ataxia. See also **Frenkel exercises**, under **exercise**.

frequency The number of cycles (q.v.) or vibrations, usually expressed in hertz (Hz), i.e., cycles or vibrations per second.

• **sound frequency.** The height, or pitch, or a sound, expressed in vibrations per second. Examples:

Range of the human ear	16 to 20,000
Range of musical instruments	16 to 20,000
Range of the human voice	100 to 12,000
Range of telephone transmission	300 to 3,000
Range of ordinary speech	200 to 2,000

• **ultrasonic (or ultrasound) frequency.** Frequency of acoustic vibrations beyond the range of the human ear, i.e., above 20,000 Hz. The frequency of ultrasonic instruments is always far above this level and may reach 15 MHz.

friction One of the standard maneuvers of massage, also called rubbing. It is either a rubbing of more or less superficial tissues, more forceful than stroking, or a moving of superficial layers over deeper-lying tissues (deep friction).

frog breathing Glossopharyngeal breathing (q.v.).

fulguration A technique of tissue destruction by electric sparks. Used mostly in dermatology.

functional assessment A method for describing abilities and limitations to measure an individual's use of the variety of skills included in performing tasks necessary to daily living, leisure activities, vocational pursuits, social interactions, and other required behaviors.

functional capacity evaluation An evaluation to determine an individual's current level of function and to establish behavioral and attitudinal assets and deficits.

Functional Communication Profile A standardized test to evaluate language disturbances in adults.

functional electrical stimulation (FES) The use of low current electricity stimulation on intact peripheral nerves, to achieve purposeful movements substituting for inadequate function of specific paretic or paralytic muscle groups.

Functional Independence Measure (FIM) A measure of function to indicate levels of dependency in clinical rehabilitation.

functional limitation A restriction or lack of ability to perform an activity that results from an impairment and may constitute a disability.

functional residual capacity (FRC) See **lung volumes and capacities**.

functional training or therapy Therapeutic motions or exercises in the form of purposeful activities, such as balancing, walking, eating, dressing, in which a combination of motions is practiced rather than isolated motions of individual muscle groups or body parts.

fundamental negative bias A bias that steers perception, thought, and feeling along negative lines to such a degree that positives remain hidden.

G

G In muscle testing: Good (q.v.).

g Gram(s).

gain To build up an increase; to acquire.

• **epinosic gain.** See **secondary gain.**

• **paranosic gain.** See **primary gain.**

• **primary gain.** The alleviation of anxiety provided by a neurotic illness or symptom; also called paranosic gain.

• **secondary gain.** The additional indirect satisfaction or advantage (e.g., manipulating other people or receiving monetary reward) derived from a neurotic illness or symptom; also called epinosic gain.

gait Manner of walking or running. During the cycle of normal human gait, each lower limb goes through a stance phase and a swing phase. Each stance phase is subdivided into heel strike, foot flat (during midstance), knee bend, heel off (during push off), and toe clearance, which initiates the swing phase. The latter, with acceleration in the first half and deceleration in the second half, terminates with the heel strike.

• **abducted gait, abduction gait.** Gait with continuous abduction of the lower limbs. Often seen in a lower-limb amputee who adopts this gait for greater stability or because the prosthesis is too long

• **alternate two-point gait.** Two-point gait.

• **ambling gait.** Gait in which both limbs of the same side advance at the same time. It is sometimes used in exercises in the quadruped position.

• **ambling two-point gait.** Gait in which the crutch or cane is advanced together with the lower limb of the same side. Term proposed in 1965 by Herman L. Kamenetz.

• **antalgic gait.** A self-protective limp due to pain.

• **ataxic gait.** An unsteady, irregular gait.

• **back-jack gait.** Gait in which the crutches, from a forward position, are moved back so that their tips are in line with the toes. Then, the subject, by flexing the trunk and hiking the pelvis, lifts the feet and places them slightly backward.

• **cerebellar gait.** A staggering gait with a tendency to fall, indicative of cerebellar disease.

• **circumduction gait.** Gait in which one lower limb is swung forward in a hemicircular fashion, with knee extended. Typical of spastic hemiplegia.

• **compass gait.**

1. So called because the tracing of the path reminds one of a mariner's compass. The subject, blindfolded, upon being asked to walk alternately forward and backward for a distance of 6 to 8 steps, turns slightly to one side at every change of direction, always to the same side, thus after about 10 walks (5 in each direction) having turned a total of 180° since the start. It may be a sign of vestibulocerebellar disorder. (After Monrad-Krohn.)
2. Gait in which both knees are extended and the limbs kept abducted, comparable to the legs of a drawing compass.

• **crosslegged gait.** Scissors or scissoring gait.

• **crouch gait.** Gait with exaggerated flexion of hips and knees. Often seen in spastic paraplegia, e.g., in cerebral palsy.

• **diving gait.** A limping gait with flexion of the trunk, characteristic of unequal length of the lower limbs. The body "dives" upon weightbearing on the shorter limb.

• **double step gait.** Gait in which there is a marked difference in length or timing between the left and the right step.

• **drag-to gait.** A gait in which the patient slides the feet along the floor toward the advanced crutches or—exceptionally—canes.

• **drop-off gait.**

1. Insufficient heelrise at pushoff (due to deficient plantar flexion of the ankle or lack of control of ankle dorsiflexion), resulting in a shorter step on the opposite side (reduced amplitude of swing phase).

2. Gait deviation in persons with a lower-limb prothesis; called also drop-off at end of stance phase: after the heel of the shoe on the prosthesis has touched the floor, the rest of the shoe drops quickly instead of rolling off progressively.

• **duck gait.** Waddling gait.

• **eggshell gait.** Gait with small steps and reduced motion in the joints of the feet, as if walking on eggshells. Characteristic of metatarsalgia.

• **festinating gait.** From the Latin *festinare*, to accelerate. Walking with small steps at involuntarily increasing speed. Seen in parkinsonism. Also called festination.

• **four-point gait.** A crutch (or cane) gait with the following sequence: left crutch, right foot, right crutch, left foot.

• **gluteus medius gait.** Trendelenburg gait. See under **Trendelenburg**.

• **heel-toe gait.** Any gait in which, as in normal walking, the foot first touches the ground with the heel, then smoothly rolls over to the anterior part, then to the toes, while the heel leaves the ground.

• **hemicircular gait.** Circumduction gait.

• **hemiplegic gait.** Typical gait of a hemiplegic patient with, on the involved side, flexed elbow, stiff knee, and inverted, plantarflexed ankle, the lower limb being swung forward in a semicircular fashion.

• **hesitant gait.** Gait characterized by hesitation at its start. Seen in parkinsonism.

• **high steppage gait.** Gait in which the foot is raised high and brought down suddenly, the whole sole striking the group in a flapping fashion.

• **intermittent double step gait.** Gait seen in some cases of hemiplegia (occasionally also in hip fracture). First variation: pause after the quick short step of the nonaffected foot. Second variation: pause after the step of the hemiplegic foot. Both patterns are also used in gait training in order to improve stability. Described in 1958 by American physiatrist Mieczyslaw Peszczynski.

• **kangaroo gait or walk.** Walking on hands and feet, knees kept extended.

• **lumbering gait.** A gait with heavy and clumsy movements due to the great weight and bulk of the individual.

• **magnetic gait.** A gait in which the feet seem heavy and difficult to lift, as if magnetized to the floor.

• **marche à petits pas.** French for "walking with small steps." A gait with very short steps, as in parkinsonism.

• **mincing gait.** Gait with very small and rather quick steps, often exhibited by women in high-heeled shoes.

• **pacing gait.** Walking with slow, measured steps.

• **pigeon-toe(d) gait, pintoe(d) gait.** See **toeing-in gait**.

• **pivot gait or walk.** The mode of progression of a paraplegic person in a pivot-ambulating crutchless orthosis. By rotary motion of the trunk the subject pivots together with the support, alternately to the right and to the left, thus advancing or retreating. The axis of rotation is lateral to the feet, and both feet move together with the support.

• **plantigrade gait or walking.** Walking on all fours, the floor being touched only by the palmar aspect of the hand (or its digits) and the plantar aspect of the foot or toes.

• **point gait.** General term for four-point or two-point gait as opposed to swing gait (swing-to and swing-through gaits).

• **propulsive (or propulsion) gait.** Acceleration in walking because of tendency to fall forward. Similar to, but more pronounced than, festinating gait; also observed in parkinsonism.

• **quadruped (or quadrupedal) gait.** Walking on hands and feet, or hands and knees. Rarely are the forearms used instead of the hands.

• **reeling gait.** Gait with staggering or swaying from one side to the other. Seen in drunk subjects.

• **retropulsive (or retropulsion) gait.** Walking backward involuntarily. Seen in parkinsonism.

• **rocking-chair gait.** A crutch gait: the subject advances the crutches (usually only a few centimeters) then rocks back and forth to produce the effort necessary to bring the feet forward, overcoming inertia and friction.

• **scissors (or scissoring) gait.** Walking with constant adduction of both thighs, typical of cerebral palsy.

• **shambling gait.** Awkward, clumsy, shuffling gait. Term rarely used. Dr. Watson in Conan Doyle's "The Adventure of the Sussex Vampire" reported: "The boy went off with a curious, shambling gait which told my surgical eyes that he was suffering from a weak spine."

• **shuffling gait.** Gait in which the feet hardly leave the ground. Often combined with short steps. Seen in parkinsonism and amyotrophic lateral sclerosis.

• **sideward gait.** Gait in which first one crutch (or cane) is moved to the side, then the foot next to it, the other foot, and finally the second crutch (or cane).

• **spastic gait.** Gait characterized by abrupt, incoordinated motions of one or several parts of the body, due to spasticity.

• **staggering gait.** Gait with incoordination in the lower limbs, manifesting unsteadiness.

• **steppage gait.** Walking with exaggerated flexion of the hip and knee because of a flaccid dropfoot, thus avoiding stumbling; typical of paralysis of the deep peroneal nerve.

• **striding gait.** Walking with long steps.

• **swing-through gait.** Gait in which first the crutches (rarely canes) are advanced, then both lower limbs are swung ahead of them.

• **swing-to gait.** Gait in which first the crutches (rarely canes) are advanced, then both lower limbs are swung to their level.

• **swivel gait or walk.** The mode of progression in a swivel walk prosthesis, a prosthesis for children devoid of lower limbs. The trunk, with the help of the upper limbs, is rotated alternately to the left and to the right, whereby one foot piece slightly leaves the floor, moving in a small arc around the other. It resembles the pivot gait but the arc of progression is smaller.

• **tabetic gait.** A slapping gait characteristic of tabes dorsalis.

• **tandem gait.** Gait in which the feet advance, one after the other, in a straight line, tandem-like. This tandem walking is also used as a test or coordination.

• **three-point gait.** Gait in which the crutches (or canes) are brought forward together with the involved lower limb, followed by the uninvolved lower limb.

• **titubating gait.** Incoordinated gait which may include staggering or stumbling in the motions of the lower limbs, or shaking of the trunk or head. Observed in drunkenness and in cerebellar disease.

• **toddling gait.** Gait characterized by instability, such as seen in small children learning to walk. Hence the term toddler for such a child.

• **toe gait.** Walking on the anterior part of the feet. It may be normal (as an exercise or in dancing) or pathologic (shortened calf muscles, as in muscular dystrophy or cerebral palsy). It may also be used as a test of balance or strength.

• **toeing-in gait, toeing-out gait.** Walking with feet or toes turned in (toeing-in gait) or turned out (toeing-out gait).

• **tottering gait.** Unsteady gait, similar to the ataxic gait, seen in very weak subjects.

• **Trendelenburg gait.** See under **Trendelenburg**.

• **tripod gait.** Gait with crutches (rarely canes) in which the feel always remain close together and behind the crutches. Thus the feet form one part of a tripod, and the crutches the other two.

• **tripod alternate-crutch gait.** Variety of tripod drag-to gait (q.v.), in which the crutches are advanced one after the other.

• **tripod alternate-step gait.** Gait in which the crutches (rarely the canes) are brought forward together, then one foot after the other while still remaining behind, thus forming the third part of the tripod.

• **tripod drag-to gait.** Gait in which the feet are dragged forward together, after the crutches (together or separately) have been advanced. Also called tripod simultaneous-crutch gait (if crutches are advanced together) or tripod alternate-crutch gait (if advanced separately).

• **tripod simultaneous-crutch gait.** Variety of tripod drag-to gait (q.v.), in which the crutches are advanced simultaneously.

• **two-point gait.** Gait in which the right crutch or cane moves with the left lower limb and the left crutch or cane with the right lower limb.

• **waddling gait.** Gait with lateral trunk flexion on each step toward the side of the supporting lower limb. Seen in bilateral congenital subluxation of the hip joint, bilateral coxa vara, muscular dystrophy, and other deficiencies of the hip abductors. For an understanding of its mechanism, see **Trendelenburg gait**, under **Trendelenburg**.

Gallaudet College The only liberal arts college in the world designed exclusively for deaf students, located in Washington, D.C. Founded in 1864 as the National Deaf Mute College. Its present name was adopted in 1894 in honor of the American clergyman Thomas Hopkins Gallaudet (1787–1851), whose son, Edwin Miner Gallaudet, was its first president, from 1864 to 1910. See also **American School for the Deaf**.

Galvani, Luigi Italian physician and physicist (1737–1798).

• **galvanic bath.** See under **bath**.

• **galvanic current.** See under **current**.

• **galvanic-faradic test.** See under **test**.

• **galvanic skin response (GSR).** The change in the electric resistance of the skin as a response to stimulation. Called also electrodermal response.

• **galvanic tetanus ratio.** See **tetanus-twitch ratio**.

galvanism The therapeutic use of galvanic current (see under **current**).

• **negative galvanism.** Local treatment by application of the negative electrode of galvanic current.

galvanometer An instrument for measuring current.

galvanopuncture Electropuncture (q.v.).

Galveston Orientation and Amnesia Test (Goat) See under **test**.

gantry Overhead pole, supporting an armsling or other device for a sitting or recumbent person. It may be attached to a wheelchair or a bed.

Garceau method Method of treatment for fractures of the surgical neck of the humerus by physical therapy and the use of a sling and swathe. Published in 1941 by Indianapolis orthopedic surgeon George J. Garceau (1896–1977) and physical therapist Shirley Cogland.

garden for the blind Also called fragrance garden. With signs in braille, it is specifically designed for the blind. Visitors can touch and smell the plants.

GED test General Educational Development test. See under **test**.

General Aptitude Test Battery (GATB) Comprises nine aptitudes considered basic in determining one's capacity for job training and performance, this instrument was developed by the Department of Labor to measure the following functions:

• **Clerical perception:** the ability to perceive pertinent detail in verbal or tabular material.

• **Fine motor coordination:** the ability to move the fingers and manipulate small objects rapidly and accurately.

• **Finger dexterity:** the ability to move the fingers and manipulate small objects rapidly and accurately.

• **Form perception:** the ability to perceive pertinent detail in objects as in pictorial or graphic material.

• **Intelligence:** general learning ability.

• **Manual dexterity:** the ability to move the hands easily and skillfully.

• **Numerical aptitude:** the ability to perform arithmetic operations quickly and accurately.

• **Spatial aptitude:** the ability to think visually of geometric forms and to comprehend the two-dimensional representation of three-dimensional objects.

• **Verbal aptitude:** the ability to understand the meaning of words and to use them effectively.

genu recurvatum (plural, genua recurvata) Hyperextended knee; a knee that extends behind the neutral position of zero degree. Lay term: back knee.

genu valgum (plural, genua valga) Also known as knock-knee, it is a knee that is placed medially in relation to the long axis of the lower limb.

venu varum (plural, genua vara) Also known as bowleg, it is a knee that is placed laterally in relation to the long axis of the lower limb.

gestation From the Latin *gestare*, to bear, to carry (hence the meaning of pregnancy). The term was used in Roman times and even as late as the end of the eighteenth century for therapeutic transportation. The patient traveled in a carrying chair, a litter, a carriage, on horseback, in a boat, or balanced on a swing, in order to be submitted to the shaking, vibration, or balancing of the vehicle, found to be physical and psychologic benefit.

Gestuno International sign language based on natural gestures, without reference to alphabetical signs. Adopted in 1975 by the World Federation of the Deaf. The name is a contraction of the terms used in several languages for "gestures" and "unification."

ghillie, gillie, or gilly See under **shoe**.

giant potential Potential of particularly high voltage seen on the electromyogram. Potentials of this type may occur spontaneously or be a sum of smaller motor unit action potentials.

Gilles de la Tourette's disease A rare form of generalized tic usually occurring in childhood; characterized by uncontrolled continuous gestures, facial twitching, foul language, and repetition of sentences spoken by other persons.

Gindler method A system of bodily education that aims at the development of consciousness of posture, muscle tone, and motion as well as of sensory acuity. It includes practice in breathing and relaxation, both aided by automassage and, during group sessions mutual massage. Probably the most profound of the modern systems to develop body awareness, "to be in contact with oneself" and to express oneself in a natural and true manner in all one does. Developed in the 1920s by Berlin kinesitherapist Elsa Gindler (1885–1961). None of her writing has been published.

glaetzel mirror A polished piece of metal serving as a mirror, used to test the patency of the nasal passages. It is held at the level of the upper lip while the patient exhales through the nose. The marks produced on the mirror reveal the patency of the nasal passages or their obstruction. Any shiny, cool metal surface may be used for this test.

Glasgow Coma Scale A rating system developed by Teasdale and Jennett and used to classify and characterize traumatic brain injury within the first two to three days after injury.

Glasgow Outcome Scale A scale designed by Jennett to categorize the clinical outcome of patients with traumatic brain injury.

glide-about chair Casterchair. See under **chair**.

glossopharyngeal breathing A technique of motions of lips, tongue, and pharynx to pump air into the lungs and thus increase the vital capacity. Used in severe weakness of respiratory muscles, such as in poliomyelitis. Published in 1951 by Clarence W. Dail, California physiatrist.

go-cart

1. A rolling walker for children.
2. A child's low carriage that can be pushed or pulled; a stroller.

• **Chailey go-cart.** Small vehicle for handicapped children who are unable to walk. Developed about 1970 at Chailey Heritage Craft School and Hospital in Chailey, Lewes, Sussex, England.

Goeckerman treatment A method of treatment of psoriasis by tar and ultraviolet radiation. A crude coal tar ointment is applied in the evening and removed the next day shortly before exposure of the skin to ultraviolet radiation in daily increasing amounts. Published in 1925 by William H. Goeckerman (1884–1954), Los Angeles dermatologist.

Golden Olympics An annual sports contest or persons of the "golden" age, i.e., 55 years old or older. Founded in 1976 in Springfield, Illinois, the movement spread to Virginia and other states. Cf. **senior olympics.**

goniometer A device to measure ranges and positions (angles) of joints.

goniometry A technique by which joint position or joint motion may be measured, using the universal goniometer (basically a double armed protractor).

Good A grade in manual muscle testing, denoting a muscle or muscle group that can move the corresponding segment through its full range against moderate resistance, i.e., less than normal power.

grab-all extension arm Device to grasp an object that is out of reach of the hand.

grab bar, grab rail A bar solidly fixed to a wall or the floor, often in a bathroom. It is used as a handhold for a person who needs a firm support.

Gradierwerk German for graduation works. A type of outdoor inhalatorium found in certain spas, notably in Germany. It consists of a wooden structure with thick layers of brushwood. The local mineral water, rich in sodium chloride, is pumped to its top from where it slowly ("gradually") drips through the brushwood. Thus the water is partly nebulized and inhaled as aerosol by patients walking inside this shedlike building. Used in asthma and other respiratory conditions.

Graham-Kendall Memory for Designs Test See under **test.**

gravity-eliminated Refers to positions or motions in which the action of gravity is more or less avoided. Examples are the immersion of a body part into water or the use of a powdered table surface for elbow flexion and extension.

guide dog A dog trained to guide a blind person, while walking, to avoid common accidents. Schools for such training also teach blind men and women how to handle the dogs. There may be no charge to the blind individual for the animal or the training program. The breeds most often used at such schools are German shepherds, Labrador retrievers, and golden retrievers.

Guillain-Barré syndrome Acute segmentally demyelinating polyradiculoneuropathy, a disease complex in which the basic mechanism appears to be an immunizing or allergic reaction commonly occurring after a minor febrile illness; inflammatory changes in the spinal cord produce bilateral weakness or paralysis, most commonly beginning in the lower extremities.

Gurdjieff movements, method, or system See under **exercise**.

gurney A wheelstretcher or wheeled cart.

Guthrie-Smith, Mrs. Olive F. London physical therapist (1883–1956), who in 1947 published her method of exercises in suspension. See next two entries.

• **Guthrie-Smith bed or apparatus.** Iron overhead frame, from which are suspended multiple springs and slings to hold a patient in horizontal suspension above a bed or plinth in order to compensate for gravity and thereby to facilitate exercises. Also used for relaxation.

• **Guthrie-Smith suspension exercises.** Exercises with elimination of gravity by suspension in a Guthrie-Smith bed. Called also weightless exercises.

Guts Muths, Johann Christoph Friedrich German founder of a system of physical education (1759–1839). This system, published in 1793 under the title **Gymnastik für die Jugend** ("Gymnastics for Youth" in the English edition), is based on movements of daily life. It was further developed by Jahn (q.v.).

gymnasium (plural, gymnasia or gymnasiums) A building, hall, or large room for sports, gymnastics, physical education, corrective therapy, or physical therapy.

gymnast A person who does or teaches gymnastics.

• **remedial gymnast.** A physical therapist, notably one whose therapy consists primarily in exercises. Term mostly used in the uk.

gymnastics Physical exercises performed with or without apparatus. A large variety exists, ranging from corrective to artistic, from calisthenics to acrobatics, from elementary movements of a single body segment to complicated combinations. For the definitions of various types, see under **exercise**.

• **curative, medical, or remedial gymnastics.** General terms indicating the medical nature and purpose of exercise. Called also therapeutic exercise. See definition of **exercise** (main entry).

H

habilitation Term sometimes used for the training of a skill an individual never had before, as contrasted with rehabilitation. Examples: gait training in a child with cerebral palsy; habilitation of the left hand of a patient who has lost his right, which was his dominant hand.

halo traction Technique of cervical traction and immobilization by a circular brace (halo) anchored in the skull and providing countertraction against another brace resting on the shoulders or the pelvis. Used in cervical vertebral fractures or fusion, and in the treatment of scoliosis and rheumatoid arthritis.

Halstead-Reitan Battery An extensive collection of psychological tests used to explore brain functioning in adults.

hammam From the Arabic, meaning a public steam bath.

hand

• **APRL hand.** See under **APRL**.

• **Becker hand.** Proprietary name of an artificial hand with voluntary opening.

• **cosmetic hand.** An artificial hand in which appearance is emphasized. It is usually covered with a thin plastic glove resembling the patient's skin. Its function of prehension is generally limited.

• **Dorrance hand.** Proprietary name of an artificial hand. See also **hook**.

• **French electric hand.** See **Vaduz hand**.

• **helping hand.** Device used to grasp an object otherwise out of reach.

• **Robin-Aids hand.** Proprietary name of a prosthetic hand with voluntary opening by a spring-loaded thumb.

• **Russian hand.** Myoelectric hand developed in the late 1950s by Popov and Yakobson, Central Institute of Prosthetics, Moscow.

• **Sierra hand.** See under **APRL.**

• **Vaduz hand.** Below-elbow prosthesis with a myoelectric hand, operated by the remaining forearm muscles, and an incorporated feedback mechanism. Developed in 1950 by Edmund Wilms, physician in Vaduz, Liechtenstein. After 1953, it was manufactured in Paris and became known as the French electric hand.

Hand Gym Exercise apparatus for the hand, consisting of a framework with five small plastic walls parallel to each other, permitting the fingers to be placed between them. Bars, rubber cushions, and rubber bands are used so as to allow various exercises and stretching. Devised for the treatment of rheumatoid arthritis by Semyon E. Krewer and published in 1974 by Doris E. Bens, OTR, and the inventor.

handicap The functional disadvantage and limitation of potentials based on a physical or mental impairment (q.v.) that substantially limits one or more major life activities, such as caring for one's self, performing manual tasks, walking, seeing, hearing, speaking, breathing, learning, working. In addition to physical and mental handicaps, there are handicaps due to economic, social, educational, and other factors.

handicapped Refers to the disadvantage of an individual with a physical or mental impairment resulting in a handicap (see preceding entry). As adjective or noun, in singular or plural, the term is interchangeably used, often incorrectly, with disabled (q.v.).

hand roll A roll of cloth (usually a wash cloth) or other cylinder-shaped object placed in the hand for the purpose of counteracting its tendency to remain closed.

handtalk Term applying collectively to fingerspelling and sign language.

Hanflig technique of neck traction Cervical traction applied in the sitting position and increased until the patient's buttocks are lifted just above the seat of the chair. While the patient is thus suspended, the shoulders are held by an assistant, and the head in the sling is rotated to the left and right. Suggested in 1936 by Boston orthopedic surgeon Samuel S. Hanflig (1901–1966).

Hanman plan, profile, system, or test See **Hanman test**, under **test.**

harness

1. A combination of leather, textile, or synthetic fabric straps, applied to a body part in order to hold the latter in a certain position (see also **restraining harness**) or to hold a prosthesis in contact with it (see **shoulder harness**).
2. A device for raising and lowering the warp threads on a weaving loom.

• **auxiliary harness.** Shoulder harness (q.v.).

• **restraining harness.** A vest or a combination of straps that holds a person securely in a lying or sitting position for protection against falling out of bed or chair and other movements possibly resulting in injuries.

• **shoulder harness.** A harness, applied to both shoulders, to provide suspension of an upper-limb prosthesis and for activation of certain of its mobile parts. More rarely it serves to attach an orthosis.

Harris footprint mat Rubber mat for the taking of footprints. It has small ridges of varying heights, which are inked with a roller and covered with a sheet of paper. The patient stands or walks on the paper. The areas of greatest pressure are revealed by the thickness of the ink in the footprint. There is also a thin variety of the Harris mat that can be cut to fit inside a shoe. Designed by Toronto surgeon Robert L. Harris and published in 1949.

Hartwell carrier Device consisting of a ceiling track, from which are suspended harnesses, tricycles, and dollies used in the locomotor education, particularly ambulation, of children with cerebral palsy and other locomotor dysfunctions. Developed in 1951 by R. Plato Schwartz (q.v.) for use by up to 12 children at the same time at Edith Hartwell Clinic, Leroy, New York. It was later transferred to Strong Memorial Hospital, Rochester, New York, and discarded in 1968.

Hauser bar See **comma bar**, under **bar**.

headache Pain or ache in the head; also called cephalagia.

• **blind headache.** A migraine.

• **cluster headache.** A recurrent unilateral headache in the orbitotemporal area; usually of brief duration, often severe, generally occurring in regular intervals of six-week cycles; usually accompanied by stuffiness of the nose and tearing of the eye on the same side as the pain.

• **histaminic headache.** See **cluster headache**

• **organic headache.** One caused by disease of the brain or its membranes.

• **tension headache.** One caused by sustained contraction of skeletal muscle about the scalp, face, and especially the neck.

• **vascular headache.** A migraine.

headpointer, headstick, headwand A dowel or similar thin wood or plastic stick, about 30 cm long, attached to a head band or cap, so that it can be used for typing, turning pages, pushing buttons by a quadriplegic person.

headwings Panels at the side of a headrest or high backrest of a chair (e.g., a wheelchair), to provide lateral support for the head.

health club, health spa An institution for physical fitness with exercise apparatuses such as stationary bicycles, rowing machines, dumbbells and barbells, striking and training bags, and facilities for showering, swimming, massage, ultraviolet radiation, etc. Users are usually more or less healthy persons. They are guided and supervised in their activities by a physical educator or therapist. In some institutions, a physician is also available; this is more often the case in a real spa or resort (see next entry).

health resort A town or other community whose climate or water is thought to be of value for the prevention or treatment of disease or for convalescence. A spa (q.v.).

hearing The capacity to perceive sound.

• **color hearing.** A subjective color sensation produced by certain sound waves; also called pseudochromesthesia.

• **conduction hearing impairment.** Reduction of hearing ability caused by interference with the conduction of sound to the end organ.

• **monaural hearing.** Hearing with only one ear.

• **sensorineural hearing loss.** Loss of hearing due to dysfunction of the end organ or nerve fibers or both.

hearing aid Any of various types of mechanical or electric devices carried in or close to the outer ear in order to improve hearing. Modern hearing aids are usually of one of the four following types.

• **body type hearing aid.** The receiver, which includes the earmold, is connected by an electric cord to a case worn on the body. This case contains microphone, amplifier, tone adjustment device, battery, and transmitter.

• **eyeglass hearing aid.** All objects are incorporated into the temple bar of the glasses, close to the ear.

• **intraauricular (or in-the-ear) hearing aid.** The entire aid fits into the external auditory canal.

• **postauricular (or retroauriculator) hearing aid.** All objects are fitted into a small box worn behind the ear.

hearing-ear dog Dog trained to respond to specific sounds such as those of sirens, car horns, cries, alarm clocks, boiling water, door or telephone bells, or smoke detectors, by nudging the deaf person, jumping, and running toward the source of the sound. Based on the concept of the seeing-eye dog (q.v.), the training of hearing-ear dogs was developed in 1973 by the Minnesota Humane Society.

hearing impairment Loss of or compromised hearing.

• **conductive hearing impairment.** A hearing defect that results in the prevention or interference of transmitted sound to the cochlea.

• **combined hearing impairment.** Hearing loss as the result of both sensorineural and conductive impairments.

• **sensorineural hearing impairment.** Hearing loss resulting from damage to the cochlea or auditory nerve or both.

• **hearing threshold level.** The reference-zero level used in audiograms. It was previously based on the ASA (American Standard Association) level of 1951. Since 1964, the ISO (International Organization for Standardization) level has been used, which is higher by a value ranging between 6 and 15 decibels, depending upon the frequency of the sound.

heat, heating

• **conductive heating.** Heating by conduction, i.e., by direct contact with a warmer object (transfer of heat from one molecule to the next). Examples: hot pack, hot-water bottle.

• **convective heating.** Heating by convection, i.e., the transfer of heat by the movement of a medium, a "vector," from the source of heat to the receiving body. Examples: moving air or water.

• **conversive heating.** Heating by conversion, i.e., the introduction of energy other than heat into the body, where it is converted into heat. Examples: diathermy in its various forms, including ultrasound therapy.

• **deep heating.** Heating by conversive heat such as produced by shortwaves, microwaves, or ultrasound.

• **infrared heat.** See under **radiation**.

• **luminous heat.** Radiant heat by a source that emits light at the same time. Examples: sun, incandescent bulb, heat cradle, electric light cabinet.

• **nonluminous heat.** heat from a nonluminous radiator, i.e., a heat generator consisting of a resistance wire. It usually glows a dull red.

• **radiant heat.** Heat issuing from a source as electromagnetic waves. Examples: heat cradle, heat lamp (of luminous or nonluminous heat), other "radiators." Heating by radiation requires no medium. Example: the radiant heat of the sun, transferred across a relatively empty space.

• **reflex heat.** Heat produced in one region of the body by local heating of another region. See also next entry.

• **reflex heating.**

1. In diagnosis: examination of a body part relative to its reaction to heat applied at a distance. Example: Gibbon-Landis test (see under **test**).
2. In therapy: application of heat to a region distance from the diseased area in an attempt to obtain vasodilation at the site of the diseased area.

• **specific heat.** Quantity of heat required to raise one gram of a given substance by one degree Celsius.

• **superficial heating.** Heating by luminous, infrared, conductive, or convective heat.

heat box Wooden or metal box for the heating of a limb by dry air. The temperature may be as high as 140°C and more. Higher temperatures may be used for a smaller body part and with appropriate ventilation. Called also hot-air box.

heat cabinet Large box of metal or other material, whose inside is studded with electric bulbs to provide a bath of hot dry air to the patient sitting or lying inside, keeping the head outside the enclosure. The temperature inside a heat cabinet may reach 80°C and more. called also hot-air cabinet, light cabinet. See also **heat box** and **fever cabinet**.

heat cradle Tunnel or hoodlike device containing electric bulbs or infrared elements for the heating of the body or part of it. Sometimes inaccurately named a baker.

heat lamp A lamp giving luminous heat, or a lamplike device generating nonluminous heat.

heat therapy Treatment used to promote temperature elevation, which in turn encourages certain physiological responses that (a) decrease joint stiffness, (b) relieve muscle spasm, (c) increase blood flow, and (d) assist in the resolution of inflammatory infiltrates, edema, and exudates.

Hébert system, Hébertism A method of physical education consisting in marching, running, walking on all fours, jumping, climbing, balancing, carrying, throwing, wrestling, and swimming. These being natural, utilitarian activities, the system, particularly known in France, was called **natural method** by its creator, the French naval officer Georges Hébert (1875–1957), who emphasized its difference from Swedish exercises (see under **exercise**). He also added moral principles to this physical education.

heel

- **negative heel.** The heel of a shoe that is lower than its sole.
- **orthopedic heel, Thomas heel.** See **Thomas heel**, under **Thomas**.

heelcord Lay term for tendo calcaneus, tendo Achillis, or Achilles tendon.

heelcord stretching Term usually doubly objectionable: (1) see preceding entry; (2) what is attempted is the stretching of muscle tissue. A better expression would therefore be stretching of triceps surae.

Heidelberg arm or prosthesis See under **arm**.

heliotherapy Treatment by exposing the body or part of it to the sun.

HELP Acronym for Help Extend Libraries to People with handicaps.

hemi- Prefix meaning half. Refers usually to one symmetric half of the body or part of it.

hemianopsia Blindness in half the visual field.

hemiparesis Muscular weakness or mild paralysis of one side of the body.

hemiparetic Weakness of one side of the body.

hemiplegia Paralysis of one side of the body.

hemisling Sling designed to support a flail upper limb affected by hemiplegia. Colloquialism.

Herodicus Greek physician, born 480 B.C., tutor of Hippocrates. Author of *Ars Gymnastica* (The Art of Gymnastics), he was the first to establish medical gymnastics.

hertz (Hz) Unit of frequency equal to one cycle or oscillation per second. Named after the German physicist Heinrich Rudolf Hertz (1857–1894), who in 1888 discovered radio waves.

Herz method or system Therapeutic system comprising baths, exercises, and walks. It combines the system of Schott (q.v.), the terrain cure according to Oertel (see **terrain cure**), and the system of mechanotherapy of Zander (q.v.). Developed by Max Herz (1865–1936), Vienna physician, who invented some additional apparatuses of mechanotherapy.

Hester evaluation system A system of vocational evaluation, developed in 1969 by industrial psychologist Edward J. Hester and sponsored by the Goodwill Industries of Chicago.

heterokinesia Performance of movements other than those a patient is told to do.

high-frequency therapy Diathermy.

high stepper Foot placement ladder (q.v.) raised to such a level that the subject must lift the knees, stepping high.

hip bath Sitzbath. See under **bath**.

hitching Locomotion by jerks. It refers especially to moving forward, backward, or sideways in the sitting position by sliding, or scooting, on the buttocks.

hohensonne From the German *Höhensonne*, meaning "high-altitude sun." The term applies to the sunrays received in the mountains and also to an artificial generator of ultraviolet radiation, an electric sun lamp.

holding glove A mitten with a T-shaped extension strap at its tip. After it is donned and the hand is flexed over a handle (e.g., of a pulley), the strap is closed by a buckle or Velcro over the wrist, so that even a paralyzed hand does not lose its grip. Used for the mobilization of an upper limb when its hand is weak.

holding sandal A sandal with web straps that hold the foot securely when attached to a pulley or other apparatus used for exercising the lower limb.

holistic A theory that focuses care on the individual's life as a whole, not solely on one's physical condition.

home lift An elevator in a private home.

hook A substitute for a missing hand, in fact the most frequent terminal device of an upper-limb prosthesis. It comprises a double hook of metal, resembling two neighboring fingers in a slightly flexed position, which can open wide to grasp objects of various sizes. Only one of these hook fingers is movable; it is operated via a steel cable by the wearer's shoulder muscles or other mechanism. Also called split hook, it was invented in 1912 by David W. Dorrance (1859–1943), an American sawmill worker who in 1909 had lost his right hand.

• **APRL hook.** See under **APRL.**

• **Dorrance hook.** Proprietary name of a prosthetic hook with voluntary opening.

• **Robin-Aids hook.** Proprietary name of a shoulder-elbow-hand orthosis that includes a prosthetic hook placed into a paralyzed hand, substituting for its lost function.

• **Sierra hook.** See under **APRL.**

• **split hook.** See above definition of **hook.**

• **two-load hook.** A prosthetic hook with two springs that can be engaged independently of each other; used to vary the force of prehension.

hooklying See **hooklying position**, under **position.**

horse, side horse, vaulting horse A thickly padded, leather-covered, firm and heavy bolster with a wooden core, shaped somewhat like the trunk of a small horse, used for vaulting (vaulting horse) and other exercises, particularly when fitted with a pair of removable handles (side horse). See also **buck.**

hospice A comprehensive unit, usually with a nurse-coordinated program and an interdisciplinary team approach to patient care;

available 24 hours a day, 7 days a week; directed specifically toward terminally ill patients.

hospital industry Various therapeutic activities of patients within the hospital, concurrently beneficial to the economy of the hospital. Now usually called industrial therapy.

hot-air box See **heat box**.

hot-air cabinet See **heat cabinet**.

HTP test House-Tree-Person test. See under **test**.

Hubbard tank See under **tank**.

huffing Forced expiration, as used in chest physical therapy.

Human Resources Center Center for the training of persons with physical disabilities in light manufacturing work on contract for large corporations. It was founded in 1952 under the name of Abilities, Inc., by Henry Viscardi, who was born without legs. It changed to the present name ca. 1965.

Huntington's disease An inherited disorder of the nervous system transmitted by an autosomal dominant gene and marked by degeneration of the basal ganglia and cerebral cortex; manifestations include choreiform movements, intellectual deterioration, and personality changes.

Hydra-Cadence See under **prosthesis**.

hydriatic Refers to hydrotherapy.

Hydrocollator Proprietary name of a small stainless-steel tank for either hot or cold packs.

1. The hot pack is a cotton bag filled with bentonite, a silicate gel. Soaked in hot water (at about 70°C), it absorbs it to form a soft heat-retaining mass. Developed in the late 1940s.
2. The cold pack (under the name of ColPac) is a similar bag filled with bentonite and a glycol solution and is maintained at ca. −6°C in a dry unit similar to the deep-freeze compartment of a refrigerator. Developed ca. 1970.

hydroelectric, hydrogalvanic Referring to electric current led through water.

hydrogalvanic bath See under **bath**.

hydrogymnastics Literally: water exercise. Treatment by exercise under water. Also called hydrokinesitherapy (see next entry).

hydrokinesitherapy Literally: water exercise treatment. Hydrogymnastics (see preceding entry).

hydrology The science of water and its uses.

hydromassage Massage by a whirlpool or other agitated water.

hydropathy Obsolete term for hydrotherapy, usually including the systematic ingestion of water.

hydrotherapy Treatment by external application of water. The term sometimes includes the therapeutic ingestion of water.

hyperextension Extension beyond the position of a joint in the neutral posture. For some joints, e.g., the shoulder, this is normal; for others, e.g., the knee, this is abnormal.

hypertherm A hot-humid-air cabinet, formerly used for the production of hyperthermia. A fever cabinet (q.v.).

hyperthermia, hyperthermy

1. Thermotherapy, fever therapy.
2. Fever, particularly artificial fever induced for therapeutic purposes.

hypertonia Excessive tension of the muscles or arteries.

hypertrophy The enlargement of an organ or part due to the increase in size of the cells composing it.

hypokinesia, hypokinesis Lack of motion.

hypokinetic Pertaining to lack of motion.

I

iatrogenic Caused by a physician; said of an illness unwittingly induced in a patient by the physician's attitude, treatment, or comments.

IC Inspiratory capacity. See **lung volumes and capacities**.

ice lollipop, lollypop, or lolly A lump of ice on the end of a stick, e.g., a tongue depressor; used for ice rubs. So called because of its resemblance to a candy lollipop.

ice rub Rubbing of an area with an ice cube or other piece of ice. It may be used either as therapy in acute injuries (in order to decrease extravasation of blood), in low back pain and similar acute conditions, or as an agent in facilitation techniques, e.g., in Rood's technique. Wrongly called ice massage.

I-D curve Intensity-duration curve. See **strength-duration curve**.

ideomotion Muscular movements influenced by a dominant idea.

idiopathic Denoting a disease of unknown cause.

IL Independent living. See also **independent living program**.

immediate postsurgical fitting Method of prosthetic replacement of a lower limb, which includes the application of a cast to the stump immediately following the amputation. A pylon is applied to the cast and used with some weightbearing within the next 48 hours. Method practiced since 1958 and published in 1961 by Michel Berlemont, surgeon at Berck-Plage, France. Cf. **early postsurgical fitting**.

impairment Any anatomic or functional abnormality or loss, such as absence of part of the body or its functions, e.g., amputation, loss of joint range, paralysis, blindness, mental retardation, psychiatric disturbance, as assessed by a physician. An impairment is a condition that is medically determined. Cf. **disability**.

impedance The opposition to transmission of electric current or of sound waves.

• **electric impedance.** The sum of electric resistance and other factors of hindrance to the flow of an alternating current. Like electric resistance, it is expressed in ohms. Its symbol is Z.

incentive therapy Industrial therapy (q.v.) that provides a patient with remuneration as an incentive for economic rehabilitation. Used for physically or psychologically handicapped persons. Called also compensated work therapy.

incoordination Inability to produce harmonious voluntary muscular movements.

independent living A service delivery concept that encourages the maintenance of control over one's life based on the choice of acceptable options that minimize reliance on others performing everyday activities.

independent living (IL) program A program established by the US Rehabilitation Act of 1978 to promote independent living for disabled persons.

Indian club A wooden object shaped like a bottle, about 35 cm high, with a knob at its top, where it is held for easy twirling by circumduction of the wrist and for other exercises of the upper limb. Used in pairs, mostly in general physical education.

Indian puzzle Fingertrap (q.v.).

Indian signs See **American Indian signs**.

inductance That property of a circuit, which is responsible for electromagnetic induction.

inductance cable or coil Single electrode ending in two plugs for the outlets of a shortwave diathermy machine, used with electromagnetic-field heating. The inductance cable is either wound around a body part or applied to it in a loop, a "pancake" coil, or a treatment "drum."

induction The appearance of an electric current or of a magnetic property in a body, due to the proximity of another electric current or a magnetic field.

inductive brace, device, or orthosis See under **orthosis.**

inductothermy Electromagnetic-field heating. Previously used in fever therapy (q.v.).

industrial therapy Therapeutic use of work that also provides benefit to the hospital or other institution in which the patient is treated. The latter may be assigned to an office, a ward, the laundry, pharmacy, laboratory, kitchen, or other department. Industrial therapy is usually prescribed as part of rehabilitation medicine and supervised by an occupational, manual arts, or educational therapist in cooperation with the supervisor of the place where the patient works. Previously at times called hospital industry, it is now also known as work therapy. See also **incentive therapy**.

influence machine See **static machine**.

infrared See under **radiation**.

infrasound Mechanical vibration of the same nature as sound waves but below the frequency range of those perceived by the human ear, i.e., below 20 Hz. **infrasonic therapy** is therapeutic vibration.

inhalation therapist, therapy See **respiratory therapist** and **respiratory therapy**.

inhalator Instrument supplying oxygen or other therapeutic gas to a patient who can breathe without mechanical assistance. The gas may be delivered via a face mask or a nasal cannula or inside an oxygen tent.

inhalatorium An inhalation room, i.e., a room in which an aerosol is produced and inhaled. Such a room can be used by several patients at the same time. It is often found in spas and institutions for the treatment of respiratory disorders.

insertion activity In electromyography, potentials evoked as the exploring needle electrode is advanced within a muscle. The amount of activity may be abnormally decreased or increased.

inspiratory capacity (IC) See **lung volumes and capacities.**

inspiratory reserve volume (IRV) See **lung volumes and capacities.**

instrumental learning Expression sometimes used as a synonym for operant conditioning (q.v.).

intelligence quotient (IQ) A numerical index of intelligence or mental functioning. It is based on the concept of relationship between the mental age and the chronologic age of an individual. Mental age divided by chronologic age and multiplied by 100 is taken as the intelligence quotient.

intensity-duration (I-D) curve See **strength-duration curve**.

INTERBOR Anagrammed acronym for the German Internaationale Union der Orthopädietechniker und Bandagisten, also known as International Association of Orthotists and Prosthetists, founded in 1958 in Brussels. Members are mostly from German-speaking and other European countries.

interdisciplinary approach A group of health care workers, representing different professional disciplines, who provide evaluation and treatment based on integrated goals that are patient-centered.

interference pattern Electromyographic pattern of the superimposition of many motor unit potentials during their normal action. Also called summation pattern.

intermediate care The medical care of patients beyond the acute phase of their conditions and prior to the phase of extended or long-term care.

intermittent catheterization This refers to a urinary catheter that is inserted only when it becomes necessary to empty the bladder. The method replaces the use of an indwelling catheter, thus avoiding or correcting shrinking of the bladder.

intermittent claudication See under **claudication**.

intermittent positive-pressure breathing (IPPB) A technique of respiratory assistance provided by an apparatus that can supply gas under positive pressure during inhalation, exhalation, or both. It may supply negative pressure at the end of exhalation. It assists in ventilation and may be used to apply aerosol medication.

Internal-External Locus of Control (I-E) scale Developed by Rotter, this scale measures the degree to which people believe there is a relationship between their behavior and subsequent reinforcers, with one end of the continuum representing those who believe that chance, luck, or fate is more important than their own behavior in determining what happens to them; at the other end of the continuum are those who perceive reinforcers to be contingent mainly on their own behavior and personal characteristics.

interpersonal theory A conceptual framework posited by Barker and his colleagues that regards the body as a value-laden stimulus to the self and others.

interpreter for the deaf A person with more or less normal hearing who, being skilled in communicating with the deaf by some type of sign language, functions as an interpreter between hearing people and deaf people.

interval training Training for general physical fitness or for competition, in which stress work alternates with nonstress work.

intrinsic muscle Muscle that originates in the part in which it functions. The intrinsic muscles of the hand, for instance, are those of the thenar and hypothenar eminences, the interossei and the lumbricals. Opposite of extrinsic muscle (q.v.).

inverse square law The intensity of radiation received by a surface from a source of light, x rays, etc., is inversely proportional to the square of the distance between the source and the irradiated surface.

inversion-eversion tread An apparatus for foot exercises. It consists of a pair of long and narrow boards on which to stand or walk, one foot on each board. Hinged together side by side, the boards can be angulated to each other so as to force the feet into inversion or eversion. They are usually fitted with shelflike projections to be grabbed by the toes, so as to exercise the muscles of the soles at the same time.

iontophoresis, ion transfer Introduction of ions into the body by means of galvanic current. Called also medical or therapeutic ionization, electroosmosis, electrophoresis, and dielectrolysis.

iron boot See **weight boot**.

iron lung Tank respirator. See under **respirator**.

IRV Inspiratory reserve volume. See **lung volumes and capacities**.

ischemia Lack of blood in an area of the body due to mechanical obstruction or functional constriction of a blood vessel.

isokinetic Refers to an exercise apparatus or to resistance exercises performed with such apparatus. See under **exercise**.

ISOM International Standard Orthopaedic Measurements. See **SF-TR method**.

isometric Literally: of equal measure. Refers to the activity of a muscle during which its length does not change. See under **exercise**.

isotonic Literally: of equal tone. Refers to the activity of a muscle during which its tension (tone) remains more or less constant while its length changes. See under **exercise**.

J

J Joule(s).

Jacobson relaxation method A method of general relaxation. The relaxation progresses by muscles or muscle groups and is enhanced by a preceding maximal contraction of the respective part. The subject is guided to consciously "contract—and relax." Published in 1929 under the name of "Progressive Relaxation" by Chicago physician Edmund Jacobson (1888–1976).

Jahn, Friedrich Ludwig German founder of a system of physical education (1778–1852), called the "Father of Gymnastics" (**Turnvater**). Based in many parts on Guts Muths' method (q.v.) and originally of military character, the system comprised exercises with and without apparatus and is still practiced with modifications. The apparatuses included the side horse, the horizontal bar, and parallel bars, all of which are still used today. The method was published by Jahn and his disciple Ernst Eiselen in 1816 under the title *Die Deutsche Turnkunst* ("Treatise on Gymnasticks" in the American edition, 1828).

jerk

1. A sudden abrupt or spasmodic movement.
2. A sudden involuntary muscular contraction following a tap on the muscle or its tendon; also called a muscular reflex.

JEVS See under **Philadelphia Jewish employment and vocational services work sample battery.**

Jewett brace A framelike thoracolumbosacral orthosis with two anterior pressure pads (one over the upper part of the sternum, the other over the pubis) and one posterior pad in the thoracolumbar area for counterpressure. Thus it restricts in particular flexion of the vertebral column. Also called hyperextension brace. Designed by orthopedic surgeon Eugene L. Jewett.

Jobst boot, sleeve Inflatable compression unit combined with an electric timing device for rhythmic inflation and deflation, thus reducing edema in a limb. Developed by Conrad Jobst, engineer in Toledo, Ohio, and published in 1955 for the treatment of lymphedema of the upper limb by physicians Brock E. Bush and Thomas J. Heldt. See also next entry.

Jobst stocking Elastic stocking for the treatment of postphlebitic edema of the leg. Invented about 1948 by Conrad Jobst, engineer in Toledo, Ohio.

jogging Slow running.

joint

- **Klenzak joint.** The proper name is that of an engineer and machinist (died in 1956) of the Pope Brace Company, after whom several orthotic devices, particularly joints, were named.
- **Klenzak ankle joint.** A type of spring-loaded metal joint, used in braces, that contains a vertical channel holding a steel rod inside a coiled spring. The spring assists motion, while the rod limits it.
- **Klenzak double-channeled ankle joint.** Metal joint that incorporates two channels with springs and rods such as described in the preceding entry. By the selective use of springs and rods and their adjustment by screws, plantar and dorsiflexion of the ankle can be limited or assisted.
- **Klenzak knee joint.** A type of self-locking knee joint used in braces.
- **Pope joint.** Proprietary name of various orthotic joints devised by the bracemaker Henry Pope or subsequently the Pope Brace Company. Some of the joints may also be labeled Klenzak joints (q.v.).

joint range Amplitude of motion in a joint. See **range of motion**.

Jolly reaction, test The test consists in repeated electric stimulation of a facial muscle, usually the orbicularis oculi, over a period of about eight minutes. The decreasing amplitude of contraction of the muscle, characteristic of myasthenia gravis, is called the Jolly reaction. Discovered in 1895 by Friedrich Jolly (1844–1904), German neurologist.

joule (J) A unit of work or energy. It is the energy expended in one second by a current of one ampere at a potential of one volt. It is equal to one watt-second or 10,000,000 ergs. Adopted in 1948 as a unit of heat, it equals about one-quarter of a calorie (1 cal = 4.19 J) and is used, among other things, to measure ultraviolet dosage. Named after james Prescott Joule (1818–1889), English physicist.

Just World Hypothesis A belief that misfortunes experienced by others do not typically occur in a random fashion and are somehow deserved by the individual.

K

K Symbol of kelvin.

k Symbol for the prefix kilo-.

Kabat method of exercise A system of therapeutic exercises for neuromuscular disabilities, based on proprioceptive neuromuscular facilitation, utilizing diagonal and spiral mass movements and other normal and pathologic reflexes. Mass patterns incorporating reflex synergies are elicited by stimulating the patient to energetic participation. This is attempted with the help of various techniques based on neurophysiologic principles such as reflexes, stretching, manual resistance by the therapist, rhythmic stabilization, reversal of antagonists, and also exteroceptive influences, notably cold. Published in 1947 by Herman Kabat, American physiatrist, the system was continued by Dr. Kabat's co-worker, Margaret Knott, and is also known as the Kabat-Knott or Knott and Voss method. See under **Knott**.

Kanavel apparatus or table See **Kanavel table**, under **table**.

kangaroo walking See under **gait**.

Katz index An instrument developed to assess competence in activities of daily living. The scale focuses on ability to perform six activities without aid. These activities can be ordered hierarchically and include feeding, continence, transferring (moving in and out of chair or bed), attending to self at the toilet, dressing, and bathing.

Kelvin Temperature scale based on the Celsius scale; the intervals are identical in both. However, the Kelvin scale indicates the absolute temperature. Thus, to give a few equivalents:

absolute zero = 0.00 K = −273.15°C
absolute temperature of 273.15 K = 0.00°C
absolute temperature of 373.15 K = 100.00°C

Named after the British physicist Sir William Thomson, Lord Kelvin (1824–1907). See also next entry.

kelvin (K) Unit of thermodynamic temperature. The formerly used "degree Kelvin" and its symbol "°K" were officially replaced by the name "kelvin" and its symbol "K" in 1967. The unit kelvin is equal to the unit "degree Celsius" (see preceding entry).

Kenny method or treatment Treatment of acute poliomyelitis by hot wet packs (to relieve muscle spasm), passive motion, and motor reeducation. Developed in the 1910s by Elizabeth Kenny (1886–1952), Brisbane, Australia, nurse, known as Sister Kenny, who in 1940 came to the USA.

Kenny self-care evaluation, rating, or score A system of numerical ratings of a patient's ability to perform 17 different activities. Six categories (bed activities, transfers, locomotion, dressing, personal hygiene, feeding) are graded on a 5-step scale (0-1-2-3-4) ranging from completely dependent (0 or zero) to independent (4). Thus the total self-care score ranges from 0 to 24. Developed at the Kenny Rehabilitation Institute, Minneapolis, and published in 1965 by Herbert A. Schoening et al.

keritherapy, kerotherapy Treatment by external use of liquid paraffin. See also **paraffin bath**, under **bath**.

keyboard rest Plate of metal or plastic, attached over the keyboard of a typewriter, with an opening over each key. It offers support to the hands and prevents the typing finger from tripping over keys not to be depressed. Used in incoordination of the hand.

KHz Kilohertz.

kilo- (k) Prefix meaning one thousand of a measure (10^3).

kilocalorie (cal, kcal, kg-cal) Large calorie, equal to 1,000 small or gram calories. It is the amount of heat required to raise the temperature of one liter of water by one degree Celsius. See also **calorie.**

kindness norm The tendency to treat and respond to persons with visible disabilities with overt kindness combined with covert behavioral avoidance.

kinematics The science of motion, particularly of the bodily parts.

kinesalgia Pain occurring during muscular movement.

kinesiatrics Kinesitherapy.

kinesiology Knowledge and science of muscular motion.

kinesitherapist Term (with variations in spelling) used in some countries as equivalent for physical therapist. See also next term.

kinesitherapy Literally, treatment by motion, that is, therapeutic exercise and massage. Term often used for physical therapy in general. See also preceding term.

kinesthesia, kinesthetic sense The sense of perception of movement and position of one's body or body parts, of tension of one's muscles, of weightbearing and resistance.

kinesthesiometer Instrument for measuring kinesthesia.

kinesthetic Referring to kinesthesia.

kinetic Relating to or produced by motion.

kinetic analysis Analysis of the forces that develop during walking.

kinetic activities In occupational therapy, activities directed mainly at the reeducation of specific motions and the development of given muscles and joint ranges.

kinetics The study of all aspects of motion and forces affecting movement.

kinetography The recording of body movements through the use of symbols. See also **labanotation**.

kink

1. A bend.
2. A muscular spasm, usually painful.

KIR self-care rating or score The acronym is a variation of kri, for Kenny Rehabilitation Institute. See **Kenny self-care evaluation, rating, or score**.

Klapp creeping exercises See **Klapp exercises**, under **exercise**.

Klenzak brace, joint See under **brace** and **joint**.

Klippel-Feil syndrome Congenital defect marked primarily by fusion of one or more cervical vertebrae, resulting in a characteristic short, thick neck with limited movements; also called cervical fusion syndrome.

kneading A maneuver of massage, also known as petrissage (q.v.).

knee

• **back knee.** Hyperextended knee. See **genu recurvatum**.

• **Bock knee.** Proprietary name of a knee for an artificial limb, which locks itself by increased friction on weightbearing, in spite of some flexion. Invented in 1950 by German prosthetist Otto Bock (1889–1953).

• **Henschke-Mauch knee.** Proprietary name of a knee for an artificial limb. See **Swing-N-Stance knee**.

• **Hydra-Cadence knee.** See under **prosthesis**.

• **Otto Bock knee.** See **Bock knee**.

• **S-N-S knee.** Swing-N-Stance knee. See next entry.

• **Swing-N-Stance (Swing-and-Stance) knee.** Knee control system of an above-knee prosthesis based on a hydraulic mechanism that controls the knee during the swing and the stance phases of ambulation. The device was developed by Henschke-Mauch Laboratories, Dayton, Ohio, and published in 1970.

• **Vari-Gait knee.** Brand name of a knee joint for an artificial limb with mechanical brake and swing-phase control. Its construction aims at imitating normal gait and affording some stability on weightbearing in spite of flexion to about 10 degrees. Developed in the 1950s by Felix Kleinekathöfer in Germany.

knee assist Elastic strap at the front of an above-knee prosthesis that helps to extend its knee joint.

knee cage A brace supporting the knee, extending from about midthigh to about mid-leg.

knee cap
1. Patella.
2. The knee pad of an orthosis. See under **pad**.

Kneipp cure or treatment, kneippism Therapeutic system consisting in cold water applications, barefoot walking in the dewy grass of the early morning (or in the snow in winter), and diet. Expounded in 1878 by its inventor, the German pastor Sebastian Kneipp (1821–1897), in his book *Meine Wasserkur* ("My Water-Cure"). It is practiced mostly in Germany, where there are several specialized Kneipp health resorts.

Knight brace See under **brace**.

Knight-Taylor brace See under **brace**.

knock-knee A deformity of the knee which, if bilateral, causes the knees to knock against each other in walking. See **genu valgum**.

knork An eating utensil combining knife and fork for a person with only one functional hand. Called also rocker knife and fork (q.v.).

Knott (or Knott and Voss) method of exercise A system of therapeutic exercise or neuromuscular disabilities. Usually known as proprioceptive neuromuscular facilitation, it is based on the Kabat method (q.v.), using proprioceptive and other reflexes and reinforcement by diagonal-spiral mass movement patterns, emphasizing energetic participation by the patient as well as the therapist. The latter guides the patient's limb through the correct movement, which covers a great amplitude, starting with a position of maximal stretch and commanding and grading direction and amount of effort in a constant interplay of give and take. Published in 1956 by American physical therapists Margaret Knott (1913–1978) and Dorothy E. Voss.

knuckle bender An orthosis that applies constant pressure to the dorsal aspect of the metacarpal bones ii to V and the corresponding proximal phalanges, thus flexing the metacarpophalangeal joints ("bending the knuckles") in case of extension contracture.

Kohs blocks See **Kohs block-design test**, under **test**.

KRI self-care rating or score The acronym stands for Kenny Rehabilitation Institute. See **Kenny self-care evaluation, rating, or score**.

Kromayer, Ernst L. F. German dermatologist (1862–1933), who is 1905 invented the water-cooled quartz lamp for ultraviolet radiation.

• **Aero-Kromayer lamp.** An air-cooled Kromayer lamp.

• **Kromayer lamp.** Mercury quartz ultraviolet generator, producing intense localized radiation, used particularly for its bactericidal spectral band of 253.7 nm in the treatment of skin ulcers. It is held in the hand and applied in contact with the lesion. Originally it was cooled by circulating water; an air-cooled type was developed later, sometimes called Aero-Kromayer lamp (see preceding entry).

kung-fu Chinese system of postures, breathing, and other exercises. The term may be translated as "work-man." Probably originating in ancient times, the system had mythical significance, was taught in religious circles, included at one time also massage, and became known in the twentieth century particularly as a martial art.

Kurzweil reading machine A computer that reads printed material aloud; used by the blind. Invented in 1975 by Raymond C. Kurzweil in Cambridge, Massachusetts.

kyphosis Abnormal posterior convexity of spine.

kyphotic Referring to kyphosis.

L

L

1. Left.
2. In measurements of volume or capacity: liter(s).
3. In the description of an orthotic or prosthetic joint, referring to its motion: lock.

l International symbol for liter(s). Since it can easily be confused with the numeral 1, the capital letter L has been recommended for United States use.

labanotation One of the better-known systems of dance notation. It can also be applied to sports, theater, physical therapy, and industry. Invented by the German dancer Rudolf Laban von Varalja—known as Rudolf von Laban—(1879–1958), who in 1928 published his method under the name of **kinetographie**. See also **movement notation**.

lallation

1. Poor articulation, especially speech sounding like the prattling of a baby; babbling.
2. Defective enunciation of words in which the phoneme (l) is substituted for (r).

Lamaze method Physical and psychologic preparation for childbirth. Based on Pavlov's findings and developed in 1949 by Ilya Velvovsky and others in Kharkov, USSR, it was introduced in France in 1951 by Fernand Lamaze (1890–1957), Paris obstetrician. The concept is that an understanding of pregnancy, labor, and delivery and an education in breathing, relaxation, and exercises decrease pain, anxiety, and the need for anesthetics. Also known as psychoprophylaxis. See also **prenatal exercises**, under **exercise**.

Lambert's cosine law The intensity of radiation received by a surface is proportional to the cosine of the angle between the direction of the rays and the perpendicular to the irradiated plane. After Johann Heinrich Lambert (1728–1777), German mathematician and physicist.

lamina (plural, laminae) A thin layer or flat plate, as of muscle or bone.

laminectomy The surgical division of the lamina of a vertebra.

lamp

• **carbon arc lamp.** A lamp with carbon rod electrodes between which an electric discharge (carbon arc) is created that gives off an intense white light. It was formerly used in ultraviolet therapy. See also entries under **Finsen**.

• **cold quartz ultraviolet lamp.** Quartz mercury arc generating ultraviolet rays, operating at low vapor pressure, low intensity (15 mA), and high potential (5,000 V). The temperature of the burner rises little, because there is little consumption of power. Most of its radiation is of shorter wavelengths, notably in the bactericidal range of about 254 nm. See also **Kromayer lamp** under **Kromayer**.

• **hot quartz ultraviolet lamp.** Quartz mercury arc lamp for ultraviolet radiation of high vapor pressure, relatively high temperature, high intensity (3 to 4 A), and low potential (65 to 70 V). Most of its radiation is of longer wavelengths, including those that produce pigmentation.

• **Kromayer lamp.** See under **Kromayer**.

• **mercury arc lamp.** A lamp in which an electric discharge is produced in mercury vapor, giving off ultraviolet radiation. Used for general irradiation of individuals or groups.

• **spot quartz lamp.** See **Kromayer lamp**, under **Kromayer**.

• **Wood lamp.** See under **Wood**.

lapboard See under **board**.

large-print typewriter A typewriter with larger than usual type; used in particular by or for persons with poor vision.

laryngectomy Removal of the larynx.

laryngismus Spasmodic contraction of the larynx.

larynx The organ of voice production, located at the upper end of the trachea.

last The wooden mold over which a shoe is constructed. See also **reversed-last shoe** and **straight-last shoe**, under **shoe**.

leader dog See **guide dog**. The term is correctly used only for dogs trained by Leader Dogs for the Blind, a school for guide dogs in Rochester, Michigan.

least restrictive environment A term included in the Education for All Handicapped Children Act of 1975, which expresses the importance of using environments for programming and treatment for persons with disabilities that maximize their vocational potential and community integration.

leg

- **air leg.** A pneumatic prosthesis for the lower limb that can be used for immediate postsurgical fitting.
- **Anglesey leg.** The first prosthesis made of wood with a steel knee joint and articulated foot, designed for Henry William Paget, first marquis of Anglesey (1768–1854). In 1839, the first prosthesis of this type was introduced in the USA.
- **bandy leg.** Genu varum.
- **bow leg.** Genu varum.
- **muley leg.** See under **prosthesis**.
- **phantom leg.** Sensation of the presence of the leg after its amputation.
- **scissor leg.** A hyperadducted lower limb, crossing the midline of the body.

leg press See under **bench press**.

leotard Elastic textile garment reaching from the toes or the ankles to the waist or higher. A rather tightly fitting leotard is used in the treatment of extended varicose veins and edema of the limbs.

Life Satisfaction Index A measure of subjective well-being and coping.

life-skill program A therapeutic program consisting of activities aimed at dealing with day-to-day problems for persons who have suffered from physical or mental disease. Examples of these activities are self-care, money management, preparation of meals, telephoning, social skills, games, and other leisure activities.

lift, lifter A cranelike device usually on rollers, used to lift completely helpless persons and to transport them from one room to another. It is operated manually. Some types are stationary, e.g., one to lift the patient in and out of the bathtub. Also called patient lifter.

• **chairlift.** Stairlift.

• **Hoyer lift.** Proprietary name of a patient lifter.

• **stairlift, stairway lift.** Chair running on a rail along a stairway inside a house.

• **wheelchair lift.** An electrically operated platform built at the entrance of a house, a van, an omnibus, etc., designed to raise a wheelchair with its occupant, thus overcoming the steps.

lift seat Catapult seat.

ligament

1. Any band of fibrous tissue connecting bones.
2. Any membranous fold, sheet, or cordlike structure that holds an organ in position.

light The visible electromagnetic waves, i.e., those whose lengths are between 400 and 760 nm. Their spectrum goes from violet to red. Therefore, ultraviolet and infrared radiations, being outside this spectrum, should not be called light.

light cabinet See **heat cabinet**.

Lightcast Proprietary name of an open-weave fiberglass bandage used for casting. It is impregnated with a photosensitive plastic resin, applied over a polypropylene stockinet, and cured by an ultraviolet lamp for 3 minutes. The completed cast is lighter and stronger than plaster and is water-resistant.

limb An extremity; an arm or leg.

• **lower limb.** The lower extremity, including the hip, buttock, thigh, leg, and foot.

• **phantom limb.** A phenomenon often experienced by amputees in which sensations, sometimes painful, seem to originate in the amputated limb.

• **upper limb.** The upper extremity, including the shoulder, arm, forearm, and hand.

limb-load monitor A device that indicates the amount of load to which a lower limb is exposed during standing and walking. This information can be read by the person concerned and by the examiner.

limp
1. To walk lamely, with a yielding step.
2. An uneven gait, favoring one leg.
3. Flaccid.

For variants of limps, see under **gait.**

Ling method of exercise See **Swedish exercises**, under **exercise**.

lipreading See **speechreading**.

LMTA Language Modalities Test for Aphasia. See **Wepman and Jones test**, under **test**.

locomotion Movement from one position, or from one place, to another. This includes moving about in bed, transfer from bed to wheelchair, traveling in wheelchair, walking, etc.

locomotor Relating to motion.

logopedics Scientific study and treatment of speech defects. Term coined by Emil Froeschels (1884–1972), Austrian-born physician (later in New York).

long-sitting See under **position**.

long-term care The prolonged medical and personal care of persons unable to take care of themselves because of locomotor or mental deficiencies or chronic diseases.

longwave diathermy See under **diathermy**.

longwave ultraviolet rays or therapy See **ultraviolet radiation**, under **radiation**.

loom An apparatus for weaving, used in occupational therapy as well as in industry.

• **floor loom.** A relatively large weaving loom with two or more treadles.

• **table loom.** Small weaving loom that can be used by a subject sitting at a table or lying in bed.

• **upright loom.** A loom standing upright on the floor, usually a loom for weaving rugs and large tapestries.

lordosis Posterior concavity of the vertebral column.

lordotic Referring to lordosis

loss resolution The successful termination of the psychological processes of bereavement and mourning.

loutrotherapy Therapeutic use of baths, especially carbonated baths. Obsolete term, from the Greek *loutron*, bath.

Lowen system See **bioenergetics**.

lower motor neuron Neuron whose nucleus lies in the anterior horn of the spinal cord or the corresponding gray matter of the brain stem (for the cranial nerves) and whose axons terminate in a muscle.

Lowman plinth See under **plinth**.

lucotherapy Therapeutic use of light. Obsolete term, from the Latin *lux*, light.

luminous heat See under *heat*.

lung volumes and capacities

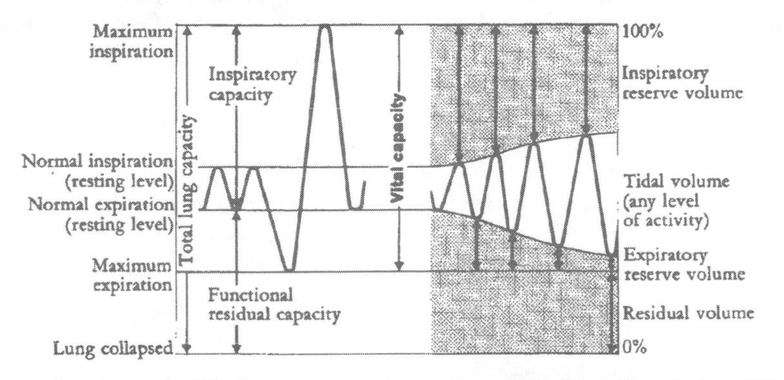

Lung volumes are the four compartments marked on the right of this schematic spirogram. **Lung capacities** are marked on the left. Each capacity is composed of two or more volumes. The total lung capacity, combining all four volumes, averages between 4 and 6 liters in the normal adult. (After *Federation Proceedings* 9:602–605, 1950, reproduced from Documenta geigy *Scientific Tables*, 7th edition, 1970, with kind permission of ciba-geigy, Basel, Switzerland.)

Tidal volume (TV): the volume of air inspired and expired during effortless breathing.

Inspiratory reserve volume (IRV): the maximum volume of air that can be inhaled in addition to an effortless inspiration.

Expiratory reserve volume (ERV): the maximum volume of air that can be exhaled in addition to an effortless expiration.

Residual volume (RV): the volume of air remaining in the lungs after a maximal expiration.

Inspiratory capacity (IC): the maximal volume of air inhaled with effort after effortless expiration.

Vital capacity (VC): the maximum volume of air inhaled after a maximal expiration (inspiratory vc) or that can be exhaled after a maximal inspiration (expiratory VC).

Total lung capacity (TLC): the volume of air contained in the lungs after a maximal inspiration.

Luria-Nebraska Neuropsychological Battery A test battery developed by Golden and based on the methods of A. Luria, designed to assess brain damage.

luxation Dislocation.

lymphdrainage (manual) Technique of massage, mainly for varicose veins of the legs. Proposed in 1936 by the German biologist Emil Vodder.

M

m Symbol for the prefix mega-.

μ Greek letter *mu*; symbol for the prefix micro-.

mA Milliampere(s).

μA Microampere(s). See Appendix.

mainstreaming The integration of persons with disabilities into society, usually used to refer to the integration of children with disabilities into schools and classrooms with nondisabled children.

major life activity A term used by the National Center for Health Statistics to describe limitations in functional tasks such as caring for oneself, performing manual tasks, walking, seeing, hearing, speaking, breathing, learning, and working. Activities are identified in terms of what is considered usual for one's age group; for example, play typical for children under 5 years of age, attending school for those 5–17 years of age, working or keeping house for persons 18–69 years of age, and capacity for independent living (e.g., the ability to bathe, shop, dress, eat, and otherwise care for oneself without the assistance of another person) for persons after age 69.

manipulation, manipulative therapy Treatment performed by the hands. As applied to the locomotor system, it consists in passive motion of a joint, aimed at increasing its range or at correcting a faulty position of one of its structures.

manual alphabet The 26 letters of the alphabet represented by different positions of the hand. Used by the deaf in fingerspelling (q.v.).

manual arts therapy The therapeutic use of tools, machines, electronic equipment, etc., in manual arts and crafts. It began under the name of prevocational shop training in US Army and Air Force hospitals during World War II. In 1947, the name was changed to manual arts therapy, a term used almost exclusively by the US Veterans Administration. Similar therapy elsewhere might be called work therapy, ergotherapy, industrial arts therapy, or it may be part of occupational therapy. In 1980, the Veterans Administration changed the name to vocational rehabilitation therapy.

manual communication or language General term for various methods used by deaf individuals to express speech, in which the hand are used either exclusively or in association with speechreading, gestures, or both. The essential methods, as applying to English, are fingerspelling, sign language, signed English, and manual English (see these terms).

manual communications module A portable "talking" typewriter that enables deaf individuals to use the telephone via a simple connecting mechanism. Its function is similar to that of a teletypewriter. See also **TDD**.

manual English Any one of several methods of communicating through the use of signs and other gestures that bear a structural relationship to English grammar and syntax.

manualism, manualist language or method Any method of communication by and with deaf persons that is based on fingerspelling or sign language. Created by the French abbé, Charles-Michel de lÉpée (1712–1789), who in 1755 in Paris founded the first public school for the deaf. It was the only method used in America before the development of the oralist method (see **oralism**).

manualist Teacher of manualism (see preceding entry).

manual muscle test (MMT) See under **test**.

manual therapy Collective term for treatment performed by the hands, such as massage, manipulation, mobilization, and manual traction.

Manuflex Proprietary name of a plastic device comprising four separate troughs, one for each of the digits ii to V of the hand. By pushing the hand forward, the fingers are passively spread; rubber bands add slight resistance.

MAPS test Make-A-Picture-Story test. See under **test**.

marche à petits pas See under **gait**.

massage Therapeutic manipulation of soft tissues. The five classical maneuvers are effleurage, friction, petrissage, tapotement, and vibration. See these terms.

• **Bindegewebsmassage.** Original (German) term for connective tissue massage (q.v.). See **connective tissue massage** below.

• **Brandt massage.** Gynecologic massage. It is performed with one hand on the abdomen while the other, in the vaginal cavity, applies counterpressure. It is aimed at correcting a faulty position of the uterus, stretching adhesions, and resorption of exudates. Developed by the Swedish masseur Thure Brandt (1819–1895), who published the method in 1868.

• **cardiac massage.** A resuscitative technique, consisting in rhythmic compression of the heart by pressure applied to the thorax (closed-chest, external, or transthoracic cardiac massage) or by direct manipulation through an opening in the chest (open or open-chest cardiac massage).

• **connective tissue massage.** A system of massage by stroking the skin and the subcutaneous tissue with one or two fingertips, following a certain order. English for **bindegewebsmassage**. Created in 1929 and published in 1948 by German kinesitherapist Elisabeth Dicke (1884–1952).

• **diathermic massage.** Electrotherapy by use of two autocondensation pads, one for the patient, the other for the therapist. The pad and the person form the plates of a condenser, the dielectric being formed by the insulating cover. Each person is charged by induction. When the therapist touches the patient a current passes between them.

• **douche massage.** Massage given to a subject sitting under a shower. Technique developed in the French spa Aix-les-Bains, hence also known as Aix massage.

• **high-frequency massage.** Electrotherapy in which a high-frequency current passes between the therapist and the patient, both being charged by induction. See also **diathermic massage**.

• **hydromassage.** Massage by a whirlpool or other agitated water.

• **Loka massage.** A massage practiced at Loka, a spa in Sweden, with a local peat, called **gytta**.

• **nerve point massage.** From the German **Nervenpunktmassage**. Technique of massage consisting mostly in deep friction by one or two fingertips in selected regions of increased sensitivity, designated as "nerve points." Developed in 1893 and published in 1909 by Berlin physician Alfons Cornelius (1865–1933).

• **plastic massage.** A kind of petrissage of the skin and subcutaneous tissue, used in the treatment of dermatologic conditions. Developed in 1908 by Raoul Leroy, physician in Paris, France.

• **reflex massage.** Massage of a region distant from or overlying the affected region, in which the effect is assumed to be due to a reflex.

• **Swedish massage.** The traditional massage, as it is practiced today in nearly all countries. Originally taught, together with therapeutic exercise, at the Central Institute of Gymnastics in Stockholm, it kept its name to emphasize its medical nature and traditional origin. See also **Swedish exercises**, under **exercise**.

• **syncardial massage.** Rhythmic compression and decompression of the lower limbs, synchronous with the heartbeat, by means of an apparatus, the Syncardon (q.v.).

• **Thiele massage.** Intrarectal massage for coccygodynia. Advocated in 1936 by George H. Thiele (1896–1978), American proctologist.

• **Thure Brandt massage.** See **Brandt massage**.

• **transverse massage.** Also called transverse friction, this is a maneuver of deep friction. It is executed with one or two digits in a direction at right angles to the fibers of a muscle, tendon, or ligament, primarily in order to loosen adhesions. Advocated by London physiatrist James H. Cyriax.

• **treadmassage.** Massage executed with the feet bearing part or the total of the masseur's body weight. It is usually applied to the back, the patient lying prone on the floor. Ancient technique, probably of Asian origin, practiced in some countries including (since 1939) Germany.

• **underwater massage.** Massage given to a subject sitting see (**douche massage**) or lying on a canvas sling spread over a bathtub while being exposed to water from one or more shower heads.

massage bath Whirlpool bath. See under **bath**.

masseur A male therapist who administers massage.

masseuse A female therapist who administers massage.

massotherapy Treatment by massage.

mat activities See under **exercise**.

mattress

• **alternating-pressure mattress.** Pneumatic plastic mattress whose parallel rows of aircells are alternately filled and emptied by an electric air pump. It provides support to the patient in alternating areas; thus, the danger of bedsores is diminished. A smaller pad is available for chairs.

• **pressurized mattress.** Alternating-pressure mattress.

• **pulsating mattress.** Alternating-pressure mattress.

• **water mattress.** A water-filled mattress. See also **water bed**, under **bed**.

maximal aerobic capacity The maximal rate at which oxygen may be utilized by the organism.

maximal voluntary ventilation (MVV) The maximal volume of air inhaled or exhaled in one minute by voluntary hyperventilation.

McCarron-Dial work evaluation A system of vocational evaluation, particularly for persons who are mentally retarded and mentally ill. Published in 1972 by Lawrence T. Mccarron and Jack G. Dial.

McKibben muscle See **artificial muscle**, first definition.

MCP joint Metacarpophalangeal joint.

mechanotherapy Therapeutic exercises with the help of apparatus.

MED Minimal erythema dose. See under **dose**.

Medcolator Proprietary brand of an electric muscle stimulator.

Medco-sonlator Proprietary brand of an electric muscle stimulator combined with ultrasound.

medical model A disease-oriented approach to the identification and treatment of physical and/or behavioral dysfunction.

medicine ball Leather-covered ball, between 20 and 40 cm in diameter and weighing between 2 and 6 kg, used for various exercises, either by one individual or with one or more partners, for strength, skill, and amusement.

mega- (M) Prefix meaning very large or, as a measure, one million (10^6).

megacycle (Mc) One million cycles. It is generally understood as "per second," which is correctly expressed as megahertz.

megahertz (MHz) One million hertz. Usual frequency of therapeutic ultrasound.

megohm (MΩ) One million ohms. See **dermohmmetry**.

Mendez, Christobal Spanish physician, born ca. 1500, who in 1553 published in Seville his *Libro del Exercicio Corporal* ("book of bodily exercises" in the English translation, 1960), the first printed book on exercise written by a physician.

meniscus (plural menisci) A crescent-shaped structure, as the fibrocartilage that serves as a cushion between two bones meeting in a joint.

mesomorph A person having a body build with prominent musculature and heavy bony structure.

Mercurialis, Hieronymus Italian physician (1530–1606), who in 1569 published the most important book on exercise at its time and for centuries to come: *De Arte Gymnastica* ("The Art of Gymnastics").

MET, Met Abbreviation for metabolic equivalent. A unit of basic metabolic energy cost. It is the amount of energy expenditure of a given person while awake and resting in the supine position. It corresponds to the consumption of approximately 3.5 ml of oxygen per kilogram of body weight (or to about 1.2 Cal) per minute. mets are a convenient way of indicating the intensity of a physical activity. Examples:

Activity	METs/min
Knitting	1.5
Walking (level), 3 km/h	2
Bicycling, 8 km/h	2
Walking, 4 km/h	3
Bicycling, 13 km/h	4
Light calisthenics	4
Walking, 6 km/h	5
Jogging, 8 km/h	7
Running, 10 km/h	10
heavy sports	up to and above 25

meter
1. A unit of length and the basic unit of the metric system. Symbol: m.
2. An instrument for measuring.

Methods-Time Measurement (MTM) A system for the analysis and time evaluation of any manual task. Its principle is that all manual work is a combination of various basic movements. It can be used to test the functional abilities of disabled persons, thus providing profiles of their work abilities. Developed about 1950.

metrotherapy Therapeutic use of repeated measurements, showing the patient the relationship between treatment, in particular his own efforts, and result. Advocated in 1920 by Fred H. Albee and A. R. Gilliland.

Meyer line The axial line of the great toe, that, in the normal foot (if shoes have never been worn) passes through the center of the heel. Expounded by Zurich anatomist Georg Hermann von Meyer (1815–1892).

μF Microfarad(s).

μG Microgram(s).

mho The reciprocal of "ohm" in spelling and meaning, it is the unit of electric conductance. It is now preferably called siemens.

micro- (μ) Prefix meaning very small or, as a measure, one millionth (10^{-6}).

microcapsule sock See **footprint slipper sock**.

micrometer (μm) One millionth of a meter or one thousandth of a millimeter.

micron μ (plural, microns or micra) One millionth of a meter. The term micron and its symbol μ have been officially replaced by the term micrometer and its symbol μm.

Microtherm Proprietary name of a microwave diathermy apparatus. Its current has a frequency of 2,450 MHz and a wavelength of 12.2 cm.

Micro-TOWER See under **tower**.

microwave apparatus Magnetron tube apparatus generating electromagnetic waves of a very high frequency, used for microwave diathermy. See under **diathermy**.

microwave diathermy or therapy See under **diathermy**.

microwave director Antenna-like reflector of a microwave apparatus, beaming its energy toward the area to be treated. The following directors are available. A: hemispheric reflector, 10 cm in diameter; B: hemispheric reflector, 15 cm in diameter; C: angulated (corner) reflector, 12 cm long; D: large angulated (corner) reflector, 50 cm long.

milli- (m) Prefix meaning one thousandth of a measure (10^{-3}).

milliliter (mL, ml) One thousandth of a liter, considered equal to one cubic centimeter. See Appendix: *Metric Measures*.

millimicron (mμ) One thousandth of a micrometer or one millionth of a millimeter. The term millimicron and its symbol mμ have been officially replaced by the terms nanometer and its symbol nm.

Millon Clinical Multiaxial Inventory Constructed to emulate the MMPI, this inventory, developed by Millon, is intended strictly for use as a clinical screening instrument for those suspected of significant personality disorders.

Milwaukee brace, corset, or orthosis See under **corset**.

miniglove A fingerless glove designed to protect the palm of the wheelchair user from soiling and rubbing by the tire while turning the handrim. Depending on the material used, it may also improve the grip. Developed by Herman L. Kamenetz in 1968.

minimal brain dysfunction syndrome A complex of symptoms that involves impairment of some or all of the following functions: learning, language, perception, memory, concentration, and motor; neurologic examination usually yields minor abnormalities if any; diagnosis rests on psychological assessment of cognitive function.

minimal erythema dose (MED) See under **dose**.

Minnesota Multiphasic Personality Inventory (MMPI) See under **test**.

Minnesota Test for Differential Diagnosis of Aphasia See under **test.**

mirror glasses A pair of spectacles with mirrors instead of lenses, enabling a person lying in bed to read printed material held upright on the chest.

Miss Wheelchair America A woman chosen in a contest held annually in the USA. The first such national pageant was held in 1972 in Columbus, Ohio, to select Miss Wheelchair America 1973.

The event developed from the first state contest, which was also held in Columbus, for Miss Wheelchair Ohio 1972. Its purpose is to show the potentials of wheelchair users by drawing attention to the achievements of some of the women in wheelchairs, their personalities, and their appearance, which are the determining factors in the adjudication of the title.

Mitchell treatment See **rest cure**.

mitella Armsling. From the Latin for headband.

mμ Millimicrons(s).

μm Micrometer(s).

MMPI Minnesota Multiphasic Personality Inventory. See under **test**.

MMT Manual muscle test. See under **test**.

mobile arm support (MAS) A functional orthosis for an upper limb with flaccid and more or less complete paralysis. It comprises a forearm trough and, depending on the extent of the paralysis, supports for the arm and hand and also, where needed, an external power source. Motions are executed essentially in the horizontal plane. Gravity is eliminated to a large extent by the attachment of the orthosis, either to the wheelchair (usually a back post) or by slings to an overhead bar, which, in turn, may be attached to the wheelchair. Rarely is it attached to a table or to the belt of an ambulatory user. Also called feeder. A frequently used mobile arm support is the balanced forearm orthosis (see under **orthosis**).

mobile stander See **wheelstand**.

mobility aid or device See **mobility aid**, under **aid**.

mobility instruction or training The teaching of a blind person of how to move around safely and effectively in various environments. It includes instruction in the use of a long cane (q.v.), topographic orientation, auditory training, and counseling.

mobility instructor, teacher, or trainer Person who teaches the blind to move around under a variety of circumstances. See also preceding entry.

mobility map Map that shows an area accessible to persons in wheelchairs, e.g., a college campus or a public building. In addition to larger areas such as parking lots, details such as elevators, toilets, and telephones may be marked.

mobilization Collective term for various types of exercises, passive motions, stretching, and other maneuvers aimed at increasing joint mobility.

modality Mode, method, or technique of applying a given physical agent or of using a given apparatus.

modular Adjective used to designate an object such as a prosthesis or part of it (leg, forearm, wrist, etc.), that comprises one or more prefabricated interchangeable parts (modules), which are standardized to be assembled.

module (foot, knee, etc.) Standardized unit, used as part of a prosthesis or orthosis.

mofette, moffette An opening in the ground from which carbon dioxide gas escapes; used in some spas for therapeutic purposes. See also **carbon dioxide bath**, second definition, under **bath**.

Moistaire Proprietary name of a cradle-shaped device for the application of moist heat.

monkey used by handicapped See **capuchin monkey helper**.

monoplegic Paralysis of one extremity.

monopolar stimulation Stimulation with only one electrode placed on the nerve or muscle. The second, called the dispersive electrode, is usually placed at a certain distance from it. Cf. **bipolar stimulation**.

Moon system, Moon type A printing system of a tangible alphabet for the blind. The embossed, rather large, letters somewhat resemble the Roman alphabet and are more readily identified by touch than braille symbols. Therefore, the system is more easily learned by older persons and others whose finger sensitivity is reduced. For finger contact without interruption the lines are printed alternately from left to right and right to left. Invented in 1845 by William Moon (1818–1894), of Brighton, England, and introduced in the US in 1880.

moor Earth from a marsh or moor; used as packs, particularly in spas close to the region of its origin.

morphosynthesis The ability to correctly organize stimuli into concepts.

motion See also under *exercise* and *movement*.

• **active motion.** A voluntary or willed movement, i.e., executed by an act of the will, without help. Opposite: passive motion.

• **confused or confusion motion.** See **confusion pattern**.

• **passive motion.** A movement imposed by a therapist or examiner upon the body or—usually—a body segment of a subject remaining passive.

• **substitution, substitutive (trick, or vicarious) motion.** See **substitution**.

motor development, stages in A child with average motor development will be able to do the following at the successive ages expressed in months. 3: lifts head when supine; 4: grasps; 5: rolls on back and abdomen; 6: sits when positioned; 7: sits alone; 8: uses thumb and index; 9: stands when held; 10: pulls up to standing; 12: walks with support; 14: walks without support; 16: climbs stairs.

motor function The observable behavioral manifestation used to achieve a purposeful outcome.

motor point The point of lowest threshold of electric stimulation on the skin of a given muscle. It corresponds grossly to the point at which the motor nerve enters the muscle.

motor unit The anatomic structure consisting of an anterior horn cell, its axon, all its branches, motor endplates, and muscle fibers.

motor unit (action) potential Electric activity of a motor unit, detectable by electromyography.

mouth-operated Refers to instruments for patients who are deprived of the use of their hands. Example: wheelchair operated by blowing into a tube or aspirating through it. See also next entry.

mouthwand A dowel or similar thin wood or plastic stick, about 30 cm long, held in and moved by the mouth. Used by persons who have no functional hand for turning pages, typing, pushing buttons, and similar activities.

movement See also under **exercise** and **motion**.

• **associated movement.** A movement produced by an individual while performing another one. There is a great variety of associated movements, notably in lesions of the central nervous system. However, many occur naturally: the eyes, for instance, moving together with the head.

movement disorders A broad group of neurological conditions characterized by involuntary disordered control of skeletal muscle movements, either excessive or insufficient. Types of movement disorders include the following:

- **akinesia.** Lack of movement.
- **ballismus.** Wild flinging or throwing movements, usually unilateral.
- **bradykinesia.** Slowness of movement.
- **chorea.** Abrupt, brief, unpredictable and irregular jerky movements that move between body parts in a continuous, random sequence.
- **dystonia.** Slow, writhing, repetitive, twisting movements that can distort the affected body part, occasionally into sustained postures.
- **myoclonus.** Rapid, brief, discrete, shocklike muscle jerks that do not blend with other movements.
- **tics.** Repetitive, irregular, stereotypic movements or vocalizations that can be temporarily inhibited by voluntary suppression.
- **tremor.** Rhythmic movement of a body part due to regular contractions of reciprocally innervated agonist and antagonist muscles.

movement notation The recording on paper of movements of the body through the use of symbols. Often called dance notation because it grew particularly out of choreography, it can also be used in physical therapy, sports, anthropology, and industry. Two systems with abstract symbols were published in 1928, each by a dancer-teacher: the English Margaret Morris (1891–1980) and the German Rudolf von Laban (1879–1958). The latter's system became known in the United States as labanotation. See **labanotation** and **dance notation**.

movement therapy Treatment by movement. Although, in a larger sense, this term includes therapeutic exercise, it usually refers to calisthenics, dancing, swimming, and other simple sports that can be practiced in groups. There is great variety in these activities, depending upon the individuals of whom such a group is composed: elderly, mentally retarded, mentally disturbed, or others.

moxa From the Japanese for "burning herb." A small tuft of vegetal matter (originally wormwood, of the genus *artemisia*), burned on the skin as a counterirritant or as a variant of acupuncture.

moxibustion The burning of moxa.

MP joint Metacarpophalangeal or metatarsophalangeal joint.

MTDDA Minnesota Test for Differential Diagnosis of Aphasis. See **Minnesota test for aphasia**, under **test**.

muff A hearing-protection device applied over the ear to deaden sound. A pair of muffs is used particularly by individuals exposed to noise reaching levels of 80 dB and above.

Müller system A method of physical fitness consisting of a sequence of eight exercises, a bath or a shower, and ten more exercises combined with self-massage. Published in 1904 by Jorgen Peter Müller (1866–1938) in Denmark and known in English as "Fifteen Minutes' Work a Day for Health's Sake."

multistation gymnastic machine See **universal gymnastic machine**.

Munster socket, prosthesis See **Munster prothesis**, under **prosthesis**.

musclebound Adjective indicating limitation in range of motion due to muscular hypertrophy and resulting shortening.

muscle endurance The ability of muscular strength to persist.

- **dynamic endurance.** The repetition of submaximal contractions.
- **static endurance.** Submaximal holding time.

muscle erotism Erotism stimulated by physical exertion.

muscle grading Measurement of muscle strength. See **manual muscle test**, under **test**.

muscle setting See **muscle setting exercise**, under **exercise**.

muscle splinting A state of contraction of a muscle or group of muscles as a reaction to pain, thus immobilizing and protecting the affected area.

muscular impairment Any physiologic limitation or deficit in muscular performance.

muscular strength The maximal voluntary resultant force, torque, or pressure that skeletal muscle can bring to bear on the environment under specific conditions.

musculoskeletal Relating to the muscles and skeleton.

mv Millivolt(s).

μv Microvolt(s).

myalgia Muscle pain.

myasthenia Weakness of muscle.

myatonia, myatony Absence of muscle tone.

myelitis
1. Inflammation of the spinal cord.
2. Inflammation of the bone marrow.

myelo- Combining form indicating a relationship to (a) the bone marrow, (b) the spinal cord.

myoatrophy Wasting away of muscles due to lack of use; also called myatrophy.

myoclonia Any disorder characterized by twitching or spasmodic contraction of muscles.

myoclonic Marked by myoclunus.

myoclonus A sudden rapid twitch resulting from the sudden contraction of one or more muscle groups.

myodynamometer An instrument used to measure muscular strength.

myodystony A succession of minute contractions during slow relaxation of a muscle following electrical stimulation.

myoelectric control of prosthesis See **myoelectric prosthesis**, under **prosthesis**.

myofascial syndrome A painful condition of skeletal muscles characterized by the presence of one or more discrete hyperesthetic areas termed trigger points, located within muscles or tendons; when stimulated by pressure, these trigger points produce pain in other areas of the patient's symptoms.

myofeedback An alternative term for biofeedback, emphasizing the role of muscle in the process, notably the attention given to muscle potentials in electromyographic biofeedback for purposes of exercise and relaxation.

myograph An instrument for graphically recording muscular contractions.

myoid Resembling muscle.

myometer Dynamometer.

myoplasty Surgical repair of a muscle.

myositis Inflammation of a muscle, usually a voluntary muscle.

myospasm Spasmodic contraction of a muscle or group of muscles.

myotonia Temporary rigidity of a muscle or group of muscles.

N

N
1. Normal (in testing of muscle power, etc.).
2. Symbol for newton.

n Symbol for the prefix nano-.

nano- (n) Prefix meaning one billionth of a measure (10^{-9}).

nanomelia Abnormal smallness of the extremities.

nanometer (nm) One billionth of a meter (10^{-9}m). Unit of wavelength of electromagnetic radiations. It replaces the previously used angstrom unit (1 nm = 10 A) and the millimicron.

naprapathy From the Bohemian *napravit*, to correct, and the Greek *pathos*, disease. A school of folk medicine, using diet, massage, and manipulation.

narcolepsy Condition characterized by paroxysmal episodes of sleep lasting from minutes to hours; frequently accompanied by transient muscular weakness, sleep paralysis, and hallucinations during the period between sleep and wakefulness; also called paroxysmal sleep and sleep epilepsy.

nascent motor unit action potential Motor unit action potential of low amplitude, appearing in the electromyogram in nerve regeneration.

nature trail for the blind See **garden for the blind**.

naturopathy A method of therapy using natural agents, such as heat, bathing, massage, sunrays, air, and diet, but rejecting the teachings of medicine and the use of drugs.

near Refers to the position of ultraviolet or infrared radiations in relation to the visible segment of the electromagnetic spectrum. Near ultraviolet rays are of longer wavelengths; near infrared rays are of shorter wavelengths. Opposite: far. See table of **electromagnetic radiation**, under **radiation**.

negative galvanism See under **galvanism**.

Nelson knife Knife-fork combination. British term.

Nemectron Proprietary name (after its inventor, Hans Nemec) or an apparatus for electrotherapy using **interference current** (see under **current**).

Neptune's girdle A wet pack embracing the abdomen.

nerve conduction test See under **test**.

nerve stimulation test See under **test**.

neural Relating to the nervous system.

neuralgia Severe pain along the course of a nerve.

neurapraxia Injury to a nerve resulting in temporary paralysis.

neurasthenia Condition marked by fatigue, irritability, and poor concentration; originally considered to be due to exhaustion of the nervous system.

neuratrophia Atrophy of the nerves.

neuraxis The central nervous system.

neurectomy Surgical removal of a nerve segment.

neurergic Of or relating to the action of nerves.

neuritis Inflammation or degeneration of a nerve.

neuro- Combining form, denoting nerve or nervous system.

neurolysis Destruction of nerve tissue.

neuromuscular Relating to nerve and muscle, such as the nerve endings in a muscle.

neuromuscular facilitation See under **facilitation**.

neuromyasthenia Muscular weakness, especially of emotional origin.

neuromyelitis Inflammation of the nerves and spinal cord.

neuromyopathy A disorder of muscle that indicates a disease of the nerve supplying the muscle.

neuromyositis Nerve inflammation complicated by inflammation of the muscles with which the affected nerve is in relation.

neuropathy Any disease of the nervous system.

• **diabetic neuropathy.** A complication of diabetes mellitus in which the peripheral nerves and the innervation of the bladder and bowel may be affected.

• **peripheral neuropathy.** A disorder of the peripheral nerves characterized by motor and sensory changes in the extremities; most commonly associated with alcoholism and/or poor nutrition.

neuropsychology The study of the relationship between the mind and the nervous system.

neuroskeleton The part of the skeleton surrounding the brain and spinal cord.

neuropathogenesis The origin of diseases of the nervous system.

neutral position See next entry and under **position**.

neutral-zero method Method of recording joint positions and motions, in which the neutral position (see under **position**) is the starting point, as presented in 1936 by Boston orthopedic surgeons Edwin F. Cave and Sumner M. Roberts. The principles of this method were accepted by the American Academy of Orthopaedic Surgeons in 1962 and, in 1964, by similar associations in other English-speaking countries.

Newton (N) A unit of force. It is the force that imparts to a mass of one kilogram an acceleration of one meter per second per second. Named after the English mathematician and physicist Sir Isaac Newton (1643–1727).

Niederhöffer method A system of exercise for scoliosis and other vertebral deviations. It consists mainly in the strengthening, by isometric contractions, of individual muscles attached to the vertebral column. Developed about 1900 by the German physician Egon von Diederhöffer and published posthumously in 1942, on the basis of his notes, by his wife and co-worker, physical therapist Luise von Egidy (1873–1946).

N-K table or exercise unit See under **table**.

nociceptor A peripheral nerve organ that receives and transmits painful sensations.

nociperception Perception of painful or injurious stimuli.

nonluminous Beyond the range of light. Referring to heat or radiation: infrared. See also under **heat**.

nonmajor life activity A term used by the National Center for Health Statistics to describe limitations in activity level. Examples of nonmajor life activities might include social, civic, or recreational endeavors that are normally less important than major life activities.

normal Conformed to an establish norm, standard, or pattern.

normalization A conceptual framework proposed by Wolfensberger that attempts to overcome the devaluation of persons with disabilities and encourages the adoption of measures that lead to a more positive view of persons with disabilities.

no-stoop shears Device to grasp an object out of reach of the hand.

O

O In muscle and range-of-motion testing: zero (q.v.).

Ω Greek letter **omega** (uppercase); symbol for ohm.

obtusion Dulling of normal sensibility.

occupational aptitude patterns Clusters of aptitudes that correlate with performance in occupations that have similar ability requirements.

occupational therapist (OT) A person trained to administer occupational therapy.

occupational therapy (OT) A system of medically prescribed activities, typically involving the use of objects to increase coordination, range of motion, power, and function, or for diagnostic, psychiatric, or other therapeutic purposes.

• **diagnostic occupational therapy.** Occupational therapy geared to evaluate the patient's posture, visual and manual coordination, skill, endurance, etc. during activities, thus aiding in diagnosis.

• **diversional occupational therapy.** Occupational therapy to occupy a patient's mind and body.

• **functional occupational therapy.** Occupational therapy aimed primarily at the achievement and improvement of purposeful motions and capacities such as eating, washing, writing, and other manual skills.

• **kinetic occupational therapy.** Occupational therapy for the reeducation of specific motions and the development of specific muscles and joint ranges.

• **metric occupational therapy.** Occupational therapy in which the performance is measured and graded for the evaluation of the patient's work capacity and progress.

• **prevocational occupational therapy.** Occupational therapy preparing for an occupation and helping in the establishment of a vocational prognosis, evaluating work capacity and employability.

• **psychiatric occupational therapy.** Occupational therapy used for various psychiatric purposes.

• **tonic occupational therapy.** Occupational therapy to stimulate the patient's mental and physical tone, interest in life, and social contacts.

occupational therapy assistant, certified (COTA) A skilled technical health worker who has completed an educational program that leads to this title and is approved by the American Occupational Therapy Association.

Oertel method See **terrain cure**.

Ohm, Georg S. German physicist (1787–1854).

• **ohm(Ω).** Unit of electric resistance.

• **ohmmeter.** instrument to measure electric resistance. See also **dermohmmeter**.

• **Ohm's law.** Relationship between electric current, voltage, and resistance, that may be expressed as follows. The intensity of an electric current (in amperes) is equal to the electromotive force (in volts) divided by the resistance (in ohms):

$$I = \frac{E}{R} \text{ or } E = ir \text{ or } R = \frac{E}{I}$$

where **I** = current (intensity), **E** = voltage (electromotive force), and **R** = resistance.

Older Americans Research and Service Center Instrument (OARS) A multidimensional assessment tool developed to yield information about functional activity in five domains: social resources, economic resources, mental health, physical health, and activities of daily living.

olympiad (or olympics) for the disabled See **Paralympics** and **Special Olympics**.

OMTRU Acronym for optimum metabolic temperature regulator unit, also called Apollo cover (q.v.).

one repetition maximum (IRM) The greatest weight that one can lift through the full range of motion one time only.

operant conditioning A technique, probably the best known, of behavior modification. It is the modification (or conditioning) of patients' behavior (or operants) through pleasant or unpleasant responses of the staff of the institution and other persons dealing with them, as well as through directly obtained results. Thus they are encouraged to respond to certain situations or tasks in the way most conducive to their rehabilitation. Based on the concept of reinforcement related to the principle of reward and punishment, it was developed in 1938 by American behavioral psychologist Burrhus Frederick Skinner (1904–1986).

opinions about mental illness scale (OMI) A scale developed by Cohen and Struening (1962) that measures attitudes toward persons with mental illness.

opponens Opposing; a qualifying addition to the names of several muscles of the hand and foot whose function is to pull the lateral digits across the palm or sole.

opponens split or brace See under **splint**.

Optacon Contraction for optical-to-tactile converter, a reading machine for the blind. A miniature camera held in one hand reads printed material, which is converted into vibrating impulses. With a finger of the other hand the user feels these vibrations, which reproduce the letters and numbers. Therefore it can also be used by persons who are deaf as well as blind. Developed in 1970 by John G. Linvill, electrical engineer at Stanford University, together with James C. Bliss.

optophone A photoelectric instrument that converts print into sounds, enabling blind persons to read. The first optophone, based on instruments similar to Alexander Graham Bell's "photo-phone," was invented in 1912–1914 by English physicist Edmund Edward Fournier d'Albe (1868–1933). A modern type (usually written Optophone) was developed in 1957–1958 at Battelle Memorial Institute, Columbus, Ohio.

oralism, oralist method A system of communication for the deaf. Also called speech-reading (q.v.), it concentrates on the recognition of lip and facial movements during speaking, without the use of signs or fingerspelling. Created by the German Samuel Heinicke (1727–1790), the system contrasts with the manualist method (see **manualism**).

oralist Teacher of oralism (see preceding entry).

organic brain syndrome (OBS), organic mental syndrome (OMS) A syndrome resulting from diffuse or local impairment of brain tissue function, manifested by alteration of orientation, memory, comprehension, and judgment.

• **acute organic brain syndrome.** Acute confusional state, characterized by a sudden onset and a high degree of reversibility.

• **chronic organic brain syndrome.** Disorder marked by an insidious onset, a progressive course, and a high degree of irreversibility; always due to focal or diffuse brain lesions.

• **psychotic organic brain syndrome.** Acute or chronic organic brain syndrome associated with psychiatric symptoms.

orientation therapist Mobility instructor for the blind.

orthesis, orthetic, orthetics Terms coined in 1956 by Robert L. Bennett, Warm Springs, Georgia, physiatrist. Based on the Greek *orthos*, "straight," they were later modified to orthosis, orthotic, orthotics (q.v.).

ortho- Prefix from the Greek **orthos**, straight, upright, correct.

orthokinetics Method of treating neuromuscular dysfunction, using exteroceptive stimulation by an orthosis made individually for any segment of the upper or lower limb, most often the forearm and wrist. Such an orthokinetic cuff has essentially two fields. The so-called stimulating field, made of elastic or "active" material, is placed over the muscle to be facilitated. As the wearer moves the limb, this material changes its shape, thus providing stimulation of the skin. The other, inhibiting or static, field made of smooth, inelastic material, is placed over the antagonist or spastic muscle, the one to be inhibited. Published 1927 in Berlin by Julius Fuchs (1888–1953), orthopedic surgeon (later in New York), who coined the term from the Greek words for "correct" and "motion."

orthopodium A variant of the Toronto standing orthosis (see under **orthosis**), with knee joints that permit sitting. Developed, like the unjointed type, at the Ontario Crippled Children's Centre, Toronto.

orthoptics Method of exercising the extraocular muscles to improve their coordination, i.e., binocular vision.

orthosis (plural, orthoses) General term for a device applied to a patient, usually with a deficiency of the locomotor system, for a supportive, assistive, adaptive, preventive, or corrective purpose. This excludes prostheses, which replace missing parts, but includes objects that may be known as braces, splints, collars, corsets, supports, bandages, or calipers and may be listed as such in this dictionary.

• **balanced forearm orthosis (BFO).** A swivel type of mobile arm support (q.v.). It often consists only of a carefully balanced forearm trough or tray, a disk for the elbow to prevent the forearm from slipping out of the trough, and a swiveled attachment to the wheelchair. Also called ball-bearing feeder and link (or linkage) feeder.

• **ball-bearing forearm orthosis or feeder.** Balanced forearm orthosis.

• **Craig (or Craig-Scott) orthosis.** See **Scott-Craig orthosis**.

• **crutchless orthosis.** See **pivot ambulating crutchless orthosis**.

• **double adjustable ankle orthosis.** An ankle-foot orthosis in which dorsi- and plantar flexion can be assisted or limited at various levels.

• **dynamic orthosis.** An orthosis in which there is at least one part that moves in relation to another part, thus allowing movement as well as providing support. The orthosis is activated either by the wearer's own power, or by rubber bands, a wire, or other means of external power; designed to correct or prevent deformity or to assist function. Called also lively orthosis.

• **flexible orthosis.** An orthosis made of textile or other flexible material. Examples: certain corsets (flexible spinal orthoses), certain belts (flexible abdominal orthoses), trusses, certain elbow, wrist, knee and ankle supports, elastic stockings.

• **flexor hinge (hand) orthosis.** A dynamic orthosis for a paralyzed hand, which incorporates the so-called flexor hinge. The latter is the finger piece, i.e., the most distal part of the orthosis. It hinges with the rest of the orthosoes at the level of the metacarpophalangeal joints and keeps the two distal joints of the index and middle fingers in flexion. Flexion of the flexor hinge brings the pads of the two digits in contact with that of the thumb in the manner of a three-jaw chuck. The flexor hinge may be part of a flexor tenodesis orthosis (see following entry). It may also be activated by a shoulder movement, or by an external power source.

• **flexor tenodesis orthosis.** A dynamic wrist-hand orthosis whose function is similar to that of surgical tenodesis, i.e., tendon fixation: after attachment of the flexor tendons to the radius, extension of the wrist produces their relative shortening, hence flexion of the fingers. Thus, the thumb being kept in the appropriate position of abduction and opposition, the three first digits, even if paralyzed, grasp in the manner of a three-jaw chuck. The extension of the wrist is achieved either by the action of still functioning muscles or by artificial means such as a carbon-dioxide-powered muscle or a micromotor. The tenodesis orthosis may incorporate a flexor hinge. See preceding entry: **flexor hinge hand orthosis**.

• **functional orthosis.** A device used to improve function through the use of levers, pulleys, movable joints, and external power storage devices such as springs, rubber bands, batteries, and tanks of compressed gas.

• **genucentric knee orthosis.** A plastic knee orthosis with supracondylar support and a special type of polycentric joint—named genucentric joint by the designers—in which the center (i.e., the axis) of motion changes according to the angulation of the knee. Developed in 1979 at the Veterans Administration Prosthetics Center (see **VAPC** or **VAREC**) by orthotist Robert Foster and orthotist/prosthetist John Milani.

• **inductive orthosis.** Appliance used in certain postural problems, "inducing" the wearer to assume a certain posture or to avoid a harmful posture or movement. An abdominal belt and a Spitzy button (q.v.) are examples of inductive orthotics.

• **lively orthosis.** Dynamic orthosis (q.v.).

• **passive orthosis.** Static orthosis (q.v.).

• **penile orthosis.** Splint providing rigidity to the penis.

• **Perlstein orthosis.** Ankle-foot orthosis for children. It has a single (lateral) upright with a cam ankle joint at the level of the sole for dorsi- and plantar flexion control (Perlstein joint). Developed by Meyer Aaron Perlstein (1902–1969), Chicago pediatrician.

• **pivot ambulating crutchless orthosis (PACO).** A standing device for the paraplegic, sturdy and high enough to hold the person without crutches, and which allows some progression by a pivoting motion of the body (see **pivot gait**, under **gait**).

• **pneumatic orthosis.** A garment-like support of synthetic fabric incorporating tubes that, when inflated, give support to the lower limbs of a paraplegic patient for standing and walking with crutches. Developed in 1965, originally for a child with osteogenesis imperfecta, by G. Morel in Berck-Plage, France, and introduced in USA in 1975.

• **powered orthosis.** An orthosis activated by an external source of energy, e.g., a motor or an artificial (carbon-dioxide-powered) muscle.

• **Scott-Craig orthosis.** A hip-stabilizing knee-ankle-foot orthosis with posteriorly offset knee joint and adjustable solid ankle joint. Used in pairs, it is designed to allow a person with paraplegia to balance in the standing position without support from the upper limbs, by leaning into it. Developed in the 1960s by orthotist Bruce A. Scott and Coworkers at Craig Hospital, Englewood, Colorado.

• **shoe-clasp ankle-foot orthosis.** An orthosis comprising a calf-band and a posterior upright that ends in a clasp (q.v.) attached to the posterior part of a low shoe. Thus the heel of the shoe is kept down and the toebox up, which counteracts an existing footdrop.

• **SKAO or SKA orthosis.** Abbreviations for supracondylar knee-ankle orthosis. A knee-ankle orthosis with plastic extension taking hold above the femoral condyles.

• **spiral ankle-foot orthosis.** A plastic orthosis winding in a spiral curve from just below the knee around the leg to the heel and fitting inside the shoe and under the arch. Used most often to counteract footdrop. Developed in 1968 at the Institute for Rehabilitation Medicine, New York University, New York. See also **leaf footdrop splint**, under **splint**.

• **standing orthosis.** A support holding a patient, usually a child, in the upright position. It holds the feet, lower limbs, pelvis, and, if necessary, part of the trunk in a fixed position by means of a footplate, uprights, and interconnected parts. Thus, the hands of a subject with paraplegia are free for various activities, in some cases even for the use of crutches.

• **static orthosis.** An orthosis in which, once it is in place, no part moves. Its main purpose is to support and maintain one or more segments in a determined position for rest or protection. Called also passive orthosis.

• **tenodesis orthosis.** See **flexor tenodesis orthosis**.

• **thoracic suspension orthosis.** A corset-like plastic thoracic orthosis attached by hooks to the uprights of the wheelchair back so that the patient is suspended above the seat. Thus the weight of the pelvis and lower part of the trunk acts as a corrective distracting force in cases of deviations of the vertebral column.

• **thoracolumbosacral orthosis.** Support of trunk, reaching from the level of the lower angles of the scapulae or higher to the midlevel of the pelvis.

• **Toronto standing orthosis or brace.** Supportive device, usually for the child unable to stand. It consists of two or more vertical supports, three or four horizontal straps attached to them, as well as special supports for the shoes. Probably the first of a series of standing orthoses, it was developed in the 1960s at the Ontario Crippled Children's Centre in Toronto, Canada. Cf. also **standing orthosis, vertical loading orthosis, orthopodium**, and **parapodium**.

• **Verlo or vertical loading orthosis.** A standing frame for children, consisting of a baseplate with shoe guides, two uprights with double-channel ankle joints, back panel, and several straps. By a swing-to gait between parallel bars or with a walkerette, or by pivoting from one side to the other, the child may even achieve some locomotion. Developed by Neal Taylor in 1972.

orthostatic hypotension An inability to tolerate the upright position, resulting in nausea, lightheadedness, and even syncope.

orthotherapy A program of physical fitness comprising a variety of exercises. Published in 1971 by New York orthopedic surgeon Arthur A. Michele (1911–1973).

orthotic Adjective referring to orthosis.

orthotics The field, knowledge, art, and making of orthoses.

orthotist A person who constructs orthoses. Formerly named brace maker. Term coined in 1956 by Robert L. Bennett, Warm Springs, Georgia, physiatrist.

oscillometer Instrument for measuring the amplitude of arterial pulsations as they are transmitted through a pneumatic cuff encircling a limb.

oscillometric index (plural, indices) Amplitude of arterial pulsations, as determined by an oscillometer.

oscillometrics, oscillometry Measurement of the amplitude of arterial pulsations by an oscillometer.

oscilloscope Instrument that displays the shape of the waves of an electric current on the screen of a cathode ray tube.

ossification The replacement of cartilage by bone.

ossify To change into bone.

ostealgia Pain in a bone.

osteotomy Cutting of a bone, usually with a saw or chisel.

otologist A physician who is a specialist in otology, i.e., the field dealing with the ear, its function, and its pathology.

overflow Spreading of a stimulus, be it voluntary, reflex, or electric, to other muscles or nerves. In electrodiagnosis, the extension of the flow of current to excite neighboring muscles.

overhead ambulation trolley A trolley running in a ceiling rail, from which a harness is suspended to hold a person during ambulation. See also **suspension walker**, second definition, under **walker**.

overhead pulleys Pulleys attached above the head of the patient, used to stretch the cervical spine or other structures; to raise a limb for greater mobility; or to lower a limb against the resistance of another limb.

Oxford classification Grading in manual muscle testing, that ranges from 0 (no contraction) to 5 (normal).

Oxford (oxford) shoe See under **shoe**.

Oxford technique of progressive resistance exercises See **regressive resistance exercises**, under **exercise**.

P

P In muscle testing: Poor (q.v.).

Pa Symbol for pascal.

PACE An acronym, Promoting Aphasic's Communicative Effectiveness, for a therapeutic approach to the treatment of persons with aphasia.

PACE II: physical function Developed by the US Department of Health, Education, and Welfare in 1978, this measure allows assessment of activities of daily living.

pace A step in walking or running. In ancient Rome, a pace was a double step (now correctly called a stride), and the term **milia passuum** (1,000 paces) is the source of the term "mile" (ca. 1,600 m). The United States Army regulation pace is 75 cm long; the fast pace, called double time, is 90 cm long.

pack Towel, blanket, sheet, or other material, either dry or wet (water, mud, peat, fango, etc.), cold or hot. It is applied to the entire body (full pack) or part of it (partial or local pack). Also called compress.

PACO Acronym for pivot ambulating crutchless orthosis (see under **orthosis**).

pad

• **butterfly pad.** A gluteal pad attached to a pelvic band. See under **butterfly**.

• **dancer pad.** A relatively thick metatarsal pad that reaches across the entire width of the sole.

• **hernia pad.** A cushion incorporated in a hernia truss.

• **kidney pad.** A cushion, usually incorporated in a flexible orthosis, designed to support a kidney, e.g., in nephroptosis.

• **knee pad.** A pad, usually of leather, attached to an orthosis in front of the knee. It restricts the forward displacement of the knee inside the orthosis.

• **metatarsal pad.** A triangular pad with rounded corners and thinned edges, made of soft rubber. It is applied to the sole of the foot or the inside of the shoe behind some or all of the metatarsal heads in order to relieve pain in that area by redistributing weightbearing.

• **navicular pad.** A firm but soft elliptic pad glued to an arch support, or to the insole of a shoe, so as to prevent the navicular bone from dropping. Called also cookie because of its shape.

• **scaphoid pad.** Navicular pad (see preceding entry). The bone to which it refers is no longer called scaphoid.

Paget (or Paget-Gorman) sign language A sign language for the deaf, using signs as in spoken English, without fingerspelling. The signs are based on 21 standard hand positions. Developed in Britain in the 1930s by Sir Richard Paget (1869–1955), a physical scientist, and later revised and expanded by Lady Grace Paget and Dr. Perre Gorman of Australia. The method is also known as systematic sign language.

Paget's disease A bone disease of unknown cause; characterized by localized areas of bone destruction followed by replacement with overdeveloped, light, soft, porous bone and associated with deformities, such as thickening of portions of the skull and bending of weight-bearing bones.

palliative
1. Alleviating.
2. A medicine or treatment that affords temporary relief but does not effect a cure.

palpate To examine by touching or pressing with the fingers or the palms of the hands.

palsy Paralysis.

• **ataxic cerebral palsy.** Cerebral palsy characterized by inability to coordinate voluntary muscular movements.

• **Bell's palsy.** See **facial palsy.**

• **cerebral palsy.** Condition marked by disturbances of voluntary motor function caused by damage to the brain's motor control centers; it is characterized primarily by spastic paralysis or impairment of control or coordination over voluntary muscles; it is often accompanied by mental retardation, seizures, and disorders of vision and communication. It may be either congenital or acquired.

• **dyskinetic cerebral palsy.** Cerebral palsy characterized by inability to coordinate voluntary muscular movements.

• **facial palsy, Bell's palsy.** Paralysis of the facial muscles on one side caused by a usually self-limited lesion of the facial nerve.

• **spastic cerebral palsy.** Cerebral palsy characterized by increased muscle tension and exaggerated reflex activity in an arm and a leg of the same side (hemiplegia) or arms and legs on both sides (tetraplegia or quadriplegia).

pancake coil A diathermy cable wound in two or three concentric circles. It may be enclosed in a container.

papaverine A nonnarcotic alkaloid of opium that has vasodilator properties; used to assist impotent males in achieving erections.

parafango A mixture of paraffin and fango, a volcanic mud. Particularly used for such mixture is the fango from Battaglia, an Italian spa. Used for packs like other types of peloids (q.v.).

paraffin The substance used for a paraffin bath (see under **bath**) is a mixture of cake paraffin and mineral oil. Its melting point is between 51° and 57°C. Also called wax (British term).

paraffin bath See under **bath**.

parallel bars See under **bar, bars**.

Paralympics Name formed by the contraction of "Paraplegics' Olympics." An international sports contest founded in 1952 as an outgrowth of the Stoke Mandeville Games (q.v.). Originally an annual event, it has been held every four years since 1960 in conjunction with the regular Olympic Games. In addition to wheelchair athletes, persons who are blind and those who have amputations have been admitted as contestants since 1976.

paralysis

1. Loss of voluntary muscular function.
2. Loss of sensation.
3. Loss of any organic function.

• **acute ascending paralysis.** Paralysis, often fatal, beginning in the lower extremities and ascending rapidly to involve the trunk, arms, and neck.

• **ascending paralysis.** Paralysis progressing from the periphery to the nerve centers, or from the lower limbs upward.

• **Brown-Sequard's paralysis.** Paralysis of the lower extremities occurring in certain disorders of the urinary tract.

• **Duchenne's paralysis.** Childhood muscular dystrophy.

• **familial periodic paralysis.** Periodic paralysis.

• **global paralysis.** Paralysis affecting both sides of the body completely.

• **paralysis agitans.** Parkinson's disease, a disorder characterized, in its fully developed form, by stiffness and slowness of voluntary movement, stooped posture, propulsive gait, rigidity of facial expression, and rhythmic tremor of the limbs; usually has an insidious onset in individuals between 50 and 65 years old.

• **periodic paralysis.** Recurrent abrupt episodes of paralysis of extreme muscular weakness, lasting from a few minutes to a few days, occurring in otherwise healthy individuals.

• **Todd's paralysis.** Temporary paralysis sometimes occurring after a grand mal epileptic convulsion and usually lasting from several minutes to hours after the seizure.

paralytic
1. Relating to paralysis.
2. A person afflicted with paralysis.

Paralyzed Veterans of America An association of veterans who have incurred an injury or disease affecting the spinal cord and causing paralysis. Founded in 1947.

paraplegia Paralysis of the lower extremities and all or a portion of the trunk.

parapodium A standing frame mounted on a small podium, designed to support a paraplegic subject, usually a child. Securely attached, the user may be able to progress either with crutches or by pivoting the whole body together with the device, turning alternately to the left and right, using the trunk and upper limbs. Developed in 1970 at the Ontario Crippled Children's Centre in Toronto.

parathesia An abnormal sensation, such as burning, tingling, or numbness.

Parcours Jogging trail, about 1 to 2 km long, leading through scenic areas, punctuated with logs, chinning bars, and other gymnastic equipment; instructional signs inform how to use these, what exercises to do, and how often. Such health paths were first designed and built in 1971 under the name of Vita Parcours by the Vita Life Insurance Company of Zurich to encourage people to get out-of-doors and exercise. From Switzerland, similar health tracks spread to other European countries. The term is French for route, run, itinerary. Peter C. Stocker, a San Francisco real-estate broker, introduced the concept to the USA in 1973 under the name Parcourse. See also **circuit training** (first definition) and **terrain cure**.

parkinsonian Relating to paralysis agitans.

parkinsonism A group of nervous disorders marked by muscular rigidity, tremors, lack of facial expression, akinesia, and postural abnormalities.

paroxysm

1. A sudden onset or recurrence of symptoms of a disease.
2. A convulsion.

pascal (Pa) A unit of pressure. It is equal to the newton per square meter (1 Pa = 1 N/m^2). Named after the French mathematician and philosopher Blaise Pascal (1623–1662).

patellar-tendon-bearing (PTB) Refers to a prosthesis or orthosis in which there is close contact with the patellar tendon (correctly, patellar ligament), so that a large amount of weight is borne on it.

Patient Appraisal and Care Evaluation (PACE) An assessment system designed to assist in managing individual patients, administering long-term care within an institution and within the community, policymaking, epidemiologic research, and evaluation.

patient lifter See **lift, lifter**.

pattern, motor pattern A complex motion, usually of an entire limb or more than a limb, that occurs purposefully or reflexly. See **proprioceptive neuromuscular facilitation**, under **facilitation**.

patterning therapy See **Doman-Delacato patterning therapy**.

PaVaEx Proprietary name of a negative-pressure boot for passive vascular (or veno-arterial) exercise in peripheral vascular disease.

PB list List of phonetically balanced (pb), i.e., monosyllabic, words that include all the common speech sounds of the English language. Examples: does, off, cap, me, else, too, bind. Used in hearing tests to assess a subject's degree of word discrimination.

peat A partially decomposed and carbonized vegetable matter found in wet spongy ground. It may be used for packs and baths.

pediluvium Footbath. From the Latin.

pedobarograph Apparatus for displaying and recording the distribution of pressure under the soles of the feet while standing or walking on a transparent plate. Developed in 1978 by Joseph D. Chodera, physician, and Marilyn Lord, engineer, in Roehampton, England.

pedograph

1. A footprint or imprint of the plant of the foot, usually on paper.
2. A device using inked paper for taking such footprints.
3. An instrument for analysis of gaits.

Pedo-Graph A device for taking footprints (see preceding entry, second definition), invented ca. 1917 by William M. Scholl (1882–1968), Chicago physician, podiatrist, and founder of a manufactory of footcare products bearing his name.

pedorthics The field of prescription footwear. A certified pedorthist (C Ped) is a shoefitter certified by the American Board for Certification in Pedorthics (established in 1975) and qualified to fill a physician's shoe prescription.

peg leg Pylon.

peloid Collective name for mud, peat, and fango. From the Greek *pelos*, mud.

pelotherapy Treatment by the use of a mud, peat, or fango bath or pack. See preceding entry.

pelvic band, belt See under **band** and **belt**.

pelvic roll Motion of the pelvis around its transverse axis. The additional direction of "anterior" or "posterior" refers to the cranial (upper) part of the pelvis. Thus, an anterior pelvic roll increases lordosis, a posterior roll flattens the lumbar spine or, if flat, makes it convex. Often called "pelvic tilt" (see next entry).

pelvic tilt Motion of the pelvis around its sagittal axis. The term is also used, less correctly, for pelvic roll (see preceding entry).

penile implant, penile prosthesis See under **prosthesis**.

percussion A maneuver of massage, also known as tapotement (q.v.).

percussor A device that delivers low-frequency vibrations. It is usually applied to the chest wall to mobilize bronchial mucus before or during postural drainage.

perineometer A pneumatic dynamometer. Inserted in the vaginal cavity, it measures the force of muscular contraction and the effectiveness of Kegel exercise (see under **exercise**).

period Referring to alternating current, the duration of one cycle.

peripatologist A mobility instructor for the blind. From the Greek *peripatein*, to walk about.

peripatology Orientation and mobility of the blind. See preceding entry.

PERLA Acronym for pupils equal and reactive to light and accommodation.

Perlstein brace, joint, orthosis See under **orthosis**.

perseveration A repetitive and involuntary motor or verbal response that possibly was appropriate to a first stimulus but continues to be repeated even after the first stimulus has been removed and other new stimuli or instructions have been introduced.

petrissage French for kneading. A maneuver of massage. It has many variants: pressing, squeezing, rolling, wringing, etc. Also known as kneading.

phantom sensation The phenomenon associated with the presence of perceived sensation in an absent or anesthetic limb, which is most commonly seen following amputation but may be present following any neurologic damage resulting in complete anesthesia.

Phelps method of exercise A method of treating patients with lesions of the central nervous system, particularly children with cerebral palsy. It combines a great variety of exercises with massage, manipulation, and occupational therapy. Usually starting with massage and passive motions, the therapist guides the child to progressively more active participation through active-assisted to active and resisted motions. Reflexes are utilized in automatic or confused motions and songs to condition the child for voluntary motions (see **conditioned exercise**, under **exercise**). Orthoses preventing undesired postures and motions are gradually reduced as control is gained. Developed in the 1940s by Winthrop Morgan Phelps (1894–1971), Boston and Baltimore orthopedic surgeon, who coined the term cerebral palsy.

Philadelphia Jewish Employment and Vocational Services Work Sample Battery (JEVS) A work evaluation system designed to assess work habits, readiness for employment, and tolerance for work.

phocomelia From the Greek *phokē*, seal, and *"Melos,"* limb. Congenital absence of part of a limb.

phon Unit used to express the subjective loudness of a sound.

phoniatrics The branch of medicine concerned with vocal disorders. Speech pathology and therapy.

phonophoresis Introduction of medication through the skin by ultrasonic energy.

phot-, photo- Referring to light.

photarium Room for the administration of preventive ultraviolet radiation.

photochemotherapy A combination of photo- (i.e., light-) and chemo- (i.e., drug-) therapies. It usually refers to the treatment of psoriasis by photoactive psoralen and ultraviolet irradiation, also known as puva (q.v.).

photodermatosis, photodermia Generic terms for skin lesions due to exposure to light.

photomotograph A photoelectric measuring device of the amplitude of a motion.

photosensitivity Exaggerated sensitivity to light.

photosensitization Sensitization to light.

phototherapy Literally: treatment by light; refers usually to ultraviolet, occasionally to infrared radiations.

physiatrics The branch of medicine concerned with diagnosis and treatment of disease of the neuromusculoskeletal systems with physical elements (heat, cold, water, electricity, etc.) to bring about maximal restoration of physical, physiological, social, and vocational function; also called physical medicine or rehabilitation.

physiatrist A physician who specializes in physiatrics.

physiatrist (preferred pronunciation: fee-zee-at-rist) From the Greek *physis*, nature, and *iater* or *iatros*, physician. A physician who specializes in physical medicine and rehabilitation.

physiatry (preferred pronunciation: fee-zee-at-ree) Physiatrics.

physical agent See **physical therapy**.

physical conditioning As applied to patients who are deconditioned because of disease, injury, surgery, or other reasons, it consists of a slowly progressive program of simple calisthenics, breathing exercises, walking, or the use of simple apparatus such as a stationary bicycle, depending upon the weakness and tolerance of the individual.

physical education See **adapted physical education, corrective therapy, gymnastics**, and **remedial physical education**.

physical medicine or physical medicine and rehabilitation The branch of medicine that has developed from the preponderant use of electrotherapy and other physical agents. The first residency of this medical specialty was established in 1936 by Frank H. Krusen (1898–1973) at the Mayo Graduate School of Medicine of the University of Minnesota. Since 1947, specialists have been certified by the American Board of Physical Medicine (and Rehabilitation, since 1949). In the United Kingdom, an important step in the establishment of the specialty was the fusion in 1931 of the Section of Electrotherapeutics of the Royal Society of Medicine with the Section of Balneology and Climatology, to form the Section of Physical Medicine. The specialty includes physical, occupational, and other restorative therapies as well as the services of other medical and paramedical disciplines for the sake of the patient's best possible rehabilitation. Hence the increasing frequency of its synonym, rehabilitation medicine (q.v.).

physical therapist A person trained to administer physical therapy and to educate patients in the appropriate way of using their bodies from the medical point of view.

• **qualified (or registered) physical therapist.** In the USA, a person who is a graduate of a program in physical therapy approved by the Council on Medical Education of the American Medical Association or who has the equivalent of such education and training, and who is licensed or registered in one of the states.

Physical Therapy The official journal of the American Physical Therapy Association. Founded in 1921 as *The Physical Therapy Review*.

physical therapy (PT) Treatment by physical agents and physical methods. Examples are heat, cold, water, electric current, ultraviolet rays, exercise, traction, massage, manipulation, mechanical devices. The four primordial elements that the ancient Greeks considered to be the constituents of all matter were also the four basic physical agents they recognized in therapeutics: fire, air, water, earth.

• **active physical therapy.** Activities performed by the patient under the direction of a physical therapist, such as exercises of various types, gait training, and wheelchair practice.

• **chest physical therapy.** Physical therapy used in pulmonary emphysema and other conditions of respiratory insufficiency; in the preparation for surgical interventions, notably of the thorax, as well as after surgery. It embraces breathing education or reeducation (including segmental breathing), relaxation, massage (notably vibration and tapotement), postural drainage, and progressive exercises to increase pulmonary tolerance.

• **passive physical therapy.** The administration of physical agents such as heat, water, massage, passive motion, which the patient receives without active participation.

physical therapy assistant A skilled technical health worker who has completed an educational program that leads to this title and is approved by the American Physical Therapy Association.

physiotherapist, physiotherapy British terms for physical therapist and physical therapy.

picture board See **communication board**, under **board**.

pilot dog See **guide dog**. The term is correctly used only for dogs trained by Pilot Dogs, Inc., a school for guide dogs in Columbus, Ohio.

pinch gauge, pinch meter An instrument to measure the strength of finger pinch. A finger dynamometer.

pivot walk or walking See **pivot gait**, under **gait**.

plastic massage See under **massage**.

plastic tone See **tonic perseveration**.

play therapy Educational activities of elementary level by means of simple objects, usually applied to severely retarded individuals—children or adults.

plethysmogram Recording made by a plethysmograph. From the Greek *plethysmos*, enlargement.

plethysmograph Instrument for recording changes in the volume of a digit, a limb, or another body part.

plethysmography The recording of volume changes in parts of the body or the whole body, as achieved by a plethysmograph. See preceding two entries.

plint, plinth A padded table for examination, massage, and other therapies.

• **Lowman plinth.** A stainless steel support attached below the water surface of a therapeutic pool, for exercise. It is rather narrow and tapers in width to allow free movements of the lower limbs in the prone position. Developed by Los Angeles orthopedic surgeon Charles Leroy Lowman (1879–1977).

PLISSIT model A conceptual scheme frequently employed in sex counseling and therapy for persons with disabilities. Acronym stands for permission, limited information, specific suggestions, intensive therapy.

plumb line A string suspending a small heavy object, the plumb bob (like any ordinary plumb line). Used in postural examination.

ply As referring to socks for amputee stumps, one of the twisted strands in the yarn from which the sock is woven. Stump socks are made from 1-ply to 6-ply yarn, usually cotton or wool, and most frequently from 3-ply or 5-ply yarn. As a new stump shrinks with appropriate use of a prosthesis, the thickness of the sock must increase by changing from a 3-ply to a 5-ply sock; later, one or more socks are added. The maximum of plies for an above-knee stump is usually 15.

pneumatic boot, sleeve Boot or sleeve of various lengths, rhythmically inflated for compression of the limb in order to decrease swelling. The boot is also used for the prevention of postoperative thrombophlebitis.

pneumatic muscle See **artificial muscle**, first definition.

pneumatotherapy Treatment by rarefied or by condensed air.

pneumobelt A beltlike device, worn around the waist, that applies intermittent abdominal pressure, replacing the function of the diaphragm in respiratory paralysis or insufficiency.

podiascope A device to examine the weightbearing parts of the feet in standing. It consists of a boxlike metal frame with a thick plate glass platform on top and an inclined mirror below it. The subject stands on the glass, and the soles of the feet are seen in the mirror.

podiatrist A specialist in podiatry (see next entry). Formerly and in some countries still called chiropodist.

podiatry The field of the study and care of the foot, including diagnosis, medical, and certain types of surgical treatment. Formerly and in some other countries still called chiropody.

Pohl, method of System of locomotor habilitation, notably of children with cerebral palsy, based on three principles: conscious relaxation and awareness of muscle tone; movements that progress from passive to active; and global utilitarian movements such as rolling from side to side, crawling, sitting up, standing up, walking, climbing, falling. Developed in 1950 by Minneapolis orthopedic surgeon John F. Pohl (1903–1981).

poker back, poker spine See under **back**.

polecat A vertical grab bar, fixed both to the floor and to the ceiling, that gives support to a person when getting up from bed, chair, etc. A common type consists of a telescoping column, about 4 cm in diameter.

polygraph An instrument that records simultaneously two or more functions, such as respiratory chest expansion, cardiac frequency, blood pressure, electric skin resistance, etc.

polyphasic potential A motor unit potential, detected by electromyography, characterized by an increased number of wave peaks and a rough sound.

pool

- **Hubbard pool.** Hubbard tank. See under **tank**.

- **therapeutic pool.** Pool large enough for one or more patients together with one or more therapists. The depth is usually appropriate for a standing person.

Poor A grade in manual muscle testing, applied to a muscle or muscle group that cannot move the corresponding segment against gravity. When gravity is negligible ("gravity eliminated"), the segment can be moved actively through its full range. Grade between Trace and Fair.

Porch Index of Communicative Ability A standardized test commonly used by speech/language pathologists to evaluate language disturbance by measuring communicative behavior in the gestural, verbal, and graphic output modalities.

Porteus Mazes A test used to assess judgement, planning and foresight.

position See also **posture**.

• **Adam position.** A position in which the subject stands with the back to the examiner, the trunk moderately flexed, knees straight, head and upper limbs hanging relaxed. Used to detect thoracic asymmetry and slight lateral deviations of the vertebral column. Origin of term obscure.

• **anatomic position.** Position of the erect standing body, toes pointing forward, upper limbs by the sides, forearms supinated. This latter fact is the most characteristic difference from the neutral position. Cf. **neutral position**.

• **crouch, crouching position.** Position of stooping or low bending of the trunk and flexion of the hips, the feet being on the ground. While there are variations, notably as far as the limbs are concerned, the knees are not completely flexed as they are in squatting.

• **Fowler position.** The position of a subject who, from lying on his back, has raised his trunk to an angle of 45° and flexed his thighs similarly, without raising his feet. Named after George Ryerson Fowler (1848–1906), New York surgeon.

• **frog position.** A position seen in the newborn. The child lies prone, thighs in external rotation and abducted to about 90°, knees also at right angles. Known also as spread-eagle position.

• **genucubital position.** Knee-elbow position.

• **genupectoral position.** Knee-chest position.

• **hand-knee position.** Position on hands and knees, whereby the legs and feet usually also touch the ground.

• **hooklying position.** Supine position with hips and knees bent, soles flat on the same level as the trunk. From this position the entire body may also turn 90° to the side, i.e., to the hooklying position on the left or right. Term mostly used in the uk.

• **knee-chest position.** Position on chest, head, upper limbs, knees, and legs, the buttocks being the most elevated part.

• **knee-elbow position.** Position on elbows and knees, whereby the legs and feet usually also touch the ground.

• **long-sitting position.** Sitting position with lower limbs straight and supported on the same level as the buttocks.

• **neutral position.** Position of the erect body with bare feet, upper limbs by the sides, longitudinal axes of all four limbs parallel and in the same plane, toes, thumbs and radial border of the forearms directed forward. This position is assumed as the recommended point of departure in range-of-motion and other tests and is therefore also called zero position or neutral-zero position. Cf. **anatomic position**.

• **prone position.** Horizontal position of the body, abdomen and face down.

• **quadruped position (pronounce KWOD-roo-ped).** Position on hand and feet, or hands and knees, or comparable position.

• **recumbent position.** Lying on a horizontal surface.

• **semiprone position.** Position in which one side of the body is strictly prone, while the head is turned to the other side and the limbs of that same side are slightly curled up, flexed at the shoulder, elbow, hip, and knee.

• **squatting position.** Position with feet flat on the ground, knees and hips in complete flexion.

• **supine position.** Horizontal position of the body, abdomen and face up.

• **Thomas position.**

1. Lying supine, one lower limb in complete extension, the other flexed in hip and knee, the thigh pressed against the trunk. This is the position used in the Thomas test (see under **test**) and for stretching tight hip flexors.
2. Lying supine, both lower limbs flexed with hips and knees at right angles, the legs resting on a stool or other support. This is a position used for relaxation (notably of the lower back) and for pelvic traction.

• **tripod position.**

1. Sitting position in bed, in which the trunk is supported by the hands placed in a plane posterior to the pelvis. Seen in abdominal weakness or meningeal irritation.
2. Sitting position with hands placed anterior to the frontal plane. Seen in respiratory insufficiency.

• **tuck position.** Kneeling with feet in plantar flexion, buttocks on heels, trunk completely flexed, and head close to knees. While maintaining this position, the subject may also turn to the side.

• **zero position.** The starting position, be it real or assumed, for range-of-motion and other tests, in which every joint is considered at point zero. The zero position most generally accepted is the one described under neutral position.

positioning The placing of a patient—in bed, on a chair, or elsewhere—in a position that corrects faults and minimizes the dangers of faulty posture, such as contractures, compression, impairment of breathing or circulation, etc.

positive end-expiratory pressure (PEEP) A technique of respiratory assistance administered with a mechanical device, in which at the end of expiration the airway pressure remains positive, never reaching the zero or atmospheric level.

positive sharp wave An abnormal potential, detected by electromyography, occurring at rest in denervated muscle, assumed to have the same significance as a fibrillation potential.

positivity bias The tendency of individuals to evaluate persons with disabilities with more lenient criteria than typically extended to others and to subsequently behave in a manner that appears to convey positive, accepting, and favorable opinions of persons with disabilities.

POSM, POSSUM Abbreviations for patient-operated selector mechanism (*possum* also being the Latin for "I can"). A system that enables quadriplegics to operate various devices with a minimum of energy such as light touch, sipping air, or blowing (cf. *sip-and-puff control*). Developed in the 1960s at the Polio Research Foundation, Stoke Mandeville Hospital, Aylesbury, England.

postexertional Adjective meaning: after physical exercise.

postural drainage Positioning of a patient so as to favor drainage of the tracheobronchial tree, bringing its secretions, pus, etc. close to the mouth to facilitate their elimination by expectoration or suction. Often combined with vibration or other procedures to loosen the secretions.

posture See also **position**.

• **dynamic posture.** Posture in action or in preparation for action; a posture that does not exclude mobility (as opposed to static posture). Posture of activity.

• **Meyer posture.** Normal posture of upright subject with fully extended hip and knee joints, as described in 1853 by Zurich anatomist Georg Hermann von Meyer (1815–1892).

• **static posture.** Posture of relative immobility. It can apply to lying, sitting, standing. Posture of inactivity (as opposed to dynamic posture).

posture chart A sheet of graph paper for the recording of body contours, notably of a subject's postural asymmetries or deviations from the normal. The recording may be made after examination of the subject behind a posture grid (see next entry).

posture grid An upright glass or plastic panel, about 2 m in height, 1 m in width, with vertical and horizontal lines at intervals of between 2 and 10 cm. Used to evaluate posture by inspecting the subject standing behind the grid. In combination with a posture mirror, notably a triple mirror, it can be used for self-examination and education of posture. See also next entry.

posture mirror An upright mirror, sometimes consisting of two or three hinged panels, used for posture training, sometimes in combination with a posture grid. There are posture mirrors marked like posture grids (see preceding entry).

posture panel Board attached to a chair or wheelchair, to give posterior or lateral support to the trunk. For lateral support a pair of panels is needed.

potentiometer An instrument for measuring voltage.

poultice After the Latin for pap, referring to any of various soft, moist masses spread on the skin for heating or counterirritation. Also called cataplasm.

prehension The precision grip resulting between the thumb, index, and middle fingers.

prelingual deafness Loss of hearing before the learning of language. It includes deafness at birth.

preorthotic education or training A program of motor education or reeducation in preparation for the use of an orthosis.

preprosthetic education or training A program of motor education or reeducation in preparation for the use of a prosthesis. It may include psychologic preparation.

press, pressing See under **bench press**.

press-up British term for push-up.

prevocational training The physical and psychologic preparation of an individual to a more-or-less specific work situation, after assessment of the potentials and inclination to work in general and to the respective activities in particular. It may be followed by enrollment in a course or school.

Priessnitz method of treatment A therapeutic system consisting mainly in the external use of cold water as baths, showers, affusions, and packs; the latter became known as Priessnitz compresses. Fresh air, exercise, work (e.g., sawing wood), and diet were other agents used in specialized institutions encountered particularly in Germany and Austria. Developed by Silesian peasant Vinzenz Priessnitz (1799–1851). Certain forms of his system were later adopted by Kneipp (q.v.).

prism glasses A pair of spectacles with prisms instead of lenses, which enable a person in the supine position to read printed material held upright on the chest.

procedural terminology Procedures and services performed by a physician (or in some instances, by a therapist) are listed in **Physicians' Current Procedural Terminology** (CPT) of the American Medical Association and identified with five-digit codes. Neuromuscular procedures, including manual muscle tests, range-of-motion measurements, elecromyography, and nerve conduction studies, are coded between 95831 and 95999. Section number 96900 is assigned to ultraviolet radiation, listed under dermatologic procedures. Section numbers 97000 to 97799 are given to all other physical medicine services and procedures.

Prod Acronym for prevention of deformity. See **PROD splint**, under **splint**.

pronation The act of lying face downward or of rotating the forearms so that the palm of the hand is turned backward or downward.

prontor-supinator A handle, usually mounted on the wall, that is turned for pronation and supination exercises. It is usually combined with a device providing adjustable resistance.

prone See **prone position**, under **position**.

prone board, prone stander See **prone board**, under **board**.

prone scooter A low board on rollers allowing easy moving in any direction. The patient, usually a child, lies prone on it, hands against the floor for self-propulsion. The lower limbs are usually also supported by the board, notably when they are in a cast, as, e.g., in congenital dislocation of the hips. Called also scooting board, crawler, crawl board, and turtle board.

proprioception The sensation of position and change of position of the body and its parts. It is transmitted through special organs, mostly in muscles, tendons, and joints.

proprioceptive Refers to proprioception. For proprioceptive neuromuscular facilitation, see under **facilitation**.

propulsion See under **gait**.

prosthesiology The subject of prosthesis; prosthetics.

prosthesis (plural prostheses) From the Greek, freely translated as "placed instead." Artificial part of the body: tooth, eye, joint, digit, limb, breast, etc.

• **adjustable prosthesis.** A temporary prosthesis for either above-knee or below-knee amputation, in which the parts between the socket and the foot are made of metal and allow adjustments in all dimensions and directions including rotation. Once the optimal adjustments have been achieved during a sufficiently long period of trial and training, the prosthesis is placed in an alignment duplication jig for the replacement of the adjusted temporary segment by the permanent one.

• **Beaufort prosthesis.** A jointed prosthesis constructed from leather and wooden splints for either the upper or lower limb. Introduced in 1867 by the Comte de Beaufort.

• **bent-knee prosthesis.** Prosthesis for a very short below-knee stump. It is fitted with the knee in slight flexion, and most of the weight is borne on the tibial tuberosity.

• **Canadian hip prosthesis.** Prosthesis for hip disarticulation, above-knee amputation with very short stump, or hindquarter amputation (hemipelvectomy). Its hip joint is far anteriorly to the position of the anatomic joint. Named for the Department of Veterans Affairs of Canada, where it was originally devised in 1954.

• **conventional below-knee prosthesis.** Prosthesis that includes a thigh corset attached to the leg piece by hinge joints.

• **crustacean prosthesis.** So called in order to specify that its shell provides solid support. Also called exoskeletal prosthesis (q.v.).

• **early postsurgical prosthesis.** A prosthesis for the lower limb, similar to an immediate postsurgical prosthesis, except that walking is initiated between 10 and 30 days after the amputation.

• **electronic prosthesis.** A prosthesis, almost always for the upper limb, that operates electronically. See **myoelectric prosthesis**.

• **endoprosthesis.** An artificial internal body part, which is implanted surgically. Examples: knee joint, vascular segment. Also called internal prosthesis.

• **endoskeletal prosthesis.** A limb prosthesis whose supporting structure (which may be articulated) is inside, as is the case in a human limb. In order to match the appearance of the normal limb, the endoskeleton is covered with an outside ("cosmetic") cover that does not need to be as rigid as in an exoskeletal prosthesis (see next entry).

• **exoskeletal prosthesis.** A limb prosthesis of the usual structure, in which the material that reproduces the shape of the normal limb serves at the same time as support. So called in order to differentiate it from an endoskeletal prosthesis (see preceding entry).

• **extension prosthesis.** Prosthesis that equalizes a limb deficient in its length as compared with its counterpart. It may also support abnormal joints such as found in congenital deformities.

• **external limb prosthesis.** An artificial replacement of a limb or part of a limb. So called to exclude prostheses of other parts of the body (tooth, eye, breast) as well as inner parts of a limb (bone, joint).

• **fluid-controlled prosthesis.** Prosthesis with hydraulic control. Most frequently it is a prosthesis with a hydraulic knee.

• **Heidelberg prosthesis.** See under **arm**.

• **Hydra-Cadence prosthesis.** Proprietary name of an above-knee prosthesis with a hydraulic unit that controls the swing of the lower limb and coordinates knee and ankle motion.

• **immediate postsurgical prosthesis.** A prosthesis for the lower limb, the socket of which is applied to the stump immediately after the amputation or within the next few days. It has an alignment device for easy attachment and removal, and a rigid support (usually of tubular metal) that ends in a foot-ankle assembly. The immediate use of the prosthesis with weightbearing and walking is believed to decrease edema and pain, helping in the patient's rehabilitation.

• **interim prosthesis.** See **temporary prosthesis**.

• **internal prosthesis.** An artificial internal body part that is implanted surgically. Examples: femoral head, interphalangeal joint, cardiac valve. Also called endoprosthesis.

• **KBM prosthesis.** The abbreviation stands for the German Kondylen Bettung Münster, meaning "nestling of condyles, Münster," which refers to the city where the prosthesis was developed by the orthopedic surgeon Götz Gerd Kuhn, about 1960. In the USA, this below-knee prosthesis is usually called supracondylar tibial prosthesis (q.v.).

• **kneeling-knee prosthesis.** See **bent-knee prothesis**.

• **modular prosthesis, modular assembly prosthesis.** A prosthesis in which modules, i.e., commercially available, standardized, and interchangeable components, are used. These can be assembled and disassembled quickly and easily, for immediate postsurgical fitting for instance.

• **muley prosthesis or leg.** Below-knee prosthesis of older type, attached to the thigh by a leather cuff just above the condyles, with two expansions fixed medially and laterally to the brim of the socket. Whether the term muley is corruption of a German proper name (Mühle) or designates a hairless or hornless animal, most often a hornless cow, the reference to the prosthesis is obscure.

• **Munster prosthesis.** Prosthesis for a very short below-elbow amputation stump with an intimately fitted suction socket extending above the condyles of the humerus. It eliminates the need for a harness or an intermediary slip socket. Developed in 1954 by Oscar Hepp, and Götz Gerd Kuhn, orthopedic surgeons in Münster, Germany.

• **myoelectric prosthesis.** Prosthesis that uses the electric potentials generated by the contraction of intact muscles to move some of the parts of the prosthesis. Electrodes and microtransmitters carry impulses that are amplified by an electronic device. The use of myopotentials in a prosthesis was first published in 1948.

• **OHC prosthesis.** Prosthesis with polycentric knee joint for knee disarticulation and long above-knee amputation. Developed at the Orthopedic Hospital, Copenhagen, whence the abbreviation.

• **patellar-tendon-bearing (PTB) prosthesis.** A below-knee prosthesis made for weightbearing on the patellar ligament (patellar tendon). Other areas participate to a smaller extent in the bearing of weight, notably the tibial condyles and the stump end. Only a small leather strap, the knee cuff or suprapatellar suspension strap, reaches above the knee, to hold the prosthesis in place. Developed in 1958 by the Biomechanics Laboratory of the University of California in Berkeley.

• **penile prosthesis.** Contrary to its name, which would imply the replacement of a missing part, this is strictly speaking a penile splint, i.e., an orthosis providing rigidity to the penis. It may also be an inflatable implant.

• **permanent prosthesis.** A prosthesis that after a trial period has been checked and found appropriate for the individual in its components, measurements, alignment, fit, functions, workmanship, and appearance.

• **pneumatic prosthesis.** A prosthesis for the lower limb with an air-filled socket, usually in form of an air sac inserted into a socket. It is used as a temporary prosthesis.

• **preliminary prosthesis.** Adjustable prosthesis.

• **preparatory prosthesis.** See **temporary prosthesis** and **adjustable prosthesis**.

• **PTB prosthesis.** Patellar-tendon-bearing prosthesis.

• **PTB SC/SP prosthesis.** Patellar-tendon-bearing prosthesis with supracondylar and suprapatellar suspension. See **supracondylar/suprapatellar prosthesis**.

• **PTS prosthesis.** Originally the abbreviation for the French *prothèse tibiale à emboiture supracondylienne*, meaning below-knee prosthesis with supracondylar socket, developed in 1960 by Guy Fajal, prosthetist in Nancy, France. It has also come to stand for the English patellar-tendon supracondylar prosthesis. In the USA it is usually known as **supracondylar/suprapatellar prosthesis** (q.v.)

• **pylon prosthesis.** See **pylon**.

• **SC/SP prosthesis.** Supracondylar/suprapatellar prosthesis.

• **Seattle foot prosthesis.** Developed in 1986, this prosthesis was designed to control and store energy that is available at heel strike and foot flat, releasing it during push-off to increase the forward movement of the foot and eliminate "drop-off." Use of this device allows single- or double-foot amputees to run and engage in other sports.

• **self-contained prosthesis.** A prosthesis, essentially for below-elbow amputations, that contains a battery and other components, thus not requiring a harness.

• **simulated arm prosthesis.** Training arm. See under **arm**.

• **skeletal prosthesis.** Endoskeletal prosthesis (q.v.). that has not as yet received its cosmetic cover.

• **step-in prosthesis.** Prosthesis for a phocomelic lower limb that is too short or in another way unfit for walking. Thus, although the limb may include a foot, it is fitted with a prosthesis into which it steps. Hence its name.

• **STP**

• **Supracondylar tibial prosthesis.**

• **supracondylar/suprapatellar (SC/SP) prosthesis.** A variant of the patellar-tendon-bearing prosthesis. Its socket extends in front, medially, and laterally, so as to fully encompass the patella and both femoral condyles, thereby obviating the need for a suspension strap. The higher socket increases knee stability, which is particularly valuable if the knee is unstable or the stump is short.

• **supracondylar tibial prosthesis (STP).** A variant of the patellar-tendon-bearing prosthesis in which the socket, while cut low in front, extends medially and laterally above the femoral condyles.

• **supracondylar wedge-suspension prosthesis.** A variant of the patellar-tendon-bearing supracondylar prosthesis. After the prosthesis is donned, a wedge is inserted above the medial or lateral femoral condyle, or both, ensuring the tightness necessary to keep the prosthesis in place.

• **swimming prosthesis.** A lower-limb prosthesis that can be used for swimming as well as for walking, being impervious to water.

• **swivel walk prosthesis.** Prosthetic device for children with bilateral amputations or severe deficiencies of the lower limbs. It consists of a pelvic socket, two pylons, and two foot pieces, rotating about a vertical axis. The child progresses with a swivel gate (see under **gait**). Developed by the Ontario Crippled Children's Centre in Toronto, Canada, and published in 1966.

• **Syme prosthesis.** Prosthesis for Syme amputation, an amputation of the foot and the two malleoli. This type of amputation was developed by James Syme (1799–1870), Scottish surgeon.

• **temporary prosthesis.** Any of a variety of prostheses of a relatively simple type for the upper or lower limb. It is used in order to assess the physical and psychologic capacities of the amputee for an artificial limb, to help him or her in getting accustomed to one, and to hasten the shrinkage of the stump, before deciding on a permanent prosthesis. Particular types of temporary prostheses are the adjustable prosthesis and the immediate postsurgical prosthesis.

• **tilting table prosthesis.** A prosthesis of the conventional type for hip disarticulation.

• **visual prosthesis.** Artificial eye that conveys visual images, e.g., with the aid of a miniature television camera.

• **voice prosthesis.** A device designed to restore speech after laryngectomy. A type developed in 1979 by otolaryngologist Mark I. Singer and speech pathologist Eric D. Blom in Indianapolis consists of a silicone tube introduced through the tracheostoma into a surgically created tracheoesophageal fistula. Air from the trachea enters the esophagus through a one-way valve that prevents aspiration. This air is used for phonation.

• **wedge suspension prosthesis.** Supracondylar wedge suspension prosthesis.

prosthetic Referring to prosthesis.

prosthetics The field, knowledge, art, and making of prostheses.

prosthetic training Training in the use of a prosthesis.

prosthetist A limb maker or a maker of other prostheses.

psammotherapy Treatment by sandbaths. Also called ammotherapy. From the Greek *psammos* or *ammos*, sand.

psychogalvanic reflex A decrease in the electric resistance of the skin by an emotional reaction to a stimulus which may be physical or psychologic. It is related to an increase in perspiration.

psychogalvanometer An apparatus used to measure the electric resistance on the surface of the skin.

psychogenic Originating in the mind.

psychogogy A word coined by Maslow to mean psychosocial intervention strategies based on an educational model.

psychoprophylaxis A system of physical and psychologic preparation to natural childbirth, also known as the Lamaze method (q.v.).

psychro- Referring to cold, having the same meaning as cryo-.

psychrotherapy Treatment by the application of cold.

puff and sip, puff and suck Expressions referring to exhaling and inhaling in the breath control of a wheelchair or other device operated by a quadriplegic patient. See **breath control**.

pulsating mattress or pad See **alternating-pressure mattress**, under **mattress**.

pulses A scale that measures the ability to perform activities of daily living or physical functioning, wherein "P" refers to a rating of physical condition; "S" refers to a rating of social factors, including emotional and intellectual adaptability, social support from family and financial ability; "U" represents upper limbs, self-care abilities; "L" refers to lower limbs (amputation); and "S" stands for sensory abilities.

Pultibec system A grading system for the medical assessment of the functional capacities of handicapped children. These capacities are placed under 8 main headings whose code letters form the acronym: physical capacity, upper limbs, locomotion, toilet, intelligence, behavior, eyes, communication (hearing and speech). Each quality is graded between 1 (normal) and 6 (without practical function). Published in 1963 by R. L. Lindon, of Middlesex County, England.

pummeling A maneuver of massage, consisting of mild pounding, thumping, or beating with the fist.

punching bag See **striking bag**.

punting The verb to punt refers to the maneuver of propelling, by pushing with a pole, a flat-bottomed boat called a punt. Similarly, punting a rolling chair or stretcher can be done by pushing with one or two canes against the floor.

Purdue pegboard A device used for testing and training in manual dexterity. It consists of a rectangular board, 30 by 45 cm, for the sequential insertion of pegs and the assembly of pegs, collars, and washers. Developed by the Purdue Research Foundation, Purdue University, Lafayette, Indiana, and published in 1941–1948.

pursed-lip breathing Slow and prolonged expiration through the lips pursed as in whistling.

pushchair A chair on wheels or casters that is designed to be pushed by a person other than the user.

push glove, pusher mitt, or mitten A glove, usually without digits (mitt, mitten), of leather, textile, or similar material, for protection of the hand against dirt and friction and for better grip of the handrim of a wheelchair.

push-up Pushing up one's body by the power of the upper limbs; the elbows, flexed at the start, straighten to full extension. The starting position may be sitting in a chair, with the hand on the armrests, or the prone position, the body supported only by the hands and toes.

PUVA Acronym for psoralen plus ultraviolet A. A treatment method, originally used for vitiligo, now particularly for psoriasis. It consists in the oral administration of psoralen and the irradiation by longwave ultraviolet rays type A.

pylon A replacement for an amputated lower limb or part of it, consisting of a socket for the amputation stump, a sturdy wooden or tubular metal support, and at its end a large rubber tip or a foot. It is sometimes used as a temporary prosthesis.

pyretotherapy, pyrotherapy Fever therapy, i.e., therapeutic use of fever.

Q

quadrantanopsia Blindness in approximately a quarter of the visual field; also called quadrantic hemianopsia.

quadriplegia Paralysis of both upper and lower extremities and all of the trunk; also called tetraplegia.

quadruped gait Walking on hands and feet, or hands and knees. Rarely are the forearms used instead of the hands.

quadruped position Position on hands and feet, or hands and knees. Rarely are the forearms used instead of the hands.

quarter The posterior part of the upper of a shoe. The two quarters form the sides posterior to the vamp and cover roughly the posterior half of the foot. Cf. upper and vamp.

qualified handicapped person A term used in the Rehabilitation Act of 1973 and incorporated into the Americans with Disabilities Act of 1990 to describe persons who are qualified to perform a job or benefit from a service because they meet all qualifications for the job or services if reasonable accommodation was made to permit that person to participate in the program, receive the service, or perform that job. Reasonable accommodation may involve changing policies, practices, or services, and using auxiliary aids such as interpreters for persons with hearing impairments; readers or taped texts for persons with visual impairments; modifying existing facilities to be readily accessible and usable by employees, and job restructuring.

quality of life (1) Aspects of daily life that collectively are construed as positive and render a feeling that life is worth living. (2) A person's ability to perform ordinary activities of daily living. (3) The ability to realize life plans.

quick test (QT) See under **test.**

R

R

1. Right.
2. In the description of an orthotic or prosthetic joint, referring to its motion: resist.
3. In electricity: resistance.

rachial Spinal.

rachialgia Pain in the spine; also called spondylalgia.

rachiopathy Any disease of the spinal cord; also called spondylopathy.

rachis The vertebral column.

radiation

• **actinic radiation.** The rays producing chemical effects, essentially ultraviolet rays.

• **bactericidal radiation.** Rays lethal to bacteria. The maximum of bactericidal ultraviolet rays has a wavelength of ca. 265 nm.

• **burning radiation.** Although radiations that produce heat (thermal radiations) have wavelengths longer than those of light, the term is used as a synonym of tanning radiation and refers to ultraviolet rays with wavelengths shorter than 320 nm.

• **caloric radiation.** See **thermal radiation**.

• **electromagnetic radiation.** Radiation of associated electric and magnetic waves. Its spectrum ranges from cosmic and gamma rays at wavelengths smaller than one millionth of a nanometer to television and radio waves measured in meters and kilometers. All electromagnetic radiations (or waves) travel at the speed of light, which is a small segment of the electromagnetic spectrum. Therefore, they can be identified either by their wavelength or their frequency, the product of both being equal to that speed, i.e., 300,000 km/s.

Electromagnetic Radiation (Approximate Values)

Frequencies			*Wavelengths*
	Cosmic Rays		
10^{20} Hz	Gamma Rays		10^{-12} m
10^{18} Hz	Roentgen (X) Rays		10^{-10} m
			180 nm
	short	C	
	far		
10^{17}	Ultraviolet Rays	B middle	
	near		
	long	A	
			390 nm
10^{15} Hz		violet	
		indigo	
	Light Rays	blue	
		green	
		yellowa	
		orange	
		red	
			760 nm
	near	short	
10^{14} Hz	Infrared Rays		
	long far		
			15 000nm
2 450 MHz	Microwaves (Diathermy)		122 mm
27.32 MHz	Shortwaves (Diathermy)		11 m
1 MHz	Longwaves (Diathermy)		300 m
100 KHz	Television and Radio Waves		3 km
	Electric Power		

• **germicidal radiation.** Rays destructive to pathogenic microorganisms. The strongest germicidal ultraviolet rays have a wavelength of ca. 265 nm.

• **heat radiation.** See **thermal radiation.**

• **infrared radiation.** Thermal radiations "below the red," referring to their position in relation to the visible spectrum in which the red is at the lower end. While their frequencies are likewise below those of the red, they are usually identified according to their wavelengths, which range between 760 and 1,000,000 nm (1 mm). All bodies (unless at absolute zero temperature) radiate in this range. The physicists distinguish three zones referring to their relative distance from the visible spectrum: near infrared (760 to 3,000 nm), middle infrared (3,000 to 30,000 nm), and far infrared (30,000 nm to 1 mm). The therapeutically used infrared radiations are in the range between 760 and 15,000 nm. These are grouped as near infrared (760 to 1,500 nm) and far infrared (1,500 to 15,000 nm). All incandescent bodies, such as the sun and luminous heat lamps, emit near and far infrared rays. Bodies of lower temperature, such as hot-water bottles and electric heating pads, emit only rays of the far infrared. Infrared or so-called nonluminous heaters emit also some visible rays; they usually glow a dull red. The more intense the incandescence, i.e., the closer to white the color, the higher is the temperature, the shorter the wavelength, the "nearer" (to the visible band of the spectrum) the rays, and the deeper their penetration into the tissues.

• **luminous radiation.** The rays that make up the visible part of the electromagnetic spectrum, roughly between 400 and 760 nm. Also called visible radiation.

• **nonluminous radiation.** See **nonluminous heat**, under **heat**.

• **tanning radiation.** Ultraviolet rays shorter than 320 nm.

• **thermal (or thermogenic) radiation.** Radiation emitted by hot bodies such as used in thermotherapy. Its wavelengths are roughly between 700 and 15,000 nm.

• **ultraviolet (UV) radiation.** Radiation of the electromagnetic spectrum beyond the violet light rays, i.e., between the extreme of the visible rays and the longest x rays. Its wavelengths range between 400 and 13 nm. The therapeutically used ultraviolet radiations are of wavelengths roughly between 400 and 200 nm. These are grouped as near ultraviolet with wavelengths between 400 and 300 nm and far ultraviolet with wavelengths between 300 and 200 nm. Another classification is the following.
UVA: longwave rays, 400 to 320 nm, used in the treatment of psoriasis (see also **PUVA**);
UVB: middlewave rays, 320 to 290 nm, known for their tanning effect;

UVC: shortwave rays, 290 to 100 nm, which include the strongest germicidal rays, the wavelength of which is ca. 265 nm.

- **visible radiation.** Luminous radiation or light.

radiation therapy Treatment by roentgen rays, radium, cobalt, or similar agents. The term almost never refers to the other radiations mentioned above.

radicular Relating to a root.

radiculopathy Disease of the spinal nerve roots.

Rancho Los Amigos feeder, orthosis, splint, etc. The name refers to Rancho Los Amigos Hospital, Downey, California, where various orthoses and orthotic components were developed.

Rancho Los Amigos Level of Cognitive Functioning Scale A widely used behavioral rating scale which uses 8 levels of functioning used to describe the progression of recovery of cognitive capacities following traumatic brain injury.

range (grade)/strength grade Refers to manual muscle testing, where a muscle or muscle group is unable to complete its full range (therefore graded below Fair) but is able to take resistance (therefore graded above Fair). Example: P/G = range grade Poor/strength grade Good.

range of motion Amplitude of a joint or a series of joints, i.e., the arc through which a given segment moves in a given direction. The motion is either carried out by the individual (**range of active motion**) or by the examiner (**range of passive motion**).

range-of-motion test A test of the various ranges of motion in one or more joints, usually expressed in angles. See **zero position**, under **position**.

Rappaport Disability Rating Scale A scale designed to measure levels of functioning on a single continuum following traumatic brain injury.

raptus Any sudden seizure.

Rathbone relaxation method Method of relaxation applied in physical education, mostly taught and used in groups. Developed by Josephine Langworthy Rathbone-Karpovich (1899–1982), American physical educator.

ray, rays See under **radiation**.

RCBA Reading Comprehension Battery for Aphasia.

reacher Orthotic device that includes a forearm cradle or elbow support and one or more swivel arms. It is usually attached to a wheelchair or a table and allows a patient with a paralyzed upper limb to reach forward and sideward. It does not include external rotation of the arm, as a feeder does. Cf. **feeder**.

• **folding reacher.** Device, usually made of metal, which is lengthened by a closing motion of one hand in order to grasp an object otherwise out of reach.

reaching tongs A pair of tongs used to pick up objects otherwise out of reach.

reaction

• **Jolly reaction, myasthenic reaction.** See under **jolly**.

• **myotonic reaction.** Delay in the relaxation of a muscle after contraction initiated by a voluntary, electric, or mechanical stimulus.

reaction of degeneration (RD) Refers to electrodiagnostic findings characteristic of denervation.

• **absolute RD.** On stimulation of nerve and muscle with faradic and galvanic currents, no response is observed. Indicative of absence of viability of muscle tissue, e.g., of fibrotic replacement of muscle fibers following denervation.

• **full RD.** On stimulation of nerve and muscle with faradic and galvanic currents, the only response observed is a sluggish contraction on stimulation of muscle with galvanic current. Indicative of total denervation.

• **partial RD.** On stimulation of nerve and muscle with faradic and galvanic currents, diminished responses are observed, particularly with the faradic current. Indicative of partial denervation.

Read exercises or method See **prenatal exercises**, under **exercise**.

Reading Comprehension Battery for Aphasia (RCBA) A reading test for aphasic patients. Developed in 1979 by speech pathologists Leonard L. Lapointe and Jennifer Horner.

reading machine One of various instruments for blind persons, converting print either into sounds (see **Kurzweil reading machine, optophone,** and **stereotoner**) or into palpable vibrations, as in a tactile reading machine (see **Optacon**).

ReadiSplint Trade name of an inflatable plastic splint for emergency use in fractures and as a compression bandage in bleeding.

reality orientation A modality of supportive therapy to counteract confusion and disorientation in elderly and brain-damaged patients, used notably in psychiatric hospitals, nursing homes, and similar institutions. It consists in repetitive orientation as to person, time, place, and other environmental facts, aided by clocks, calendars, and notices in large print, and is applied by the entire health care personnel day and night, whenever appropriate. Systematized in 1965 by psychiatrist James C. Folsom and coworkers at the Tuscaloosa, Alabama, Veterans Administration Hospital

reasonable accommodation A term introduced with the Rehabilitation Act of 1973 and incorporated into the Americans with Disabilities Act of 1990, which require employers, governmental agencies, and other public entities to make reasonable accommodation to individuals with disabilities in employment situations and with respect to public accommodations. Such accommodation refers to the adaptation of a program, facility, or work place that permits a person with a disability to participate in the program, receive the service, or perform a job. Reasonable accommodation may involve changing policies, practices, or services, and using auxiliary aids such as interpreters for persons with hearing impairments; readers or taped texts for persons with visual impairments; modifying existing facilities to be readily accessible and usable by employees, and job restructuring.

reciprocal Referring to motions or exercises, it usually means crosswise combinations of one upper limb with the opposite lower limb, alternating with the two other limbs.

reconstruction therapy A term used for a short time during and after World War I for occupational therapy and physical therapy. Only women were accepted as therapists; they were called **reconstruction aides**.

recreation therapist A person licensed to administer recreation therapy.

recreation therapy The therapeutic use of recreational activities for physically or mentally handicapped individuals. It includes the provision of opportunities to improve the quality of their lives and aid them in their reentry into the community after disease or injury.

recumbency The position of lying down.

recumbent Lying down.

reduce To return a part to its normal position; e.g., the ends of a fractured bone.

reeducation

• **audio-neuromuscular reeducation.** Reeducation of muscular function with the use of audible signals of an electromyograph. Proposed in 1960 by physicians Alberto A. Marinacci and Marcel Horande.

• **motor (or neuromuscular) reeducation.** Systematic education and strengthening of a weakened muscle by conscious exercise. It may start with massage or other passive therapy.

reflex heat, reflex heating See under **heat, heating**.

reflex massage See under **massage**.

reflex therapy Therapeutic utilization of reflexes, e.g., the use of reflex contraction of muscles that have lost volitional control.

refractory (1) Not responsive or readily yielding to treatment. (2) Not responsive to stimulation, said of a muscle or nerve; immediately after responding to an initial stimulation, it enters a period of functional inactivity, during which it does not respond to a second stimulation.

refracture The breaking again of a bone that was improproperly set.

regimen A systematic procedure or regulation of an activity (exercise, diet) designed to achieve certain ends, usually hygienic or therapeutic in nature.

rehabilitation (1) Restoration of form and function following an illness or injury. (2) Restoration of an individual's capability to achieve the fullest possible life compatible with his abilities and disabilities.

rehabilitation The development of a person to the fullest physical, psychological, social, vocational, avocational, and educational potential consistent with his or her physiological or anatomical impairment and environmental limitations.

rehabilitation center An institution with professional services in rehabilitation medicine and other medical and surgical specialties, in clinical psychology, social work, and vocational guidance, which cooperate for the rehabilitation of the physically disabled.

Rehabilitation Codes System of classification of information relative to the rehabilitation process. A coding system of physical and mental disability including psychosocial and communicative functions. The system covers all ages and types of impairments, services, and agencies and provides a serial case record of an individual within the context of his or her family and community. Code numbering is designed for use with punch card systems. Developed in the years between 1957 and 1968 by Maya Riviere and coworkers and published by the former in 1970.

rehabilitation counselor A trained individual who counsels persons who have physical and mental disabilities, helping them to improve their ability to function optimally in society, using medical, social, and other resources as needed. He or she may administer vocational tests and procure prevocational or vocational training to those with potential for employment, providing occupational information to help them select an occupation best suited to their interests, abilities, and general life situations.

rehabilitation (or rehabilitative) engineering The field of technology and engineering serving disabled individuals in their rehabilitation. It includes the construction and use of a great variety of devices and instruments designed to restore or replace function, mostly of the locomotor and sensory systems. Thus it applies to prosthetics, orthotics, communication, seeing, hearing, the control of the individual's residential and work environment, the operation of vehicles, etc. For examples, see **artificial muscle, environmental control system, visual communication system, voice control**, as well as under **aid, orthosis, prosthesis**.

Rehabilitation Evaluation System (RES) A type of medical record that is particularly disability-oriented, replacing the traditional medical history and physical examination format or complementing the usual problem-oriented medical record. Developed in 1975 by Leon Reinstein, William E. Staas Jr., and Carl H. Marquette.

rehabilitation medicine A physician's specialty concerned with all aspects of medical rehabilitation. Also called physiatrics, physiatry, physical medicine, or physical medicine and rehabilitation, since physical agents and physical methods have traditionally been its predominant means in diagnostic procedures and in physical, occupational, and related therapies. The growing importance of the rehabilitative aspect of this branch of medicine and its value in guiding patients toward the fulfillment of their physical, mental, social, and vocational capabilities are reflected in the increased use of the term, as compared with its synonyms.

rehabilitation therapist A therapist usually working in the field of educational therapy or manual arts therapy (vocational rehabilitation therapy).

rehabilitative medicine A synonym of rehabilitation medicine. This variant is used in analogy with preventive medicine and curative medicine.

reinforcement patterns A system of exercise therapy in which one part of a composite motion is facilitated by the motion of another part.

relaxation State or action of diminution of muscular tonus or psychologic tension.

• **isometric relaxation.** Relaxation of a muscle without change of its length.

• **progressive relaxation.** See **Jacobson relaxation method**.

• **Schultz relaxation.** See **Schultz autogenic training**.

relaxation therapy Conscious education of the muscular tonus, aimed at achieving relaxation of the body, hence of the mind. William James (1842–1910), American psychologist and philosopher, was one of the first in modern times (1892) to use relaxation in the management of psychiatric disorders. See also **Gindler, Jacobson, Rathbone**, and **Schultz**.

rem-daw sheath A nylon stump sock impregnated with lanolin, worn under a regular stump sock in order to reduce friction. Known mainly in the UK.

remediable Capable of being cured or remedied; also called curable.

remedial gymnast A therapist who practices remedial gymnastics. Title mostly used in the UK, Canada, Australia, etc. It may be likened to that of corrective therapist in the USA. See also next entry.

remedial gymnastics A designation, used mostly in countries other than the USA, that may be likened to those of remedial physical education, corrective therapy, medical gymnastics, kinesitherapy, or therapeutic exercise. It may include athletics, dance, games, and other recreational activities. See also preceding entry.

remedial helper Physical therapy assistant or aide. Term used mostly in countries other than the USA.

remedial physical education Physical education applied to children and adults with special needs because of poor posture, minor deficiencies in any body part, or minor dysfunction of the locomotor system. It is most frequently administered in schools by physical education teachers. Also called corrective physical education.

remedial therapist Remedial gymnast (q.v.). A designation that in the UK has a tendency to be applied collectively to remedial gymnasts, physiotherapists, and occupational therapists.

remission A diminution of the severity of a disease or abatement of its symptoms.

rentschlerization Destruction of bacteria by ultraviolet radiation of a wavelength of 253.7 nm. Suggested by Harvey C. Rentshler (1881–1949), American physicist.

repetition maximum (RM) Refers to the maximum weight that can be lifted for a specified number of repetitions in progressive resistive exercises. Example: 10 RM.

replantation Replacement of a bodily part to its natural position.

resectable Amenable to surgical removal; capable of being cut off.

resection The surgical removal of a portion of any part.

RES Rehabilitation Evaluation System.

resettlement British term referring to vocational and social rehabilitation of a patient.

residual volume (RV) See **lung volumes and capacities**.

resistance, electric The opposition to the flow of electric current. Its unit is the ohm, its symbol: R.

resonance, electric Maximum transfer of high-frequency energy from one circuit to another.

respirator An apparatus that provides mechanical pulmonary ventilation (artificial respiration). Also called ventilator.

• **chest respirator.** A mechanical device tightly attached to the trunk, either to the chest or the chest and abdomen, and connected to a pump. Designed to produce alternately positive and negative pressure to facilitate breathing.

• **cuirass respirator.** A chest respirator in form of a shell or cuirass applied to the front of the trunk.

• **Drinker respirator.** See **tank respirator**.

• **Emerson respirator.** Proprietary name of a tank respirator. Developed in 1937 by John H. Emerson.

• **negative-pressure respirator.** A respirator (such as the old so-called iron lung) in which negative pressure pulls the chest wall outward and sucks air into the lungs from outside the apparatus.

• **positive-pressure respirator.** A respirator that pushes air into the lungs. Expiration is triggered at a predetermined pressure, volume, or duration in various types of ventilators called accordingly **pressure-cycled, volume-cycled,** or **time-cycled**.

• **tank respirator.** Metal cabinet designed to enclose a recumbent patient with the head protruding and an air-tight seal around the neck. An electric pump empties and fills the lungs through alternation of negative and positive pressure, thus supporting respiration in case of paralysis of respiratory muscles. Invented in 1928 by Philip Drinker, then a student at Harvard University. Also called iron lung.

respiratory therapist One who administers respiratory therapy as prescribed and supervised by a physician. Associated with this activity are usually the administration of certain pulmonary function tests or assistance in these tests as well as instructions given to patients with respiratory insufficiencies. See also following entry.

respiratory therapy Treatment consisting primarily in the use of various respirators, oxygen apparatuses, aerosol dispensers, nebulizers, and other devices to give mechanical assistance with or without medications for respiration. Since 1978 the term has officially replaced the previous term of inhalation therapy (and the still earlier term of oxygen therapy) to indicate the enlarged scope of the field. See also preceding entry.

respite care Temporary, short-term supervisory, personal, and nursing care provided to give temporary relief or respite to persons with caregiving responsibilities.

rest cure Therapeutic system published in 1874 by Silas Weir Mitchell (1829–1914), Philadelphia neurologist. Applied particularly in neurasthenia, hysteria, and for convalescence, it consisted mainly of bedrest, high-calorie diet, massage, exercise, and electrotherapy. Its purposes were to improve muscle tone and circulation, increase body temperature, and foster relaxation.

restless legs syndrome A feeling of creepiness, twitching, and restlessness deep in the legs, usually occurring in older individuals after lying down; the cause is unknown.

restorator Exercise apparatus consisting essentially of a pair of mounted bicycle pedals. It can be used while sitting in a chair or lying on a plinth or in bed.

restrainer A vest, belt, strap, or combination of straps designed to prevent a patient from moving; used where movement might interfere with a therapeutic or diagnostic procedure or may result in injury to the patient or others.

retropulsion Walking backward involuntarily. Seen in parkinsonism. Also called retropulsive gait.

reversal of antagonists An exercise method in which the patient is asked to move a body segment against the manual resistance of the therapist who applies that resistance alternately to agonists and antagonists. See **Kabat method of exercise**.

revulsion The local application of an irritant (counterirritation) to an area away from a diseased area in order to diminish its hyperemia.

revulsive Referring to revulsion.

rheobase The minimum intensity (expressed in milliamperes) or the minimum tension (expressed in volts) of an electric current (usually of 300 ms duration) able to provoke a contraction in a given muscle. Proposed in 1909 by French physiologist Louis Lapicque (1866–1952). See also **chronaxy**.

rhythm method (or technique) of travel See **cane travel of the blind**.

RICE An acronym for first-aid treatment for athletic injuries; R stands for rest and immobilization, I for ice, C for compression, and E for elevation.

rigid dressing A postoperative dressing of the amputation stump, made with plaster bandages. Used to control edema and prepare the stump for a prosthesis.

rigidity Stiffness, immobility; the quality of being rigid or inflexible.

• **cerebellar rigidity.** Stiffness of the body and limbs due to an injury or lesion of the vermis of the cerebellum.

• **cogwheel rigidity.** Rigidity of a muscle that, when passively stretched, gives way to a series of small jerks, as seen in Parkinson's disease.

• **lead-pipe rigidity.** The diffuse tonic contraction of muscles as seen in paralysis agitans.

ripple bed, mattress, pad See **alternating-pressure mattress**, under **mattress**.

risk factor An element that influences the likelihood of an occurrence.

Risser jacket A scoliosis plaster jacket, also called localizer cast, because pressure pads are localized over the highest points of the deviation for correction. Advocated in 1955 by California orthopedic surgeon Joseph C. Risser.

Rochester method for the deaf Fingerspelling, i.e., the use of the manual alphabet for communication.

rocker knife A knife with a convexly curved edge. Thus, meat can be cut by a rocking motion without the use of the other hand to hold a fork.

rocker knife and fork A rocker knife (see preceding entry), ending in three or four prongs, thus also for use as a fork.

rolfing See **structural integration**.

rollator A walkerette whose front legs are fitted with rollers.

roller shoe See under **shoe**.

roller skate See **skate**.

Rollier's formula Formula regulating the progressive exposure of the body to natural or artificial ultraviolet radiation. The exposure, beginning with the feet, extends progressively toward the head by adding daily a new segment and prolonging the exposure of all previously exposed segments. Proposed in 1913 by Swiss physician Auguste Rollier (1874–1954).

rolling stand See **wheelstand**.

Rood method of exercise A system of therapeutic exercise enhanced by cutaneous stimulation for patients with neuromuscular dysfunctions. In addition to proprioceptive maneuvers such as positioning, joint compression, and joint distraction and the general use of reflexes, stretch, and resistance, more than in any other comparable method of facilitation and inhibition, greatest emphasis is given on exteroceptive applications such as stroking, brushing, icing, warmth, pressure, and vibration in order to achieve optimal muscular action, even of the lips and tongue. Developed in 1954 by Margaret S. Rood, American occupational and physical therapist.

rotator A muscle that rotates a part, such as one of several muscles that rotate the vertebral column.

rotatory force That component of the muscle tension that produces angular motion about the joint.

running A mode of locomotion that, in contrast to walking, is characterized by a period of so-called floating during which there is no contact with the ground.

rupture
1. Hernia.
2. The bursting or tearing of a part.

Russell traction A weight-and-pulley arrangement for a supine patient, which provides an upward pull to the knee by using a sling laced in the popliteal area, together with longitudinal traction to the leg. Devised in 1924 by Melbourne surgeon R. Hamilton Russell.

S

S

1. In electricity: siemens.
2. In the description of an orthotic or prosthetic joint, referring to its control: stop.

s In measurements of time: second(s).

ς Greek letter **sigma** (lowercase).

1. In measurements of time: obsolete symbol for millisecond(s).
2. In statistics: standard deviation.

SACH foot See under **foot**.

salt glow A rub of the body with moistened salt. Administered in times past in hydrotherapy institutions, it was usually followed by a shower or other application of water as a means of stimulating the functions of the skin and hardening the body.

Sandow apparatus Elastic extensor apparatus for exercises, mostly of the upper limbs and shoulder girdle. Named after Eugene Sandow (1867–1925) of Königsberg, Germany. See next entry.

Sandow method or system Method of muscular training and development by the use of the Sandow apparatus (see preceding entry). The method became known in the USA especially after the inventor's exhibit at the Chicago World's Fair in 1893.

sauna, sauna bath See under **bath**.

• **facial sauna.** Boxlike apparatus producing warm air saturated with moisture, for inhalation. Used to mobilize bronchial secretions.

Sayre head sling See under **sling**.

Scamp Hand-operated vehicle for paraplegic children between 4 and 9 years of age. Its levers, which steer and propel it, require normal function of the upper limbs.

scanning speech Prolonged phonation of each syllable with slow and slurred articulation of the consonant sounds. Characteristic of multiple sclerosis.

Schanz collar A narrow tube of soft material such as stockinette stuffed with cellulose, which is wound in three loops around the neck so as to form a collar. Used to reduce movement of the cervical vertebrae. Designed by German orthopedic surgeon Alfred Schanz (1868–1931).

Schnee bath See under **bath**.

Schott system System of treatment of heart disease by the use of Nauheim baths (see under **bath**), graded walks (see **terrain cure**), and progressive exercise against resistance given by the therapist. Developed by the brothers Schott—August (1839–1886) and particularly Theodor (1852–1921)—physicians in Bad Nauheim, a German spa.

Schultz autogenic training System of general relaxation and awareness of one's body parts and their degree of warmth. Developed in the 1920s and published in 1932 under the title *dad autogene training* by Berlin neurologist and psychiatrist Johann Heinrich Schultz (1884–1970).

Schwartz method System of locomotor habilitation of children with cerebral palsy or similar conditions, in which psychologic, intellectual, and physical stimulation of the child's own effort, unhindered by bracing, is emphasized. Hence the preference of work and play in a group with other children. Also included was the use of the Hartwell carrier (q.v.), a locomotor device developed in 1951, together with the method, by the orthopedic surgeon R. Plato Schwartz (1892–1965).

scissoring Refers to the tendency of the lower limbs during walking to cross the midline because of spastic adductors of the thighs.

sclerosis Hardening of tissues due to proliferation of connective tissue, usually originating in chronic inflammation.

• **amyotrophic lateral sclerosis.** A disease characterized by degeneration of the lateral motor tracts of the spinal cord, causing progressive muscular atrophy and exaggerated reflexes.

• **multiple sclerosis (MS).** Disease of the brain and spinal cord affecting mostly young adults and characterized by loss of the fatty sheaths (myelin) that surround nerve fibers; its name is derived from the plaques or patches of scarred nervous fibers that dot the central nervous systems; symptoms vary but frequently include weakness, incoordination, scanning (halting, monosyllabic) speech, involuntary oscillation of the eyeballs, and coarse tremors.

• **tuberous sclerosis.** A familial disease marked by progressive mental deterioration, epileptic convulsions, and sometimes sebaceous adenomas of the skin.

scoliosis A rotary lateral curvature of the spine.

• **congenital scoliosis.** Scoliosis resulting from malformation of the spine or chest.

• **idiopathic scoliosis.** Lateral spinal curvature for which the cause is unknown; constitutes 80% of all cases of scoliosis.

• **myopathic scoliosis.** Scoliosis due to weakness of the spinal muscles.

• **osteopathic scoliosis.** Lateral curvature resulting from pathologic conditions of the vertebrae, such as tuberculosis, rickets, and tumors.

• **static scoliosis.** Scoliosis due to difference in the length of the legs.

scoliotic Referring to scoliosis.

scooter See **prone scooter**.

Scotch douche See under **douche**.

Scultetus bandage or binder See under **bandage**.

S-D curve Strength-duration curve.

seatboard See under **board**.

seat shell Molded seat, usually of plastic, designed to give better support, particularly during prolonged sitting, to a person with severe deficiency of the pelvis or lower trunk.

Seattle foot prosthesis See under **prosthesis.**

sec In measurements of time: second(s).

secondary gain Indirect physical or psychological benefits derived from a disability or illness.

section numbers Numbers assigned to codes of procedures and services. See **procedural terminology**.

seeing-eye dog See **guide dog**. The term is correctly used only for dogs trained by The Seeing Eye, Inc., the oldest school in the USA for guide dogs and their users, established in 1929 (now in Morristown, New Jersey).

Seeing-eye machine A vision aid for the blind. A miniature television camera mounted on a pair of glasses is wired to an apparatus that transmits vibrations to a plate attached to the user's body, where the hand can feel them. Developed at the Pacific Medical Center in San Francisco.

segmental breathing Breathing into a given area of one or both lungs. It is part of a program of breathing reeducation, when ventilation in one particular region should be developed.

Seguin formboard A board, 30 by 45 cm, with 10 cutouts into which the subject is asked to place correspondingly shaped blocks of simple geometric forms such as circles, squares, triangles. Probably the first in a long series of psychologic kits used in the testing and education of the mentally deficient. Invented by Edouard Séguin (1812–1880), French-American psychiatrist. It was later modified as Seguin-Goddard formboard.

seismotherapy, sismotherapy Treatment by mechanical vibration or shaking.

self-care Refers to activities such as washing, bathing, toileting, dressing, grooming, and eating.

self-concept Perception of the self as an object based on reflections of one's attitudes, beliefs, values, body image, and experiences.

self-esteem A judgment of one's own value or worth considered to be an important factor affecting mental health, interpersonal relations, and competence in activities such as work/leisure, as well as general outlook on life.

self-help clothing Clothing designed for disabled persons, for easy dressing and undressing as well as for other needs.

self-help device See **self-help aid**, under **aid**.

self-help groups Groups composed of persons who want to cope with a specific problem or life crisis that meet for the purpose of exchanging information, providing social support, discussing mutual problems, and improving psychological functioning.

Semantography See **Bliss symbols**.

semiflexion The position of an extremity midway between extension and flexion.

senescence The process of aging or growing old.

senescent Aging; growing old.

Senior Olympics An annual sports contest of persons 65 years or older. Developing in the 1970s, it became best known in California. Cf. **Golden Olympics**.

sensorimotor Both sensory and motor; said of certain nerves.

sensorimotor technique of treatment Any of several methods of treatment using proprioceptive and exteroceptive stimulation, facilitation, and inhibition to achieve the desired muscular response in patients with neuromuscular dysfunctions. For examples of such techniques, also called proprioceptive neuromuscular facilitation, see **Bobath, Brunnstrom, Doman-Delacato, Fay, Kabat, Knott, orthokinetics, Phelps**, and **Rood**.

sensory integration therapy A therapeutic approach, usually applied by occupational therapists, that aims at improving sensorimotor coordination in patients with disturbances of such coordination. It uses movements and postures as well as tactile, visual, auditory, and olfactory stimuli and may be applied to communication, expression of emotions, activities of daily living, play, and games.

setting Refers to muscular contraction not accompanied by joint motion. See also **muscle setting exercise**, under **exercise**.

SFTR method Method of measuring and recording joint motions and positions. The motions start at the neutral position (see under **position**) and are executed in the sagittal, frontal, and transverse planes or as rotation. The combination of the neutral-zero method (q.v.) with the measurement in various directions was proposed as sftr method in 1964 by Otto A. Russe, Austrian orthopedic surgeon, and John J. Gerhardt, Oregon physiatrist. It became also known as International Standard Orthopaedic Measurements.

shank

1. Lay term for tibia or leg.
2. The leg part of a prosthesis. More correctly called leg.
3. The posterior part of the sole of a shoe, i.e., its narrow part, that reaches as far posteriorly as the breast of the heel and does not touch the ground. It often contains a steel shank, i.e., a piece of flat steel between the insole and the outsole.

shaping (of the amputation stump) Application of bandages or of a shrinker, or other procedures to make an amputation stump more appropriately shaped for a prosthesis.

sheltered workshop A place of work in which people with various disabilities may be able to fulfill productive jobs, thanks to the selection of occupations and the help provided. The disabilities may stem from mental and emotional disorders and retardation as well as deafness, blindness, and other physical impairments. The work is generally obtained by subcontracting with manufacturers. Wages and salaries are usually below the minimum federal rates. A sheltered workshop may also provide vocational evaluation, adjustment, and training and prepare its workers for further rehabilitation.

shiatsu From the Japanese *shi*, finger(s), and *atsu*, pressure. Technique of massage of Asian origin, possibly 500 years old. Great pressure is applied for a few seconds with the pads of the fingers, notably of the thumbs, on key points of the body similar to those of acupuncture.

shin Colloquial term designating the anterior part of the natural or prosthetic leg or of the entire leg of a prosthesis, i.e., the part between the knee and the ankle. Thus, the term is often used instead of tibia or (prosthetic) leg.

shin splints Irritation or inflammation of the extensor muscles of the lower lateral area of the legs caused by an unusually great adduction of the legs and aggravated by overexercise.

shoe

- **Bal (bal) shoe.** Abbreviation for Balmoral shoe.

- **Balmoral (balmoral) shoe.** A laced shoe in which lace stays, tongue, and vamp are sewn together at the throat. Introduced in 1853 by Queen Victoria's consort Prince Albert and named after Balmoral Castle, Scotland, then the center of world fashion. Also called by its abbreviation Bal (or bal) shoe.

- **Blucher (blucher) shoe.** A laced shoe in which the lace stays are not sewn together at the throat. Thus, they can be opened fully, allowing the foot to enter more easily. Named after the Prussian field marshal Gebhard von Blücher (1742–1819), who in 1810 introduced a high boot with side pieces lapped over the front.

- **chukka, chukka boot or shoe.** Shoe with a three-quarter upper: the upper covers the malleoli without being as high as in a high (high-quarter) shoe.

• **depth shoe.** See **in-depth shoe**.

• **Derby (derby) shoe.** Similar to the Blucher shoe, the quarters overlapping the vamp. Named after Edward Stanley (1752–1834), 12th Earl of Derby, England.

• **Earth shoe.** Proprietary name of a shoe with a large toe box and a heel that is lower than the sole. Invented in 1957 by Anne Kalsø in Denmark, it has been marketed in the USA since 1 April 1970, Earth Day, whence its name.

• **extra-depth shoe.** See **in-depth shoe**.

• **ghillie (gillie, or gilly) shoe.** A low-cut shoe that is open from throat to instep.

• **Gibson shoe.** A variant of the Blucher or Derby shoe, the quarters overlapping the vamp.

• **gillie (or gilly) shoe.** See **ghillie shoe**.

• **high-quarter shoe or boot.** Shoe whose upper reaches about two or three fingerbreadths above the malleoli.

• **in-depth shoe.** A shoe with more than the usual vertical space for the foot. The toe box is particularly high and wide, and there is space for an extra insole, an arch support, other orthosis, or extra padding. Sole and heel may be of one piece, with no sharp delimitation between the two: the heel has no breast, so as not to catch on objects.

• **lace-to-toe shoe.** A shoe that is laced as far as the toes. Also called convalescent shoe, it is used after operations on the foot, since it can be opened widely, thus admitting the foot more easily.

• **Murray shoe.** The prototype of space shoes (q.v.), devised about 1940 by Allen E. Murray, later manufactured by the Murray Space Shoe Company, Bridgeport, Connecticut.

• **open-toe shoe.** A shoe without a toe box. Thus the lace stays can be widely opened to admit the foot, and the toes are free and visible.

• **orthopedic shoe.** As opposed to fashion or regular shoes, it is of heavier construction, has a toe box of good width and height, a long counter, particularly on the medial side, and a large, low heel, extending usually farther forward in its medial half (Thomas, or orthopedic, heel).

• **Oxford (oxford) shoe.** A stout, low shoe in which the quarters extend to just below the malleoli. It is laced over the instep and has a low heel. Reportedly introduced about 1715 by students at Oxford University, who until then had worn high shoes or boots.

• **prewalker shoe.** Shoe for infants, worn before the walking age. It is laced to the toe, having no toe box, thus allowing the foot to enter easily.

• **reversed-last shoe.** Shoe in which the medial border is convex instead of concave, thus giving the impression as if it were made for the other foot. Used in the treatment of certain foot deformities, notably metatarsus varus. Cf. **straight-last shoe**.

• **rocker shoe.** Shoe with a rigid sole that is much thicker about midway between the breast of the heel and the heads of the metatarsals. Thus, on walking, the shoe rocks like a sea-saw. Used to diminish weightbearing on the metatarsal heads.

• **roller shoe.** A shoe or other footwear on rollers to diminish friction for easy exercising of a lower limb on a board or other smooth surface or to counteract a tendency to contracture. See also **skate**.

• **space shoe.** A shoe molded over a cast of the individual foot, making "space" for any deformity, yet providing a snug fit. The sole is thick and has usually little flexibility. Used most frequently in deformities due to rheumatoid arthritis.

• **straight-last shoe.** Shoe built on a symmetric last to be worn on either foot. Used in certain cases of mild foot deformities. Cf. **reversed-last shoe**.

shoe clasp Posterior clasp. See under **clasp**.

shortwave diathermy or therapy See under **diathermy**.

shortwave ultraviolet rays or therapy See **ultraviolet radiation**, under **radiation**.

shoulder control System of activating an apparatus, designed for a person with absent or functionless upper limbs: the shoulder mobilizes a switch. It may be used for the control of a wheelchair or of an upper limb orthosis or prosthesis.

shoulder-hand syndrome Pain and stiffness of the shoulder and hand, sometimes with late atrophy of hand muscles; usually associated with neck or upper arm injuries or with myocardial infarction.

shoulder harness See under **harness**.

shoulder ladder, shoulder abduction ladder A gymnasium device resembling a small ladder, fixed to the wall, upon which the fingers climb, thus affording shoulder flexion or abduction.

shoulder loom Weaving frame placed vertically and raised or lowered according to the desired degree of elevation of the patient's upper limbs.

shoulder press See under **bench press**.

shoulder saddle Part of the harness for an upper-limb prosthesis. It is made of leather or rigid plastic material and covers the shoulder on the prosthetic side.

shoulder wheel An exercise wheel for the upper limb. Usually mounted by its axle on the wall (less often on a movable stand), it is turned by a handle attached to one of the spokes. The circular motion of the upper limb varies according to the height of the axle attachment and the level of the handle. The resistance to the motion can be varied by a braking mechanism.

shrinker See **stump shrinker**.

sick role behavior Any activity undertaken by persons who consider themselves sick, for the purpose of getting well.

side-joint thigh corset suspension Method of attachment of a below-knee prosthesis, consisting of a thigh corset and one, or usually two, metal knee joints connecting with the socket.

side rail A metal rail attached to the side of the bed, protecting the patient from falling out and offering a hold for moving about.

siemens (S) The unit of electric conductance, formerly called mho. Named after British inventor Sir William (German-born Karl Wilhelm von) Siemens (1823–1883).

Sierra hand, hook See under **APRL**.

Siglish Contraction of signed English. See next entry.

signature The part of a pharmaceutical prescription containing instruction to the patient for the use of the medication; also called transcription.

signed English (Siglish) English in sign language for the deaf. It uses the signs of the American sign language (q.v.) but follows the English grammatical order, has extra signs to express grammatical variations, and includes fingerspelled words. For these reasons, it is also called grammatical sign language.

signer A person who communicates in sign language.

signing Communicating in sign language.

sign language Communication by the use of gestures, mostly of the hands and fingers, for words and concepts. Used by people who are deaf or cannot talk. In the USA, there are two main systems: American sign language (q.v.) and signed English (q.v.). See also **manualism**, and **Amer-Ind**.

sign language interpreter See **interpreter for the deaf**.

Silesian band or bandage See under **bandage**.

sinew A tendon.

Singer Vocational Work Sample A work evaluation system designed to assess work habits, readiness for employment, and tolerance for work.

sip-and-puff control See **breath control**.

sitting press See under **bench press**.

sitzbath See under **bath**.

SKA orthosis, SKAO See under **orthosis**.

skate Support on casters or wheels for a foot, hand, or elbow, used to decrease friction during exercises on a skate board (see **skating exercise**, under **exercise**). Also called roller skate.

• **Brachman skate.** Device used in clubfoot correction and other abnormalities. Developed by Philip R. Brachman, podiatrist.

skate board See under **board**.

skating exercise See under **exercise**.

skin conductance meter Dermohmmeter

skin resistance test See **dermohmmetry**.

skin temperature See under **test**.

skis, walking skis A pair of ski-like boards used in ambulation training.

• **reciprocal skis.** Ski-like boards with attached poles crossing over to the other side so that each foot advances together with the opposite hand.

• **straight skis.** Ski-like boards for ambulation training without any attachment for the hands.

sling Soft support, usually of canvas, for a body part, in some cases for the entire body, as in a hoist.

• **Glisson sling.** Sling support for the head, as used in cervical traction. Named after Francis Glisson (1597–1677), English physician.

• **overhead sling.** A sling suspended from a bar over the head to support the upper limb. The bar may be attached to a wheelchair, bed, or other object.

• **Perthes sling.** A sling made of a web strap suspended from the back of the waist belt or shoulder to the ankle in order to carry that leg in partial flexion and thereby avoid weightbearing. The patient usually walks with crutches. So called since it may be used in Legg-Calvé-Perthes disease. Other names: Perthes belt and sling, Legg-Perthes sling, Sam Brown sling.

• **Sam Brown sling.** See **Perthes sling** (preceding entry).

• **Sayre head sling.** Sling for head suspension, for distraction of the cervical vertebrae and straightening of the vertebral column. Named after the American surgeon Lewis Albert Sayre (1820–1901), who in 1877 described its use for the treatment of spinal curvature.

slip socket See under **socket**.

S-N-S knee, prosthesis, system See **Swing-N-Stance knee**, under **knee**.

SOAP An acronym (S = subjective; O = objective; A = assessment; P = plan) for a format widely used in organizing and recording information regarding treatment.

social service worker, social worker A health professional providing social services.

socket (of prosthesis) The part of a prosthesis that contains the amputation stump. See also under **prosthesis**.

• **adjustable socket.** A socket made of a more or less flexible and adjustable material, which allows its form to be changed easily.

• **air-cushion socket.** A prosthetic socket, notably for a patellar-tendon-bearing prosthesis (see under **prosthesis**), with an elastic sleeve that encloses an air chamber, providing contact with the distal stump area, for better support.

• **diagonal socket.** Pelvic socket for a hip disarticulation prosthesis, a variant of the socket for a Canadian hip prosthesis (see under **prosthesis**). Developed by 1962 by Colin A. Mclaurin, Toronto, Canada.

• **Dundee socket.** Prosthetic total-contact socket for below-knee amputation, developed about 1964 at the Prosthetics Research Department in Dundee, Scotland.

• **hard socket.** The usual rigid (laminate) prosthetic socket without a soft liner as opposed to the soft socket (q.v.).

• **non-total-contact socket.** Partial-contact socket (see next entry).

• **partial-contact socket.** A socket constructed in such a way that only part of its inner surface is in contact with the amputation stump.

• **plug fit socket.** Socket of above-knee prosthesis of the old type. It has a grossly horizontal and circular brim and is conical in shape, compressing the stump about equally from all sides. It has been supplanted by the quadrilateral socket (see next entry).

• **quadrilateral socket.** The universally adopted type of above-knee socket. The lumen of its brim is of grossly quadrangular shape. Thanks to the small anteroposterior dimension and the high anterior wall, the posterior border of the brim is maintained directly under the ischial tuberosity, so that the amputee sits on it during weightbearing. For this reason the socket (in its upper part) is also used for orthoses, when weightbearing on a more distal part of the limb is to be avoided.

• **rigid socket.** A socket made of rigid material such as metal, wood, or glass fiber.

• **segmental socket.** Prosthetic socket for knee disarticulation, consisting of two separate parts, the socket brim and the distal socket section. The parts are jointed by the external uprights of the knee hinges and can be further separated from each other to accommodate a growing child. Developed in 1977 at Children's Orthopedic Hospital, Seattle, Washington.

• **semirigid socket.** A rigid socket with a soft lining.

• **slip socket.** A socket containing a second socket designed to maintain contact with a very short stump. Otherwise the contact might be lost on pronounced flexion.

• **soft socket.** A prosthetic socket with a soft insert, or liner.

• **split socket.** An intermediary socket between a very short amputation stump, usually of the forearm, and the prosthesis itself. Jointed with the latter by a step-up hinge, it ensures better contact between stump and prosthesis, thus providing a larger range of motion than that of the stump.

• **suction socket.** Prosthetic socket, particularly for the thigh, which is held in place by suction, i.e., by negative pressure between stump and socket. Invented in 1863 by Dubois Parmelee, it came into general use only 90 years later.

• **total-contact socket.** A socket whose entire inner surface is in contact with the amputation stump.

somatopsychology The study of the impact of physical disability and chronic illness on personality and interpersonal behavior.

SOMI Sternal-occipital-mandibular immobilizer, a rigid cervical orthosis, designed particularly for injuries of the cervical spine.

sonogram The graphic result of a diagnostic examination by ultrasound.

SOREFI program Acronym for social, recreation, and fitness, indicating the factors emphasized in a program aimed at weaning patients with long-term diseases from unnecessary therapies and accepting self-maintenance in the community. It is usually administered by a physical or corrective therapist and a recreational therapist. Developed at the Veterans Administration Medical Center, West Roxbury, Massachusetts, and published in 1979 by the physiatrist Margarete Di Benedetto.

sound waves Longitudinal pressure waves. The waves audible by the human ear have frequencies ranging from 20 to 20,000 per second. See also **infrasound** and **ultrasound**.

spa A place in which water, notably from mineral springs, is extensively used for therapeutic purposes by ingestion, bathing, or both. Named after the Belgian town of Spa, which is such a watering place. More rarely, the term is used to designate a health resort in which water does not play a role. See also **health club**.

spark gap Gap in a circuit between two conductors.

spasm An involuntary, sudden, violent contraction of a muscle or a group of muscles.

• **carpopedal spasm.** A spasm of the feet and hands.

• **clasp-knife spasm.** Spasticity of the extensor muscles induced by passive flexion of a joint that suddenly gives way on exertion of further pressure, allowing the joint to be easily flexed; the rigidity is due to an exaggeration of the stretch reflex; also called clasp-knife rigidity.

• **clonic spasm.** One characterized by alternate rigidity and relaxation of the muscles.

• **intention spasm.** One occurring when voluntary movements are attempted.

• **nictitating spasm.** Involuntary winking.

• **tonic spasm.** A spasm in which the muscular contraction is persistent.

spasmodic Relating to or characterized by spasm.

spasmogenic Causing spasms.

spasmolysis The arrest or elimination of spasm.

spastic Convulsive.

spasticity An involuntary velocity-dependent increase in the response of muscle to passive stretch (hypertonia) that sometimes accompanies lesions of the brain or spinal cord.

special education General term for education that is different from that for the great majority of children, most often because it is applied to those with blindness, deafness, other physical disabilities, or learning, behavioral, or other psychologic problems. It may be given at home, at school, in a hospital, or in another institution, instead of, or in addition to, the regular school program. Special education is also given to gifted and talented children. See also **exceptional child**.

Special Olympics Program of physical fitness, sports training, and athletic competition for mentally retarded children and adults, created in 1968 by the Joseph P. Kennedy Jr. Foundation. Meets and games are held year-round in all States of the USA. The **International Special Olympics**, since their Fourth Games in 1975, are held every fourth year. In 1979 there were 3500 contestants from over 20 countries. Special Olympians must be 8 years old or older (there is no upper age limit), have a maximum iq of 75—with rare exceptions, such as an additional handicap. There are 14 sports offered: track and field, swimming, diving, gymnastics, basketball, volleyball, soccer, floor hockey, poly hockey, bowling, frisbee-disc, wheelchair events, and—for the Winter Special Olympics—skiing and ice skating.

spectrum, electromagnetic The range of electromagnetic waves in the order of frequencies or wavelengths. See **electromagnetic radiation** (definition and table), under **radiation**.

speech The production of articulate sounds to convey ideas.

• **esophageal speech.** Speech produced by swallowing air and regurgitating it; used by an individual who has had his larynx removed.

• **scanning speech.** Slow speech with pauses between syllables.

• **staccato speech.** Jerky, abrupt speech in which each syllable is pronounced separately.

• **telegraphic speech.** A sparse speech, usually consisting mainly of nouns, important adjectives, and transitive verbs, omitting articles, prepositions, and conjunctions; seen in certain types of aphasia.

speech clinician, pathologist, or therapist A health professional who evaluates and treats disturbances of communication and often also those of hearing. See also next entry.

speech disorders A disruption in the mechanics of oral language resulting from a dysfunction in the neuromuscular sequence, which produces and alters the patterns of phonation and articulation. Types of speech disorders include the following:

• **dysarthria.** A disturbance in neuromuscular apparatus that produces abnormalities in articulation and phonation.

• **hypophonia.** The presence of abnormal voice volume.

• **mutism.** Total lack of voice.

• **palalalia.** Involuntary repetition of words or phrases during verbal output.

• **stuttering.** Irregular interruptions of the normal rhythm by voluntary repetition, prolongation, or arrest or speech sounds.

speech pathology The field of human communication and its disorders. The term is used interchangeably with speech therapy (q.v.) but is preferred when its larger scope is emphasized. See preceding entry.

speechreading The process of judging the content of human speech by observing and integrating information gathered from lip movements, facial expressions, and other nonverbal cues, as well as one's residual hearing.

speech therapy Treatment of speech disorders such as aphasia due to cerebral lesions, dysarthria due to local organic lesions, speech defects after laryngectomy and other operations, and other disorders of communication. See also **speech pathology**.

spina (plural, spinae) The spine.

• **spinal bifida.** Congenital defects in which part of the vertebral column is absent; it allows the spinal membrane and sometimes the spinal cord to protrude.

• **spina bifida occulta.** Spinal bifida without protrusion of the spinal cord or its membranes.

spinal conformator An apparatus designed to record the spinal curves in the sagittal (anteroposterior) plane. A vertical bar, about 1 m long, is adjusted so as to reach from the level of the occiput of the standing subject to that of the buttocks. Horizontal slots, about 30 or more, at intervals of 2.5 cm house metal dowels, about 30 cm long. Their tips are lightly pushed against the occiput and the midline of the subject's neck and back as far down as the gluteal cleft. The other ends of the dowels thus duplicate the curves of the spine, which can be traced on a paper placed on a board directly behind the dowels.

spirogram A tracing, by a spirograph, of respiratory movements. See illustration under **lung volumes and capacities**.

spirograph Device to register the movements of pulmonary ventilation.

spirography The recording and graphic measurement of pulmonary ventilation.

spirometer An instrument for measuring volumes of air inhaled and exhaled such as vital capacity, timed vital capacity, and forced expiratory volume.

• **incentive spirometer.** An instrument to stimulate inspiration and produce maximal lung inflation. The patient inhales until a predetermined volume of air is reached, as indicated by a light or other signal. Yawning may result. Hence its colloquial name of yawn box.

spirometry The measurement of ventilatory functions by a spirometer.

Spitzy button or spike A device used to correct a postural defect due to muscular weakness or indolence. The spike is mounted on an orthosis where it provokes pain, forcing the patient to make a muscular effort, thus correcting his or her posture. Example: a spike on an arch support elicits the patient's effort to supinate the foot and elevate the arch. Devised by Vienna orthopedic surgeon Hans Spitzy (1872–1956).

splayfoot Foot with flattened transverse arch.

splint A device used to immobilize, support, and correct injured, displaced, or deformed structures.

• **air splint.** Inflatable sleeve or stocking giving rigidity and protection to a limb. Used as a first aid for fracture, burns, or other injuries or after a lower-limb amputation to help shrinkage and to prepare the stump for a prosthesis.

• **airplane splint.** One designed to hold the arm in abduction at shoulder level.

• **baseball splint.** A splint applied to the anterior aspect of the forearm and hand, holding the latter in the position in which a baseball is usually held.

• **cervical splint.** A splint for supporting the head, thus taking some pressure off the cervical spine.

• **cockup splint.** Splint that holds the wrist in a cocked-up position, i.e., in extension (dorsiflexion).

• **Cramer's splint.** A flexible splint resembling a ladder, consisting of two parallel wires connected with a series of fine wires.

• **crutch splint.** An orthosis for a paralyzed or deformed hand, enabling it to handle a crutch which it could not handle otherwise.

• **cylinder splint.** Splint of cylindrical form, applied over a limb in order to immobilize a joint, most often the knee. An additional joint (hip, ankle) may be included. It may be made of paper, cardboard, plaster, fiberglass, or other material. Depending upon the material, it may also be called cylinder cast, etc.

• **Denis Browne splint.** An attachment to the soles of a pair of shoes with connecting crossbar, maintaining the lower limbs in abduction and the desired position of internal or external rotation, while correcting talipes equinovarus. Devised in 1934 by London orthopedic surgeon Sir Dennis John Browne (1892–1967).

• **dropfoot splint.** A splint that holds a foot with insufficient voluntary dorsiflexion in a neutral or near-neutral position.

• **dynamic splint.** See **dynamic orthosis**, under **orthosis**.

• **feeding splint.** See **feeder**.

• **flexor hinge splint.** See **flexor hinge orthosis**, under **orthosis**.

• **Frejka's splint.** A pillow splint used to correct dislocations of the hip in infants under the age of 12 months.

• **Hodgen's splint.** One designed for a fractured femur, essentially used to apply balanced traction.

• **knee splint.** A splint supporting or stabilizing the knee. It may be constructed to avoid certain movements, such as hyperextension or lateral deviation.

• **knee extension splint.** A splint designed to provide continuous dynamic stress while patients are asleep or at rest.

• **leaf footdrop splint.** An ankle-foot orthosis made of one "leaf" of rigid or semirigid plastic and a calf band. It is molded to embrace calf and heel, continues under the arch of the foot, and is worn inside the shoe. Designed to counteract footdrop and give mediolateral stability to the ankle. Originally developed in 1967 at the University of Washington, Seattle. See also **spiral ankle-foot orthosis**, under **orthosis**.

• **lively splint.** See **dynamic orthosis**, under **orthosis**.

• **opponens splint.** A splint that keeps the thumb in abduction at a right angle to the plane of the palm and opposition.

• **prod splint.** Abbreviation for prevention-of-deformity splint. One of several splints slipped on one or more digits or the hand, to prevent or reduce deformity. Developed in 1969, mostly for use in rheumatoid arthritis, by physiatrist Robert L. Bennett, Warm Springs, Georgia.

• **Readisplint.** Trade name of an inflatable plastic splint for emergency use in fractures and as compression bandage in bleeding.

• **rocker splint.** See **feeder**.

• **tenodesis splint.** See **flexor tenodesis orthosis**, under **orthosis**.

• **Thomas's splint.** One used to immobilize the leg, consisting of an iron ring that fits on the upper thigh and is connected to a continuous iron bar with a W shape on the upper side.

splinting The application of a rigid device to a limb to prevent motion of a dislocated joint or the ends of a fractured bone.

splinting of muscles See **muscle splinting**.

split hook See **hook**.

spondylitis Inflammation of one or more vertebrae.

• **ankylosing spondylitis.** Ossification of the ligaments of the spine with involvement of the hips and shoulders; also called Strumpell-Marie arthritis.

spondylolisthesis A structural abnormality of the spine.

spondylolysis A structural abnormality of the spine.

spondylolysis Abnormal immobility and fixation of a vertebral joint.

spondyolysis Breaking down or destruction of a vertebra.

spork A spoon that ends in three or four tines, thus combining spoon and fork. Used by persons who have difficulty changing from one to the other.

spotting The watchful stand-by of a therapist, teacher, or trained helper ready to assist a patient, athlete, or any person during the performance of an exercise, in order to prevent injury.

spot trainer See **bolster**.

spray-and-stretch therapy Treatment that consists in passively stretching a muscle while cooling it with a spray, such as ethyl chloride or Fluori-Methane (q.v.). Used in the treatment of tight and painful muscles.

spread The tendency to overgeneralize the effects of a disability as limiting a person in functions that are actually unrelated to the disability.

squat, squatting See **squatting position**, under **position**.

squeezer Wheelchair narrower (q.v.).

stairlift, stairway elevator, stairway lift Chair running on a rail along a stairway inside a house.

stall bars See under **bar, bars**.

stance phase The period in ambulation during which the foot remains in contact with the ground. Cf. **swing phase**.

Stand-Alone Proprietary name of a wheelstand (q.v.).

stander (mobile or rolling) See **wheelstand**.

standing (or stand-in) table See under **table**.

Stanford-Binet test, Stanford test See under **test**.

static machine A machine, previously used for electrotherapy, delivering powerful contractions by direct current of very high voltage (about 100,000 V) and very low amperage (about 1 ma or less). Called also influence machine.

stationary technique Refers to the administration of ultrasound therapy in which the soundhead is kept more-or-less in place during its application.

stay Long and thin support of various dimensions to reinforce a corset or similar flexible orthosis. A corset may have several rigid or flexible stays made of steel, aluminum, or plastic.

Stebbins system of gymnastics or physical training See **Delsarte system**.

step The walking distance covered from one foot to the other, or the corresponding motion. See also **stride**.

step test See **two-step test**, under **test**.

Stereotoner A stereophonic reading machine for the blind. A miniature camera reads printed material. Each letter is converted into a musical tone and received through a pair of earphones. Developed in 1972 by Hans A. Mauch, Dayton, Ohio.

stick, walking stick Cane, usually but not necessarily used for support during walking. See also **cane** and **crutch**.

stirrup A U-shaped, stirrup-like device made of steel, for the attachment of an ankle orthosis to the shoe. The middle piece is attached to the outsole of the shoe, the lateral parts reach to the level of the ankle joint to articulate with the uprights of the brace. See also **stirrup brace**, under **brace**.

stockinette, stockinet A soft, washable cloth, usually of cotton, machine knitted, in tubular form. It is used under a cast, for bandages, and for similar purposes. Term probably derived from the earlier stocking net.

Stoke Mandeville Games An annual sporting event for wheelchair users, which takes place at Stoke Mandeville Sports Stadium for the Paralysed and Other Disabled, Aylesbury, England. Inaugurated in 1948 by the director of the Stoke Mandeville National Spinal Injuries Centre, German-born neurosurgeon Ludwig Guttmann (1899–1980), later Sir Ludwig.

stooping Flexion of trunk and head.

strap

• **ankle strap.** A strap, usually of leather, attached to a shoe below the malleolus and used in combination with an orthosis in order to support the ankle. Depending upon its shape it is either a T strap or a Y strap. The former covers the malleolus, the latter does not. Depending upon its attachment, it has one of two opposite functions.

1. **Lateral T or Y strap**. The single branch of the strap is attached to the lateral side of the shoe. The forked branches pull the ankle toward the medial upright of the brace, around which they are buckled, thus counteracting a varus deformity of the ankle (supination or inversion of the foot). Less desirable synonyms are: outside, outer, varus, anti-varus, varus-correction, and eversion T or Y strap.
2. **Medial T or Y strap**. Attached to the medial side of the shoe and buckled around the lateral upright of the orthosis, it counteracts a valgus deformity (pronation or eversion of the foot). Inside, inner, valgus, anti-valgus, valgus correction, and inversion T or Y strap are less desirable synonyms.

• **inverted Y strap.**

1. A strap in the form of an inverted Y on the anterior aspect of a lower limb prosthesis. Used as a suspension aid for a below-knee prosthesis, the single branch of the strap is attached to the belt, the forked branches to the prosthesis. A similar device may be used in an above-knee or an upper limb prosthesis.
2. A kick strap with a forked lower end. See next entry.

• **kick strap.** An elastic strap of webbing that is attached to an above-knee prosthesis. It extends from the front part of the belt or the socket to the leg just below the knee. Its lower part may be forked. During the swing phase of walking, after knee flexion has stretched the strap, its recoil assists in knee extension before heelstrike.

• **T strap.** See **ankle strap**.

• **Y strap.** See **ankle strap** and **inverted Y strap**.

strength-duration (S-D) curve The tracing of an electrodiagnostic test. The curve is plotted from the points in which the ordinates represent the strength (intensity), and the abscissae, the duration of the electric current necessary to provoke the contraction of a given muscle. Also called intensity-duration (I-D) curve.

stretch-and-spray therapy See **spray-and-stretch therapy**.

stretcher

• **prone stretcher.** A wheelstretcher with one pair of wheels large enough so that its user, being in the prone position, may turn them (they have handrims) for self-propulsion. Called also self-propelled stretcher.

• **self-propelled stretcher.** A wheelstretcher that can be propelled by its user, almost always lying prone on it (see preceding entry: **prone stretcher**). Rarely, the propelling wheels are higher than the stretcher, in which case self-propulsion in the supine or sitting position may be possible.

• **water stretcher.** Frame spanned with canvas for the support of a patient. It is placed on a wheelstretcher and hooked onto a trolley to lower the patient into the water of a therapeutic tank.

• **wheelstretcher.** A carriage for the transportation of a patient in a recumbent position. It consists of a litter mounted on a frame with four or six wheels.

stretch glove A tightly fitting glove of elastic textile or similar material. It is worn throughout the night to reduce swelling and stiffness in arthritic hands, as suggested in 1971 by Philadelphia rheumatologist George E. Ehrlich and osteopath Alfred M. Dipiero.

stretching

• **active stretching.** Stretching done by the patient through contraction of opposing muscles (antagonists).

• **active assisted (or active-assistive) stretching.** Stretching done by the patient through contraction of the antagonists of the muscles to be stretched and aided by the therapist or other person, by pulleys or other mechanical device.

• **passive stretching.** Stretching done by the therapist or other person, or by a mechanical device, without active participation by the patient.

• **self-assisted stretching.** Stretching by the patient who, using one body part, stretches another part, which may either participate in the attempt or remain passive.

stride The walking distance covered between two successive contacts of the floor by the same foot, or the corresponding motion. See also **swing phase** and **step**.

strigil An instrument used in ancient Greece and Rome for removing the oil applied on the skin before exercise, together with seat and sand. A scraper.

striking bag A pear-shaped air-filled leather bag, about 25 cm in height, 20 cm in diameter, hanging on a swivel from a wooden platform. It is struck with the fist at a fast cadence, each time bouncing back from the platform. Mostly used by boxers. Also called punching bag.

strip cast A plaster cast made of narrow strips or slabs.

stroke club An association of individuals who had a stroke and of their families and friends. Its purposes are to educate its members about the nature of stroke and the means of overcoming the resulting handicaps, and to provide mutual aid and encouragement. The first stroke club was founded in 1968 in Galveston, Texas, by Ellis Williamson, a 41-year-old stroke patient, under the sponsorship of the American Heart Association. It became a national organization and in 1979 "Stroke Club International." Several hundred stroke clubs now exist in the US under various names. Most of them are sponsored by the American Heart Association; others are maintained by the Easter Seal Society, by medical centers, or as private organizations.

stroking One of the fundamental maneuvers of massage, also called effleurage.

stroking technique If applied to ultrasonic therapy, it designates the usual technique of moving the soundhead during its use, although it is habitually a circular motion.

stroller Walker or walkerette with rollers.

Strong Interest Inventory A measure of vocational interests.

Strong-Campbell Interest Inventory (SCII) A 325-item test that assess the degree to which one's interests in the areas of occupations, school subjects, activities, and amusements match with persons representing 207 different, primarily professional occupations.

structural awareness A variant of structural integration (see next entry), developed by Dorothy Nolte.

structural integration A combination of posture training and massage of large muscle groups, aiming at good body alignment, relaxation of tight muscles, and greater ease in motion. Developed by the American biochemist Ida P. Rolf (1896–1979); therefore also called rolfing. See also **structural patterning** (next entry).

structural patterning A system of posture training consisting in movements based on the principles of structural integration (see preceding entry), of which it is a simplified method that can be taught in groups. Developed in the early 1970s by Judith Aston.

stubbies Very short nonarticulated prostheses for a bilateral above-knee amputee. They allow early ambulation and are used mostly for children.

Study of Values An instrument developed by Allport, Vernon, and Lindzey that measures the relative strength of six basic motives or evaluative attitudes, including theoretical, economic, aesthetic, social, political, and religious.

stump shrinker Device applied to an amputation stump in order to shape and shrink it appropriately for a prosthesis. See also **shaping**.

stump sock A sock applied to the stump of an upper or lower limb as a buffer between stump and prosthesis. See also **ply**.

• **pressure-sensitive stump sock.** A stump sock made of polyurethane with microcapsules that break upon pressure, spilling a dye, thus producing a map of pressure distribution. Used as a test of stump pressure in a prosthesis. See also **footprint slipper sock**, which is made of the same material.

subluxation Partial dislocation.

substitution, substitutive motion Motion performed by a muscle or muscle group other than the prime mover. Example: in paralysis of the deltoid, abduction of the humerus can be achieved by the long head of the biceps. Also called trick motion or vicarious motion.

succumbing framework A paradigm that highlights the negative aspects of disablement. The perceptual orientation of this framework leads to major consequences regarding how people think about and act on wide-ranging disability-related matters, such as the adjustment process, interpersonal relations, role playing, fundraising, health care messages, language usage, and civil rights legislation.

sudomotor test See **sweat test**, under **test**.

summation pattern See **interference pattern**.

supine Lying on the back.

supine press See under **bench press**.

supporter Flexible orthosis designed to support a body part. examples: breast supporter (brassiere), testicular, abdominal, lumbosacral supporter.

surfboard A padded board consisting of two hinged parts of about equal length, placed over a wheel chair from the footrests to the backrest. The user, lying prone on it at an oblique angle, faces the rear, the hands on the large wheel for self-propulsion

suspension In prosthetics, suspension refers to the method of attachment of the prosthesis to the body. Examples: suction, cuff suspension, side-joint thigh corset suspension.

suspension ambulator See **suspension walker**, under **walker**.

suspension feeder Feeder suspended from above, usually from a metal rod attached to a wheelchair. See **feeder**.

suspension sling A sling hanging from above, usually from a metal rod attached to a wheelchair, in order to support the upper limb of a patient.

suspension walker See under **walker**.

sweat test See under **test**.

Swedish exercises, gymnastics, or movements See under **exercise**.

Swedish massage See under **massage**.

Swedish walking A program of walking preceded and interspersed by simple exercises in the upright position. With three sessions per week, the program spans a 12-week period during which the walks lengthen from 1 to 3.5 km, their speed increasing from slow to brisk as defined by the individual's physical condition. Developed in 1967, primarily for the elderly, by attorney Harry Kaufmann (1906–1978) of the Maryland Commission on Physical Fitness, who named it to denote the combination of walking with exercises of Swedish type.

swing control system, hydraulic Hydraulic system incorporated into the knee joint of a lower limb prosthesis, designed to enable the amputee to walk at various speeds in a rather natural manner.

swing phase The period in ambulation between two successive contacts with the floor by the same foot. Normally, the swing phase begins when the toes leave the ground and ends when the heel touches it again. It corresponds to the distance of a stride, except for the length of the foot itself. Cf. **stance phase**.

swivel walk or walking See **swivel gait**, under **gait**.

symbol for access See **accessibility symbol**.

symbol for deafness See **deafness symbol**.

Syncardon Proprietary name of an apparatus for the treatment of peripheral vascular insufficiency. Pneumatic pressure impulses are transmitted to cuffs applied to the limbs to be treated. These impulses are synchronized with the heartbeat by monitoring the patient's R wave of the electrocardiogram, transmitted to the apparatus. Invented in 1945 by Maurice Fuchs (1890–1969).

synergist A muscle that enhances the action of another one. See **agonist**.

synkinetic Refers to a motion occurring more or less involuntarily together with another motion.

systematic sign language See **Paget sign language**.

T

T In muscle testing: Trace (q.v.).

tabes Progressive wasting away.

table

• **Baruch table.** A table for hydrotherapy. Developed by Simon Baruch (q.v.).

• **bed table.** A platform on four legs for use while in bed. In some models the table top or its center part can be tilted for easier reading.

• **Chandler table.** A plinth with an opening at one end, through which the patient, lying prone, lets one upper limb hang down for pendulum and circular motions, thus eliminating the need to move against gravity. Designed in the early 1930s by Boston orthopedic surgeon Fremont A. Chandler (1893–1954).

• **chimney table.** Stand-in table (q.v.).

• **Delorme table.** Universal exercise table equipped with adjustable parts, pulleys, weights, and other devices, to be used in a sitting, prone, supine, or sidelying position for simple or progressive resistive exercises. Named after Thomas L. Delorme, (see **DeLorme exercises**, under **exercise**.). Called also Elgin table.

• **Elgin table.** Proprietary name of a universal exercise table. See preceding entry.

• **Kanavel table or apparatus.** Table equipped with cords, pulleys, and weights for resistance exercises of fingers, wrist, and forearm. Description published in 1921 by its inventor Allen B. Kanavel (1874–1938), American orthopedic surgeon.

• **N-K table or exercise unit.** Table for progressive resistance exercises, mostly of knee flexors and extensors, performed in the sitting position. Devised, published in 1954, and named after them, by physical therapists Royce P. Noland and F. Albert Kuckhoff.

• **stand-in (or standing) table.** Table with an enclosure that secures a patient in a standing position. Used mostly for children with cerebral palsy.

• **tilt table.** Support with table top on which the patient lies and which can be tilted up to the vertical position. Used in particular for patients who cannot assume the upright position actively or who must be brought to it progressively.

table chair A combination of rolling armchair and tabletop. Frequently called geriatric chair.

tactual map Map for the blind, with a palpable relief, generally of areas such as a park, college campus, public building. The legends are usually in braille, but tactual maps may also be designed for sighted persons.

t'ai-chi ch'uan Chinese system of exercise, having possibly started as a martial art many centuries ago. The three individual words may be translated as "supreme," "ultimate," and "fist," respectively. In this system, which has also been called circular gymnastics, all segments of the body participate, at times several segments simultaneously, in slow circular motions. During an entire session, which may last 15 minutes, there is a steady, uninterrupted flow of movements. The exercises are taught as a psychophysical and spiritual discipline aiming at harmony of body and mind.

Talent Assessment Program (TAP) work evaluation A system of vocational evaluation, published in 1973 by Talent Assessment Programs, Des Moines, Iowa.

talipes General term that denotes a deformity involving the ankle and foot.

talking book Record of text taken from a book, magazine, or newspaper, for use by persons who are blind on a record player.

tank A container, such as a tub, usually of stainless steel, for hydrotherapy. Fitted with one or two agitators, it provides hydromassage and is also called whirlpool tank. See the following examples.

• **arm tank.** A whirlpool tank for the upper limb.

• **full body tank, fully body immersion tank.** See **Hubbard tank**.

• **half tank, half body tank.** Hydrotherapeutic tan similar to a bathtub, for the immersion of the lower limbs and the pelvis. It usually includes an agitator, as do other whirlpool tanks.

• **Hubbard tank.** A keyhole-shaped tank for full-body immersion. It usually includes two agitators, has a capacity of about 1,500 L, and is large enough to permit abduction of upper and lower limbs. Named after Chicago engineer Carl P. Hubbard, who in 1928 built the first such tank. Also called full body tank.

• **leg tank.** A whirlpool tank for the immersion of one or both legs; the patient usually sits on a high stool outside the tub. Using a removable seat across the inside permits the immersion of both legs and thighs.

• **wading (or walking) tank.** A Hubbard tank (q.v.) with a removable perforated base plate in its floor. Removal of the plate opens a troughlike lower section (also called walking trough) with parallel bars for walking. A filled tank contains about 2,600 L.

• **whirlpool tank.** See above definition of **tank**.

tap-key electrode, tap-Key stimulator Electrode for the stimulation of a muscle or nerve. A flat contact switch spring, attached to the handle, allow interruption of the flow of current without removing the electrode, by simply releasing the spring.

tapotement French for tapping. A maneuver of massage. It has many variants—tapping, clapping, hacking, hammering, pounding, etc.—and is performed with the fingertips, fingers, flat hand, ulnar border, or fist. Also known as percussion.

TAT Thematic Apperception Test. See under **test**.

Taylor brace See under **brace**.

TDD Abbreviation for telecommunication device for the deaf. A teletypewriter that, coupled with an ordinary telephone, transmits and receives typed messages also appearing on a roll of paper. Used by those who cannot hear or speak. See also **TV-Phone**.

team, rehabilitation A group of health care workers with backgrounds in rehabilitation who work together to provide integrated, patient-oriented care.

• **interdisciplinary team.** A team model in which communications flow freely between team members who, while understanding each other's roles, may suggest treatment goals and modalities that represent another discipline.

• **multidisciplinary team.** Individuals representing the traditional rehabilitation disciplines, each of whom acts as an individual consultant, evaluating the patient and providing discipline-specific treatment recommendations.

• **transdisciplinary team.** A model of team functioning in which rehabilitation disciplines cross over into the traditional treatment areas of other disciplines.

tenodesis hand splint Flexor tenodesis orthosis. See under **orthosis**.

tensor A muscle that makes a part tense or firm.

terminal device The substitute for the hand in an artificial upper limb. See also **voluntary-closing device** and **voluntary-opening device**.

terminal impact at knee Exaggerated and audible extension of knee in a lower-limb prosthesis at the end of its swing phase.

terrain cure A system of outdoor walking along a series of paths graded in length and degree of incline. Used in health resorts and prescribed especially for patients with obesity or cardiovascular deficiencies. The paths are numbered from 1 through 4 and marked by red, blue, purple, and yellow markers, respectively, indicating the increasing slope, for progressive training. Advocated in 1866 by Munich laryngologist Max Joseph Oertel (1835–1897). See also **Herz**.

test An examination.

• **acoustic impedance test.** A test that assesses the integrity and function of the middle ear, especially transmission characteristics, by measuring the reflected sound waves (acoustic impedance) at the tympanic membrane.

• **Appraisal of Language Disturbance (ALD) test.** Test for aphasia in adults, developed about 1970 by Lon Emerick, speech pathologist at Northern Michigan University.

• **Arthur Point Scale of Performance.** Nonverbal test of intellectual performance for children, developed in its original form in 1925 and published in 1930 by the American psychologist Grace Arthur (1883–1967). Administered by pantomime, it is particularly useful for children with impaired speech or hearing, mental retardation, emotional handicaps, and also for foreign-born or bilingual children.

• **association test.** A method for examining the content of the mind, whereby the subject is required to respond as quickly as possible to a given stimulus word with the first word that comes to mind; also called word association test.

• **Attitudes Toward Disabled Persons Scale.** See **Attitudes Toward Disabled Persons Scale.**

• **Ayres test.** One of several tests now known as Southern California Sensory Integration tests (q.v.).

• **Barthel index.** See **Barthel index.**

• **Beck Depression Inventory.** See **Beck Depression Inventory.**

• **bench step test.** See **two-step test.**

• **Bender Gestalt test.** A test of visual motor function in which the subject is asked to copy nine standard designs; its chief application is to determine organic brain dysfunction in both children and adults and level of development of visual motor function in children; secondarily used to assess personality variables; also called Bender visual-motor Gestalt test.

• **Binet test, Stanford-Binet test.** One used to determine the mental age of a child; it consists of a series of questions standardized according to the mental capacity of normal children at different ages.

• **Boston Diagnostic Aphasia Examination.** See **Boston diagnostic aphasia examination.**

• **Boston Naming Test.** A standardized test, used to evaluate language disturbances in brain-injured adults, that requires the individual taking the examination to name the objects based on stimulus and phonemic cues.

• **break test.** Technique of manual muscle test in which the patient holds a body segment in a position indicated by the examiner, who then attempts to "break" this position. Thus it is a test of power in isometric contraction. Called also holding test and yield test.

• **Bruce test.** An exercise test for patients with coronary heart disease. Developed by cardiologist Robert A. Bruce in 1971.

• **Cage Questionnaire.** See **Cage questionnaire.**

• **California Psychological Inventory.** See **California Psychological Inventory.**

• **Category test.** Psychologic test of perception based on the assumption that organic brain damage disturbs the capacity to abstract, the principle of categorization. Developed by K. Goldstein.

• **cold pressor test.** A measure of the change of blood pressure in response to the immersion of one hand in ice water. Normally, the systolic pressure rises by about 20 mm Hg and returns to the pretest level after two minutes. An excessive increase and prolonged high reading are indicative of a tendency to hypertension. Also called Hines-Brown test, after the American physicians Edgar A. Hines, Jr. (1906–1978) and George E. Brown (1885–1935), who published it in 1933 under the name of **cold stimulation test**.

• **Communicative Abilities in Daily Living Test (CADL).** A standardized test composed of 68 items; used to evaluate language disturbances in adults.

• **Comprehensive Assessment and Referral Evaluation (CARE) instrument.** See **Comprehensive Assessment and Referral Evaluation (CARE) instrument.**

• **Cornell Medical Index.** See **Cornell medical index**.

• **Differential Aptitude Test (DAT).** A widely used multiaptitude test that emphasizes abilities that are important mainly in academic activities.

• **Disabilities Factor Scales (DFS).** See **Disabilities Factor Scales (DFS).**

• **Doppler ultrasonic test.** Test for detecting the presence of an obstacle to the blood flow in a vessel. Using an ultrasonic transducer and a probe, the examiner evaluates the shift in sound from a change in ultrasonic signals to and reflected from the vessel, transmitted transcutaneously and received via a pair of earphones. The shift in sound, the so-called Doppler effect, is the apparent change in the frequency of sound and other waves reaching the observer, due to a change of the distance between source and observer. This effect was described by the Austrian physicist and mathematician Christian J. Doppler (1803–1853).

• **double-blind test.** One in which neither the person giving the test nor the one receiving it knows whether the drug used is active or inert.

• **Draw-A-Person test.**

1. A method of determining a child's level of intellectual development, based upon the "best" drawing of a human figure; also called Goodenough test.
2. A projective personality test requiring the subject to draw a person; also called Machover test.

• **Eisenson test.** An aphasia test, also called Examining for

Aphasia. Published in 1954 by California speech pathologist Jon Eisenson.

• **electric stimulation tests.** These include chronaxy determination, establishment of strength-duration curve, nerve stimulation tests, etc. They are sometimes termed collectively electrodiagnosis, though this latter term, in the opinion of some, includes electromyography.

• **Ely test.** A test for hip extension. The subject lying prone, the leg is passively flexed until the heel touches the buttock. If the patient cannot keep the hip fully extended, i.e., if the inguinal area moves away from the surface of support, it means that there is a shortening of the fascia lata or of another soft-tissue structure of the anterior aspect of the thigh. Named for Leonard Wheeler Ely (1868–1944), American orthopedic surgeon.

• **exercise (or exercise stress) test.** Examination of an individual's reactions to exercise, notably the cardiac responses as revealed by the electrocardiogram that is taken before, during, and after exercise.

• **Flack test.** Cardiopulmonary test that consists in maintaining an expiratory effort at a pressure of 40 mm Hg. The result is assessed according to endurance and cardiac rhythm. Proposed in 1919 by Martin Flack, London physiologist, as a test for pilots, it was later used in sports medicine. Called also 40-mm test.

• **Frostig test.** Developmental test of visual perception, developed by Marianne Frostig, in collaboration with Welty Lefever and John R. B. Whittlesey, and published in 1961.

• **Functional Communication Profile. See functional communication profile**.

• **Functional Independence Measure (FIM).** See **Functional Independence Measure (FIM)**.

• **galvanic-faradic test.** Electrodiagnostic test of muscles by stimulation with galvanic (impulses of 100 ms or more) and faradic current (impulses of 1 ms or less). For interpretation see **reaction of degeneration**.

• **Galveston Orientation and Amnesia Test (GOAT).** A test designed to assess amnesia and disorientation after head injury.

• **GED (or General Educational Development) test.** The official test of high school equivalency, open to persons of any age. It is frequently administered by educational therapists in hospitals.

• **General Aptitude Test Battery (GATB).** See **General Aptitude Test Battery (GATB).**

• **Gesell test.** Test of motor and language development and general adaptability in children between 1 month and 6 years of age. Developed in 1947 by Arnold L. Gesell (1880–1961) and Catherine S. Amatruda (1903–1949), physicians at Yale University.

• **Gibbon-Landis test.** A diagnostic test of reflex vasodilation in the lower limbs when heat is applied to the upper limbs, or vice versa. Published in 1932 by John H. Gibbon Jr. (1903–1973), Philadelphia surgeon, and Eugene M. Landis (1901–1970), Philadelphia physician, later Boston physiologist.

• **Glasgow Coma Scale.** See **Glasgow Coma Scale.**

• **Glasgow Outcome Scale.** See **Glasgow Outcome Scale.**

• **Graham-Kendall Memory for Designs Test.** A test of right parietal lobe functioning that requires perception of visual-spatial relationships and discrimination of the test object.

• **GXT.** Abbreviation for graded exercise test or testing (see above: **exercise test.**

• **Halstead-Reitan Battery.** See **Halstead-Reitan Battery.**

• **Hanman test, plan, profile, or system.** A method for establishing a profile of a worker's physical abilities. A list of 80 factors comprises lifting, carrying, running, kneeling, and other physical activities, as well as heat, cold, lighting, noise, and other environmental factors to which the subject may be exposed. Developed in the 1940s and 1950s and published in 1958 by Bert Hanman, Boston.

• **Hines-Brown test.** See **cold pressor test.**

• **holding test.** See **break test.**

• **House-Tree-Person (HTP) test.** A projective test (q.v.) in which the subject is asked to draw a person, a tree, and a house. It is used for the analysis and evaluation of the individual's personality and relation to the environment. Presented in 1946 and published in 1948 by Virginia psychologist John N. Buck (1906–1963).

• **HTP test.** House-Tree-Person test. See preceding entry.

• **intensity-duration test.** See **strength-duration curve.**

• **Internal-External Locus of Control (I-E) scale.** See **Internal-External Locus of Control (I-E) scale.**

• **Ishihara test.** A test for detection of color-blindness, based on the ability to see patterns in a series of multicolored plates or cards (Ishihara plates).

• **Jolly test.** See under **jolly**.

• **Katz index.** See **Katz index.**

• **Kohs Block-Design test.** A psychologic performance test in which cubes are used, each of their six sides being of a different color. The subject is asked to arrange them according to the colored designs on a set of cards. Most often used as an intelligence test. Described in 1923 by the psychologist Samuel C. Kohs (1890–1977).

• **Kraus-Weber test.** A minimum muscular fitness test. A series of six exercises used to make a rapid estimate of an individual's physical fitness, in particular flexibility and power of trunk muscles. Developed by Austrian-born New York physiatrist Hans Kraus (1905–1979) and physical therapist Sonia Eisenmenger-Weber and published in 1954 by Hans Kraus and Ruth P. Hirschland.

• **Landis-Gibbon test.** See **Gibbon-Landis test**.

• **Language Modalities Test for Aphasia.** See **Wepman and Jones test**.

• **Life Satisfaction Index.** See **Life Satisfaction Index**.

• **Luria-Nebraska Neuropsychological Battery.** See **Luria-Nebraska Neuropsychological Battery**.

• **Make-A-Picture-Story (MAPS) test.** A projective test (q.v.) in which the subject places cutout pictures of persons or animals on pictures of rooms or landscapes and tells a story illustrated by this composition. It is used for the analysis of the subject's ideals, desires, and behavior. Introduced in 1947 by the American psychologist Edwin S. Shneidman (1918–).

• **manual muscle test (MMT).** Manual evaluation of the power of individual muscles or muscle groups. Several grading scales are in use. The first systematized test, and the most frequently used in the USA, was developed by Boston orthopedic surgeon Robert W. Lovett (1859–1924) and his physical therapist Wilhelmine G. Wright (1885–1934). The latter published it in 1912. Its grades are Zero, Trace, Poor, Fair, Good, and Normal. In 1938 the Baltimore physical therapists Henry O. Kendall (1898–1979) and his wife, Florence P. Kendall, published a percentage scale, 10% corresponding to Trace, 25% to Poor, 50% to Fair, 75% to Good, and 100% to Normal. In other systems, muscles from completely paralyzed through normal are graded from 0 (zero) through 5 (see **Oxford classification**) or even in reversed order, from 4 though 0. Intermediary grades are expressed by plus (+) and minus (-) signs, except in the centesimal scale.

• **MAPS test.** Make-A-Picture-Story test.

• **MED test.** Minimum erythema dose test.

• **Methods-Time Measurement test.** See under **Methods-Time Measurement**.

• **Millon Clinical Multiaxial Inventory.** See **Millon Clinical Multiaxial Inventory**.

• **minimal erythema dose (MED) test.** A test applied to the skin, designed to establish the smallest dose of ultraviolet radiation that results in an erythema.

• **Minnesota Multiphasic Personality Inventory (MMPI).** A psychologic test in which the subject answers a questionnaire containing 550 true or false statements related to physical and mental status. It is used to assess personality, interests, emotions, and attitude toward self and others. Published in 1940 by psychologist Starke R. Hathaway (1903–1991) and neuropsychiatrist J. Charnley Mckinley (1891–1950) at the University of Minnesota.

• **Minnesota Test for Aphasia.** Also known as Schuell test, it was published in a short form in 1957 and as Minnesota Test for Differential Diagnosis of Aphasia in 1965 by Hildred Schuell (1906–1970), speech pathologist in Minneapolis.

• **Minnesota Test for Differential Diagnosis of Aphasia.** A standardized test used to evaluate language disturbances in adults by assessing five disorder areas, including (a) auditory disturbances, (b) visual and reading disturbances, (c) speech and language disturbances, (d) visual, motor, and handwriting disturbances, and (e) disturbances of numerical relationships and arithmetic processes.

• **MMPI.** Minnesota Multiphasic Personality Inventory.

• **muscle test.** See **manual muscle test**.

• **nerve conduction test.** Measurement of nerve conduction velocity, used as a diagnostic test. Normal average values for a motor or sensory nerve are between 40 and 60 m/s.

• **nerve stimulation test.** Examination of the response of muscles to the electric stimulation of their motor nerve.

• **nonprojective test.** One of several psychologic tests that evaluate personality traits quantitatively, comparing the result with statistically established norms. Cf. **projective test**.

• **Ober test.** A test to assess the degree of tightness of the fascia lata. The subject is in the sidelying position, the lower limb that rests on the table being flexed at the hip and knee. The examiner, supporting the other lower limb, abducts it and extends it at the hip and knee. Upon sudden removal of the supporting hand, a relaxed limb normally drops; a contractured fascia lata keeps it in the air (Ober sign). Described in 1936 by Frank Roberts Ober (1881–1960), Boston orthpedica surgeon.

• **Older Americans Research and Service Center Instrument (OARS).** See **Older Americans Research and Service Center Instrument (OARS)**.

• **Opinions About Mental Illness Scale (OMI).** See **Opinions About Mental Illness Scale (OMI)**.

• **PACE II: Physical Functioning.** See **PACE II: physical functioning**.

• **Patient Appraisal and Care Evaluation (PACE).** See **Patient Appraisal and Care Evaluation (PACE)**.

• **performance test.** One of many tests that require the handling of certain objects and the use of manual or other physical skills.

• **Philadelphia Jewish Employment and Vocational Work Sample Battery (JEVS).** See **Philadelphia Jewish Employment and Vocational Work Sample Battery**.

• **PICA test.** Abbreviation for Porch Index of Communicative Ability. See under **Porch**.

• **Porch Index of Communicative Ability.** See under **Porch**.

• **Porteus Mazes.** See **Porteus Mazes**.

• **projective test.** One of many psychologic tests in which the subject completes sentences, makes drawings, discusses intentionally ambiguous test material presented, or completes other tasks and answers related questions. Performance, comments, and answers are analyzed as projections, i.e., revelations, or the subject's own thinking, inner feelings, emotional and other problems, and other personality characteristics. Examples: House-Tree-Person, Make-A-Picture Story, Rorschach, and Thematic Apperception tests.

• **pulmonary function test.** One of several tests evaluating functions of the lung. See also **spirography** and **spirometry**.

• **pulses.** See **pulses.**

• **pure-tone test.** A test of the acuity of hearing simple sounds, such as beeps, at various frequencies (levels of pitch).

• **Quick Test (QT).** An instrument that provides a means of assessing vocabulary quickly; correlates well to an IQ score on the WAIS.

• **Rancho Los Amigos Levels of Cognitive Functioning Scale.** See **Rancho Los Amigos Levels of Cognitive Functioning Scale.**

• **range-of-motion test.** See under **range of motion**.

• **Rappaport Disability Rating Scale.** See **Rappaport Disability Rating Scale**.

• **Rorschach test.** Projective psychological test for evaluating conscious and unconscious personality traits and emotional conflicts through the individual's associations to a set of inkblot patterns.

• **Schuell test, Schuell's Aphasia Inventory.** See **Minnesota test for aphasia**.

• **skin resistance test.** See **dermohmmetry**.

• **skin temperature test.** A diagnostic and prognostic procedure used in peripheral vascular disease. Example: Gibbon-Landis test.

• **Southern California Sensory Integration tests.** A battery of 17 tests of kinesthesia, tactile and visual perception, etc., known since 1971 under the above name, developed in the 1960s by occupational therapist. A. Jean Ayres, and particularly used in the evaluation of perceptual deficits and educational potentials of brain-injured persons.

• **speech reception test.** A test of the acuity of hearing ordinary speech.

• **Stanford-Binet test or intelligence scale, Stanford test.** A psychologic test used to measure intelligence. Based on the original Binet-Simon test (q.v.) of 1905, it was revised in 1916, 1937, and 1960 by psychologists at Stanford University. The first revision was made by Lewis M. Terman (1877–1956), the second and third by Terman and Maude A. Merrill (1888–1978)

• **strength-duration test.** See **strength-duration curve**.

• **stress test.** See **exercise test**.

• **Strong Interest Inventory.** See **Strong Interest Inventory**.

• **Strong-Campbell Interest Inventory (SCII).** See **Strong-Campbell Interest Inventory (SCII).**

• **Study of Values.** See **Study of Values.**

• **sudomotor test.** See **sweat test.**

• **sweat test.**

1. Determination of the degree of sweating in various regions of the skin as a diagnostic aid in peripheral nerve lesions. Also called sudomotor test. Dermohmmetry is one kind of sweat test.
2. Determination of constituents of sweat as a diagnostic aid, as e.g., in cystic fibrosis.

• **TAT.** Thematic Apperception Test. See next entry.

• **Thematic Apperception Test (TAT).** Psychological test in which the subject is asked to tell stories about ambiguous pictures that may be interpreted in different ways, according to the individual's personality.

• **Thomas test.** A test for measuring the degree of hip flexion contracture. The subject lies supine, maximally flexing one hip and knee by holding that knee pressed against the trunk, thus flattening the lumbar spine against the examining table. The other limb is lowered toward the horizontal position; if the thigh reaches that position, it is considered to be in complete extension. Described in 1875 by Hugh Owen Thomas (1834–1891), Liverpool orthopedic surgeon.

• **Thomasat test.** See **Thomasat.**

• **Token Test.** A test of auditory comprehension used for patients with aphasia.

• **TOWER.** See **TOWER.**

• **treadmill exercise test.** Physiologic test of the functional capacity of the heart. It is combined with examination of the heart, notably an electrocardiogram.

• **Trendelenburg test.** See under **Trendelenburg.**

• **two-step exercise test.** Test for coronary insufficiency in which the person makes two steps, nine inches high, repeatedly for 1.5 minutes; a depression of the st segment of the electrocardiogram indicating coronary insufficiency; also called Master's test.

• **VIRO scale.** See **VIRO scale.**

• **vocational evaluation or test.** A comprehensive assessment for determining vocational aptitude and potential. For specific tests, see under **COATS, Hester, JEVS, McCarron-Dial, Singer, tap, tower, Valpar, views,** and **wrest.**

• **Weber hearing test.** The application of a vibrating tuning fork to the midline of the forehead, bridge of the nose, and against the chin, for audiologic assessment.

• **Wechsler Adult Intelligence Scale-Revised (WAIS-R).** See **Wechsler Adult Intelligence Scale–Revised (WAIS-R)**.

• **Wechsler Intelligence Scale for Children (WISC).** See **Wechsler Intelligence Scale (WISC)**.

• **Wechsler Memory Scale.** See **Wechsler Memory Scale**.

• **Wepman and Jones test.** An aphasia test, published as Language Modalities Test for Aphasia in 1961 by speech pathologist Joseph M. Wepman and psychologist Lyle V. Jones

• **Western Aphasia Battery.** See **Western Aphasia Battery**.

• **Wide Range Achievement Test, Revised (WRAT-R).** An instrument that assesses academic achievement in reading, spelling, and arithmetic.

• **Woodcock-Johnson Psycho-Education Battery–Revised (WJ-R).** See **Woodcock-Johnson Psycho-Education Battery–Revised (WJ-R)**.

• **yield test.** See **break test**.

• **Zung Depression Scale.** See **Zung Depression Scale**.

testing board See under **board**.

tetanus-twitch ratio The ratio between the intensity of an electric current required to produce a tetanic contraction and that producing a single contraction. Normal values are 4 to 6. Values between 1 and 2 are found in nerve lesions. Also called galvanic tetanus ratio.

tetra-, tetr- Combining forms denoting four.

thalassotherapy From the Greek *thalassa*, sea. The sojourn on the sea or at the beach and the use of sea water, internally or externally, for therapeutic purposes.

Thematic Apperception Test See under **test**.

therapeutic environment

1. The combination of all external conditions and influences affecting the treatment of a person's disease and/or disability.
2. The surrounding area in which the therapy takes place, including location, objects within the space and health workers' attitudes, actions, and behaviors.

therm- (or thermo-), thermic Referring to heat.

thermatology The study of heat as applied to the treatment of disease.

thermoesthesia The ability to perceive changes in temperature; also called thermesthesia.

thermoplegia Heat stroke.

thermotherapy Treatment by heat of any kind: hot air, hot water, hot pack, infrared radiation, diathermy, etc.

thigh-lacer Thigh corset for a prosthesis or orthosis.

Thomas, Hugh Owen Liverpool orthopedic surgeon (1834–1891).

- **Thomas bar.** Metatarsal bar.

- **Thomas heel.** Shoe heel whose medial part is extended forward to prevent the sagging of the shoe under the longitudinal arch. In the **reverse Thomas heel** the lateral part is extended forward: a right thomas heel is applied to the left shoe and vice versa.

- **Thomas ring.** A padded metal ring embracing the thigh (rarely the arm) at its most proximal level. It is usually attached to a Thomas splint (see next entry) to offer ischial weightbearing.

- **Thomas splint or caliper.** Knee-ankle-foot orthosis consisting of a medial and a lateral steel bar connected proximally by a padded ring (see preceding entry) and distally by a crossbar beyond the foot. Used for fracture of the limb.

- **Thomas test.** A test for determining the degree of hip flexion contracture. See under **test**.

Thomasat An individually administered timed test for the evaluation of the motor skills of the upper limbs. It appraises eye-hand coordination, the ability to grasp, to hold, to stabilize, and to manipulate objects according to size, color, and shape. Developed in 1957, and named after them, by Charles W. Thomas, vocational counselor, and Satoru Izutsu, occupational therapist, at Highland View Hospital, Cleveland, Ohio.

three-track skiing Skiing by unilateral lower-limb amputees. One ski is worn on the remaining foot, and two shorter ones are attached to the lower ends of the ski poles.

through-knee amputation Knee disarticulation.

thumb post A component of an orthosis, it supports the thumb in a generally functional position, a combination of abduction and opposition.

tidal drainage Procedure of automatic irrigation and drainage of the urinary bladder by a system of siphonage triggered at a predetermined intravesical pressure. Used as a means of bladder reeducation in spinal cord lesions.

tidal volume (TV) See **lung volumes and capacities**.

tilt table See under **table**.

timbre The characteristic quality of a sound whereby one may distinguish between two sounds of equal pitch and loudness.

tipping lever One of the two bars that protrude from the rear of a wheelchair, a few centimeters above the floor. The wheelchair pusher applies one foot on it in order to tip the chair back.

TIRR Acronym for Texas Institute for Rehabilitation and Research, in Houston, Texas, where various orthoses were developed, among which the following.

• **TIRR dropfoot brace.** A molded plastic orthosis reaching from the calf over the heel to the sole of the foot, to be worn inside the shoe in case of footdrop. See also **leaf footdrop splint**, under **splint**.

titubation Incoordination manifested during walking. See also **titubating gait**, under **gait**.

toe (of a shoe), toe box The part of a shoe, that covers the forepart of the foot. See also **box toe**.

toe cap The piece of leather or other material that covers the toe of a shoe.

token test See under **test**.

Tonar Acronym for the oral-nasal acoustic ratio. Device to measure and to help in the treatment of the nasality in speech, notably, in patients with cleft palate, various oral lesions, deafness, mental retardation, cerebral palsy, multiple sclerosis, or myasthenia gravis. Developed about 1971 by Dr. Samuel Fletcher, Director of Biocommunications Laboratory, University of Alabama, Birmingham.

tone, tonicity, tonus Applied to a muscle, these terms usually mean the degree of its consistency, elasticity, turgor, contraction, or a combination of these qualities. In a larger sense, tone refers to the physical and mental condition.

tonic A state of sustained muscular contraction.

tonicity The normal condition of tension, as the slight continuous contraction of skeletal muscles; also called tonus.

tonic perseveration Active maintenance by a conscious patient of an imposed (by an examiner) position of his body or part of it, and without apparent conscious attempt to do so. Also called plastic tone. Cf. **clonic perseveration**.

Toronto standing orthosis or brace See under **orthosis**.

Toronto swivel walker See **swivel walk prosthesis**, under **prosthesis**.

total communication Referring to communication of the deaf, it is the combination of multiple means: speech and speechreading, signing, gesturing, pantomime, fingerspelling, reading, writing, amplification by hearing aids, etc.

total lung capacity (TLC) See **lung volumes and capacities**.

Touch and See Nature Trail Nature trail, about one-half kilometer long, built in 1968 in the National Arboretum, Washington, D.C. Markers with legends in braille and large print and a rope railing invite the blind and near-blind to touch trees and other plants, to smell the bark, leaves, flowers, and soil and to listen to the rustling sound of various leaves. See also **trail for all people** and **garden for the blind**.

touch method (or technique) of travel See **cane travel of the blind**.

TOWER An acronym for a work evaluation system designed to assess work habits, readiness for employment, and tolerance for work, wherein T means testing, O means orientation, and wer represents work evaluation in rehabilitation.

• **Micro-TOWER.** A variant of tower, this simplified system of vocational evaluation was developed in 1975. It is applied to groups rather than to individuals. Total testing time is about 15 to 20 hours, so that testing of a group may be completed within three to five days.

trace In muscle testing, a grade applied to a muscle or group of muscles whose contraction is perceptible but not strong enough to result in a motion of the corresponding joint.

traction A therapeutic procedure used to distract joints (vertebral or limb joints), reduce fractures, maintain bone fragments in position, increase joint range, or overcome muscle spasm or shortening of soft tissues.

• **Cotrel traction.** See **EDF**.

• **isometric traction.** Traction in which the respective body segment is immobilized. Example: in traction to the foot in a rigid knee-ankle-foot orthosis with inguinal ring, the knee cannot move.

• **isotonic traction.** Traction in which the respective body segment is allowed to move. Example: skin traction to the lower limb.

• **skeletal traction.** Traction applied through direct fixation to bone, usually by a pin, a wire, or tongs.

• **skin traction.** Traction of a body part by the use of an adhesive bandage, usually adhesive tape or moleskin. In the recumbent patient traction is applied by a weight-and-pulley arrangement.

Trail for All People Nature trail for blind individuals. Example: Harriet L. Keeler Woodland Trail for All People in Cleveland, Ohio. Guidewires and other special adaptations make it possible for a blind person to walk the trail independently. Braille and large-print descriptions of the trail are available. See also **touch and see nature trail** and **garden for the blind**.

trailing The natural method of orientation used by a blind person while walking. The fingers keep contact with furniture, walls, or other objects.

training, autogenic See **Schultz autogenic training**.

training bag A cylinder-shaped leather bag, filled with sawdust and/or cloth, about 1 m long., 30 cm in diameter, and weighing between 20 and 30 kg. It is suspended vertically from the ceiling or other solid support and is used for boxing training.

transducer A device that converts one form of energy into another. A pressure transducer converts pressure pulsations into electric signals. A Doppler ultrasonic transducer detects the Doppler effect (change in the frequency of sound) along a blood vessel

transcutaneous nerve stimulation (TENS) The use of electrical stimulation for pain relief.

transdisciplinary approach A model of team functioning in which communication is lateral, across team members, and also between team members.

transfer A pattern of movements by which the patient moves from one surface to another.

• **lateral transfer.** Sitting transfer.

• **sitting transfer.** Transfer from sitting on one piece of furniture (chair, bed, toilet) to sitting on another next to it, without passing through the upright standing position.

• **sliding transfer.** Transfer in the sitting position, sliding along a transfer board (see under **board**).

• **standing transfer.** Transfer from sitting on one place to sitting on another next to it by momentarily using the standing position.

• **wheelchair transfer.** Transfer from and to the wheelchair.

transfer tub seat Seat attached to a bathtub for the transfer in and out of the tub as well as for use while bathing and drying.

trapeze A short horizontal bar suspended by two ropes above a bed or a chair, providing a hold to a person for rising or for a change of position. The term is also used for a metal triangle suspended from above for the same purpose.

trauma Injury or damage.

traumatic Caused by or related to injury.

traumatize To injure or wound either physically or psychologically.

traumatology The branch of surgery concerned with injuries.

travel aid Usually referring to aids used by blind people. See **mobility aid**, under **aid**.

travel trainer Mobility instructor (q.v.).

travel training Mobility instruction (q.v.).

treadmill A moving belt mechanism that permits individuals to walk or run in a stationary location under controlled conditions; used in studies of physiologic functions, particularly cardiac stress.

treatment The course of action adopted to care for a patient or to prevent disease.

• **conservative treatment.** One in which any radical therapeutic or surgical measures are avoided.

• **drug treatment.** Treatment with medicines.

• **empirical treatment.** One based on experience rather than scientific data.

• **expectant treatment.** One aimed at the relief of symptoms until the nature of the illness is known; also called symptomatic treatment.

• **heroic treatment.** The use of aggressive measures to preserve the life of the patient.

• **palliative treatment.** Treatment aimed at mitigating symptoms rather than curing the disease.

• **preventive treatment, prophylactic treatment.** Treatment instituted to prevent a person from acquiring a disease to which he had been or is expected to be exposed.

• **supportive treatment.** One aimed at maintaining the patient's strength.

treatment tank A tub or other container for hydrotherapy. For examples, see under **tank**.

tremor Trembling; rhythmic, involuntary, alternating contraction of opposing muscle groups, fairly uniform in frequency and amplitude.

Trendelenburg, Friedrich German surgeon (1844–1924).

• **Trendelenburg gait.** Gait resulting from a disturbance in the mechanism of the hip abductors. It is associated with a positive Trendelenburg test (see **Trendelenburg test**, second definition). During stance phase of the involved side, the pelvis cannot be stabilized. Therefore it drops on the side of the swinging lower limb. Also called gluteus medius gait.

Frequently the patient avoids the drop of the pelvis by lateral trunk bending to the side of the supporting limb, i.e., the involved side. This is called **compensated Trendelenburg gait**. A waddling gait results when such compensatory trunk bending occurs bilaterally.

• **Trendelenburg sign.** See **Trendelenburg test**, second definition.

• **Trendelenburg test.**

1. Test of competence of the valves in varicose veins of the lower limb (vena saphena magna). The patient lies supine and raises the involved lower limb. The examiner milks blood out of the

great saphenous vein, then compresses the vein at its proximal end about 5 cm distal to the inguinal ligament. While the vein is being compressed, the patient lowers the limb and stands up. Examiner makes sure the vein remains unfilled. On release of the compression, the vein fills either slowly (negative Trendelenburg test: venous valves intact) or suddenly and copiously (positive Trendelenburg test: valves incompetent).

2. Test of the mechanism of the hip abductors. In standing on one foot on the involved side, the pelvis cannot be fixed. Therefore it drops on the other side (Trendelenburg sign). This can be due to weakness of glutei medius and minimus, subluxation of the hip joint, coxa vara, or ununited fracture of the femoral neck.

• **Trendelenburg waddle.** Waddling gait. See above, under **Trendelenburg gait**.

trick motion See **substitution**.

trigger point Point at which pressure provokes pain or any other phenomenon to a greater degree than in the surrounding area.

trochanter roll A large towel or other textile tightly rolled and placed under the greater trochanter of a patient lying supine in bed, in order to prevent external rotation of the lower limb.

t strap See **ankle strap**, under **strap**.

tuberosity A rounded protuberance from the surface of a bone or cartilage.

turnhall, turnhalle The former is the anglicized word for the latter, German term meaning a hall for gymnastics, or gymnasium. Also a building consisting mainly of a gymnasium. See also next entry and **jahn**.

Turnverein German for gymnastic association. See also preceding entry and **Clias exercises**, under **exercise**.

TV Tidal volume. See **lung volumes and capacities**.

TV-phone A telecommunication device for persons who cannot hear or speak. Like a TDD (q.v.), it comprises a telephone and a typewriter. However, the messages, instead of being recorded on paper, appear on a television (TV) screen.

twister Also called leg rotator, it is a web strap or a metal spiral, which is attached to the waist belt and the shoe in such a way as to impose an external or internal rotation to the limb, depending upon the desired direction. If a web strap is used, it is wound around the limb. If it is a metal spiral (also called cable twister), it runs along the lateral aspect of the limb.

twitch A brief involuntary or spasmodic contraction of a muscle fiber; usually phasic.

typhlocane See under **cane**.

typing stick Adaptive device for typing, either secured to the hand or the forehead or held in the mouth. Used by persons without hand functions.

U

ultrashortwave diathermy See under **diathermy**.

ultrasonic Referring to ultrasound.

ultrasonic blood flow device See **Doppler ultrasonic test**, under **test**.

ultrasound Sound waves that vibrate at frequencies beyond the hearing power of the human ear, i.e., above about 20,000 Hz. The most commonly used frequency for deep tissue heating (ultrasonic diathermy) is 1,000,000 Hz (1 MHz). Ultrasound is also used for diagnostic purposes (see sonogram), destruction of tissues, cleansing of surgical and other instruments, in dentistry, etc.

ultraviolet cabinet A cabinet the interior of which is fitted with ultraviolet lamps. The patient sits or stands in it for total body irradiation. Most often used in extensive psoriasis.

ultraviolet radiation, rays, therapy See under **radiation**.

ultraviolet radiometer Instrument to measure intensities of ultraviolet radiation. One such instrument ranges from 1 $\mu W/cm^2$ to 199.9 mw/cm^2.

UMNL Upper motor neuron lesion.

Uniform Data System for Medical Rehabilitation (UDSMR) A system that incorporates a minimum data set for uniformly describing and communicating information about disability.

unilateral neglect A deficit resulting from central nervous system (cns) damage in which a person ignores the side of the body and/or extrapersonal space opposite to the cns lesion site.

units of measurements For International System of Units, see **SI**. For some applications, see Appendix.

universal gymnastic machine Metal structure combining various devices for resistance exercises, primarily weight lifting. Also called multistation weight training apparatus, it occupies a relatively small space and can be used by up to 12 or more persons at the same time. Developed in 1960 by Harold Zinkin, weight lifter and health club owner in California, with the assistance of Arthur Jones.

Unna (paste) boot or dressing Bandage impregnated with gelatin, zinc oxide, and glycerin, habitually applied to the foot and leg, therefore taking the form of a boot. It aims at the reduction of edema and is used in the treatment of varicose ulcers. Proposed in 1885 by Paul Gerson Unna (1850–1929), dermatologist in Hamburg, Germany.

upper The part of a shoe, that, being attached to the sole and heel, covers the foot. It consists of the vamp and the quarters.

upper motor neuron Motor neuron whose nucleus lies in the brain and which conducts impulses to the nucleus of a cranial or spinal nerve. One of the principal pathways for volitional activity.

upright Part of an orthosis or prosthesis, designed to reenforce the device, to give it some rigidity, to maintain its shape, or to support some other part. Corsets may be fitted with steel, aluminum, or plastic uprights, also called stays. Many leg braces have a medial and a lateral upright.

upright wheeler See **wheelstand**.

V

valgus Latin for turned outward (feminine, **valga**; neuter, **valgum**). This refers to the distal component of various parts of a limb: coxa valga, genu valgum, pes valgus, etc. The plural can be expressed by bilateral coxa valga, etc. Opposite: **varus**.

valgus stiffener A piece of rigid material applied to the medial side of a shoe so as to counteract the faulty position of a pronated foot (pes valgus).

Valpar work sample series A system of vocational evaluation, designed in particular for industrially injured workers by the Valpar Corporation, Tucson, Arizona.

Valsalva procedure or maneuver There are two variants. After a deep inspiration, an expiratory effort is made either against the closed glottis (contracting the abdominal muscles) or against a closed mouth and nose (inflating the auditory [eustachian] tubes). The first variant is often used during a brief muscular effort, the second to adapt oneself to a change in air pressure, e.g., in an airplane during take-off and landing. Named after Antonio Maria Valsalva (1666–1723), Italian anatomist.

vamp The front portion of the upper of a shoe, covering roughly the anterior half of the foot. Cf. **upper**.

vari-gait knee See under **knee**.

varus Latin for turned inward (feminine, **vara**; neuter, **varum**). This refers to the distal component of various parts of a limb: coxa vara, genu varum, tibia vara, pes varus, etc. The plural can be expressed by bilateral coxa vara, etc. Opposite: **valgus**.

vase stance A postural deficiency of the lower limbs: the thighs and knees are tightly adducted, while the feet are farther apart. Hence, in the standing subject, the comparison with a vase.

vaulting Gait deviation in persons with a lower-limb prosthesis. During the stance phase of the uninvolved side there is an exaggerated rise of the body, in order to clear the prosthetic foot.

Velcro Textile closure material consisting of two layers that adhere to each other by virtue of tiny hooks on one layer ("hook" section) interlocking with tiny loops ("loops," "pile," or "eye" section) on the other layer. Glued or sewn on clothing, corsets, shoes, etc. to replace buttons, zipper, buckles, and laces, the two mating surfaces are closed by simple pressure and opened by peeling one strip away from the other. Thus Velcro can be operated with one hand. Invented in 1951 by the Swiss Georges de Mestral and named after the French velours (velvet) and crochet (hook).

ventilator See **respirator**.

Verbo-tonal method A technique of teaching hearing-impaired children and adults.

Verlo Acronym for vertical loading orthosis. See under **orthosis.**

vibration

1. One of the maneuvers of massage, a quivering or trembling motion.
2. The motion performed by a vibrator, an instrument used in massage.

vibrator A hand-held device, electrically set in vibration by either a battery or main line. Depending on its shape and size, it is used over the thorax to assist in postural drainage (q.v.) or over a more or less paralyzed muscle to stimulate its contraction.

vicarious motion See **substitution**.

VIEWS Acronym for Vocational Information and Evaluation Work Samples.

VIRO scale An acronym for vigor, intactness, orientation, and relationship; scale is designed for measuring social skills among persons who are so cognitively impaired that they cannot be expected to respond to a questionnaire approach.

visual communication system Any method or combination of methods replacing the spoken word. Examples: printed or written words, charts, pictures, light signals, three-dimensional models. Used by deaf persons and those with speaking disturbances.

Vita Parcours See **Parcours**.

vocational counselor See **vocational rehabilitation counselor**.

vocational evaluation See under **test**.

Vocational Information and Evaluation Work Samples (VIEWS) A system of vocational evaluation, developed by the Philadelphia Jewish Employment and Vocational Service. See also **JEVS**.

Vocational Rehabilitation Act of 1973 A federal law prohibiting employers who receive funds from federal programs to discriminate against individuals with disabilities.

vocational rehabilitation counselor A rehabilitation counselor (q.v.), most often in a state agency, who specializes in vocational counseling, i.e., guiding handicapped persons in the selection of a vocation or occupation.

vocational rehabilitation therapy (VRT) The name given in 1980 to manual arts therapy in the US Veterans Administration.

voice control See **breath control**.

volar Obsolete term for palmar, plantar, or anterior. It is correctly replaced as shown in the following examples: palmar aspect or palmar flexion (or hand or digits); anterior aspect (of wrist or forearm); plantar aspect or plantar flexion (of foot or toes).

volition Will or voluntary power.

volitional Referring to volition; willed.

volt (v) The unit of electromotive force or the potential difference causing it. A potential difference of one volt produces a current of one ampere when the resistance is one ohm. Named in honor of Alessandro Volta (1745–1827), Italian physicist.

voltage The electromotive force, or difference of potential, as expressed in volts.

voltage-stabilized stimulator See **chronaximeter**.

voltmeter Instrument to measure voltage, i.e., the electromotive force or the difference in electric pressure between the two points it connects.

voluntary-closing device Terminal device of an upper-limb prosthesis, in which the amputee applies force to close it. To open the device, it must first be unlocked by a new motion, after which a spring opens it.

voluntary-opening device Terminal device of an upper-limb prosthesis, in which the amputee applies force to open it, by a shoulder motion transmitted via a cable. A rubber band or spring closes it.

Voss method of exercise See **Knott method of exercise**.

W

W Symbol for watt(s).

waddle Waddling gait. See under **gait**.

WAIS Wechsler Adult Intelligence Scale. See under **test**.

walker

1. Walkerette.
2. Cagelike frame on casters, with supports for the hands, designed to aid the user in standing and walking. Usually includes also a pair of crutch-like axillary supports and a bracket seat. In order to distinguish it from the less bulky walkerette (q.v.), by which it has been more and more supplanted, it is also called large walker, wheelwalker, or casterwalker.

• **casterwalker.** A walker the four legs of which are fitted with casters.

• **folding walker.** A walkerette that can be folded sideways, for easy stowing and transportation.

• **hemiwalker.** Walker-cane combination.

• **pick-up walker.** Walkerette.

• **reciprocal walker.** A walkerette articulated in such a way that either side can be moved independently. Thus, the opposite side (i.e., one pair of legs) maintains its contact with the floor, providing support without interruption.

• **rolling walker.** Any type of walker with casters or wheels.

• **Shrewsbury paraplegic walker.** This is not a walker but a pivot ambulating crutchless orthosis (see under **orthosis**). Developed in Shrewsbury, England, in the early 1970s.

• **stair walker.** A walkerette, also used on stairs, with an additional pair of handles extending backward to provide support when it is in the tilted position, at which time these extra handles are vertically above the supporting lower pair of legs. Therefore, for ascending stairs, the walker is turned around and kept behind and below the user.

• **suspension walker.**
1. A large and high rolling frame from which a harness is suspended to hold a person during ambulation.
2. A walker attached to an overhead trolley, for ambulation training.

• **swivel walker.** Reciprocal walker. The term has also been used for pivot ambulating crutchless orthosis and swivel walk prosthesis (see under **orthosis** and **prosthesis**, respectively).

• **threewheeled walker.** A threelegged casterwalker, hinged at the center post for folding.

walker-cane combination A small walkerette that is held at the side, like a cane, with one hand. The four legs are much closer together than in a regular walker. Most models are collapsible, to take even less space and to be used on stairs.

walkerette A light metal frame on four legs, providing support during standing and walking. After lifting and advancing it (it can also be slid on a very smooth floor), the user steps forward, with the feet either together or one after the other. Also used by subjects with only one foot but good function of upper limbs. So called in order to distinguish it from the larger type (see **walker**, second definition), although it is most often also called walker.

walking See under **gait**.

walking bars Parallel bars. See under **bar, bars**.

walking belt Transfer belt. See under **belt**.

walking frame Walkerette, walker. Term mostly used in the UK.

walking ladder See **foot placement ladder**.

walking parallel bars See **parallel bars**, second definition, under **bar, bars**.

walking path or track A path on the floor, marked by painted foot tracks (see **Frenkel tracks**), by tiles of a special color, or other design, for walking reeducation in locomotor disorders of the lower limbs.

walking skis See under **skis**.

walking stick Term mostly used in the UK for walking cane.

walking tank Wading tank. See under **tank**.

walking trough The lower part of a wading tank (see under **tank**).

walk'n wear footbath boot Plastic boot that holds between 0.5 and 1 L of water. It provides a footbath while its user may walk around.

Wallerian degeneration Degeneration of a motor or sensory nerve fiber, as seen in peripheral nerve disorders. Described by August Volney Waller (1816–1870), British physiologist.

wall pulleys See under **chest weights**.

Warm Springs The name refers either to Georgia Warm Springs Foundation, Warm Springs, Georgia, or to Gonzales Warm Springs Foundation, Gonzales, Texas. It is applied to various orthoses devised in one or the other institution.

Warm Springs corset See **hoke corset**, under **corset**.

waste To emaciate; to grow thin.

wasting Emaciation.

water bed, water mattress See under **bed**.

water cure Obsolete term for spa therapy, including the systematic ingestion of water.

water stretcher See under **stretcher**.

watt (W) A unit of power. In electricity, one watt is the power in a circuit when the intensity is one ampere and the difference of potential is one volt. Named in honor of James Watt (1736–1819), Scottish inventor.

wavelength The distance between two identical points in two adjacent waves.

wax bath British term for paraffin bath. See under **bath**.

Wechsler Intelligence Scale for Children (WISC) The most commonly used instrument to determined global intelligence among children.

Wechsler Memory Scale A test battery designed to measure memory function apart from intelligence.

Wechsler Adult Intelligence Scale-Revised (WAIS-R) The most commonly used instrument to determine global intelligence in an adult population.

wedge suspension Refers to the use of one (medial or lateral) or two wedges placed inside the supracondylar extensions of certain patellar-tendon-bearing prostheses.

weight-and-pulley circuit Combination of weights, pulleys, ropes, and handles, used in weight-and-pulley exercises.

weight boot A bootlike frame weighted with iron (or any other material), used for strengthening exercises, most often of the thigh muscles. Called also iron boot.

weight cuff A cuff for the ankle or the wrist, weighted with lead in amounts from 0.25 to 8 kg or more, for resistance exercises.

Weir Mitchell treatment See **rest cure**.

Wernicke-Korsakoff syndrome Disorder of the central nervous system caused by abusive intake of alcohol and nutritional depletion, especially of thiamine; characterized primarily by sudden weakness and paralysis of eye muscles, double vision, and inability to stand or walk unaided; followed by derangement of mental functions, e.g., confusion, apathy, loss of retentive memory, and confabulation; it may terminate in death.

Western Aphasia Battery A standardized test commonly used by speech/language pathologists to evaluate language disturbances by assessing fluency, information content, comprehension, repetition, and name ability.

wheelchair A chair on wheels that can be propelled by the occupant's action upon it.

• **amputee wheelchair.** Wheelchair in which the rear axle is offset posteriorly, in order to prevent the chair from tipping backwards because of the lack of counterweight in a bilateral leg amputee.

• **collapsible (or folding) wheelchair.** A wheelchair that can be folded either sideways or—more rarely—forward, for easier stowing and transportation, as compared with the chair with a rigid frame.

• **frontwheel-drive wheelchair.** Wheelchair with large wheels in front and casters in the rear.

• **growth wheelchair.** A wheelchair that can be adjusted in its measurements to fit a child during several years of growing.

• **manual wheelchair.** Any wheelchair propelled by the user's hand or hands.

• **one-arm-drive wheelchair.** Wheelchair with two handrims mounted on the same side (left or right) so that one hand can operate them both together to move forward or backward, or separately to turn left or right.

• **rearwheel-drive wheelchair.** The most common type of wheelchair: the large wheels are in the rear, the casters in front. Amputee, sports, and one-arm-drive wheelchairs belong in this category. Cf. **frontwheel-drive wheelchair**.

• **self-propelled wheelchair.** Any wheelchair propelled by the user without help by another person or a motor.

• **sports wheelchair.** Wheelchair reduced in parts and weight to the strictly necessary, so as to give freedom to the upper half of the body and allow for speed in racing, basketball, and other sports.

• **stand-up wheelchair.** A wheelchair that incorporates a support aiding the user in standing up and sitting down; it can also maintain any intermediary position.

• **transit wheelchair.** Folding wheelchair. Term used in the UK.

• **traveler wheelchair.** Frontwheel-drive wheelchair.

• **two-arm-drive wheelchair.** Any wheelchair with one handrim on each side. Its occupant propels it by using both hands.

wheelchair access symbol See **accessibility symbol**.

wheelchair dancing Rhythmic moving, to music, of a wheelchair by its occupant, usually in coordination with a partner or—as in wheelchair square dancing—with several partners.

wheelchair lift See under **lift**.

wheelchair narrower A device that allows the wheelchair user to decrease the width of the chair (even while sitting in it), thus allowing the passage through a narrow doorway. It is commonly a handle connected to the two siderails of the seat that brings them closer together.

wheelchair push-up Pushing oneself up from sitting in a wheelchair by placing the hands on the armrests and straightening the elbows.

wheelchair seatboard A board placed on the hammock seat of a folding wheelchair to overcome the sag.

wheelchair sports Sports performed by wheelchair users. Examples: archery, billiards, bowling, fencing, rifle shooting, table tennis, basketball, volleyball, and track and field sports. The latter include discus, javelin, precision javelin, shotput, dashes, distances, hurdles, and slalom, which is an obstacle course of ramps, curbs, and gates. Wheelchair athletes also compete in weight lifting, performed in the supine position on a bench, and in swimming. A few examples of international class follow; comparable results of unimpaired athletes are added in parentheses. All values are approximate.

Javelin throw, men	37 m (90m)
Javelin throw, women	28 m (60 m)
Discus throw, men	40 m (70 m)
Discus throw, women	25 m (50 m)
Dash, 100 m, men	19 s (10 s)
Dash, 100 m, women	23 s (11 s)
Marathon (42.75 km)	2:00 hrs (2:15 hrs)

For wheelchair sports contests, see **National Wheelchair Games, Paralympics**, and **Special Olympics**.

wheelchair tray Wheelchair lapboard. See **lapboard**, under **board**.

wheelie Colloquialism for tiling the wheelchair backward while sitting in it, to raise its front. A wheelie is of value for a quick change of direction and for overcoming a curb or other obstacles.

wheel peg One of several extensions (usually 6 to 8) attached to the handrim of a wheelchair, offering a better grip for its propulsion. Used in case of deformity or extreme weakness of the hand.

wheelstand A platform on wheels for self-propulsion in the standing position. Most often used by paraplegic individuals, and only indoors. Also called rolling stand or mobile stander.

whip Gait deviation in persons with a lower-limb prosthesis, referring to the motion of the heel during the swing phase. The heel deviates medially (medial whip) or laterally (lateral whip) from a straight line.

whirlpool bath Bath in which the water is swirled by a powered device, as in a whirlpool tank.

whirlpool tank See **tank**.

Wide Range Achievement Test, Revised (WRAT-R) See under **test**.

Wide Range Employment Sample Test (WREST) A system of vocational evaluation, particularly for mentally retarded and physically disabled individuals.

Williams brace See under **brace**.

Williams exercises, Williams flexion regime See **Williams flexion exercises**, under **exercise**.

Wimshurst machine An induction type of static machine (q.v.), developed by English engineer James Wimshurst (1832–1903).

WISC Wechsler Intelligence Scale for Children. See under **test**.

wogging Term formed by combining the words "walking" and "jogging," to mean walking at different rates, from brisk to rapid, as advocated in 1978 by New Jersey physician Thomas W. Patrick Jr., who coined the term.

Wood, Robert Williams American physicist (1868–1955), who in 1903 invented the filter and lamp described in the following.

• **Wood filter or glass.** Glass containing nickel oxide, opaque for most visible radiations but transparent for ultraviolet radiations between 330 and 390 nm (maximum at ca. 365 nm).

• **Wood lamp.** A mercury-vapor source of ultraviolet radiation with a Wood filter. The passing rays with wavelengths centered around 365 nm induce fluorescence in certain dermatologic diseases, especially some fungus infections. Used in the diagnosis of such lesions, in other clinical investigations, and in the treatment of vitiligo.

• **Wood light.** Ultraviolet radiations obtained from a Wood lamp (see preceding two entries). These radiations are also called near or longwave ultraviolet rays or black light.

Woodcock-Johnson Psycho-Educational Battery-Revised (WJ-R) A series of 35 subtests that assess cognitive ability and academic achievement.

work hardening A physical rehabilitation program that uses graded work tasks to progressively increase the bodily strength, mobility, flexibility, and endurance necessary to return to work.

work disability A health problem or disability that prevents persons from working or that limits the kind or amount of work they can perform.

work therapy Therapeutic use of work, with or without remuneration. In some instances it might be the same as industrial therapy.

- **compensated work therapy.** Incentive therapy (q.v.).

work tray Lapboard. See under **board**.

WREST Wide Range Employment Sample Test (q.v.).

Wright's relaxation A method of general relaxation.

wrist flexion unit A device designed to set the hook of an upper-limb prosthesis into some degree of palmar flexion. Used especially by bilateral amputees for activities close to the body.

wristlet Device of leather, canvas, or similar material, applied to the wrist in order to support or protect it or to limit its motions.

wrist roll A set of cylinders of various diameters, usually of wood and mounted on a wall, to be grasped and rolled for dorsiflexion and palmar flexion exercise of the wrist. It commonly includes a mechanism for variable resistance.

wrist unit Part of an upper-limb prosthesis that provides a means of connecting the forearm with the terminal device (hand or hook) and of rotating the latter into a position of pronation or supination.

X

XBX Abbreviation for ten (Roman numeral) basic exercises. See **Royal Canadian Air Force Exercises**, under **exercise**.

Y

yawn box Incentive spirometer. See under **spirometer**.

yoga Named after the Sanskrit word for "union" (which refers to the union of the human spirit with the infinite), this is a very old Hindu philosophy that includes religious features and the practice of mental and physical exercises. The latter are the subject of **hatha yoga**, one of several parts of the yoga doctrine. It comprises relaxation, breathing education, isometric contractions called *bandhas*, and the assumption of a certain number of positions called *asanas*, all of which are aimed at attaining physical, mental, and emotional well-being.

Y strap See under **strap: ankle strap** and **inverted Y strap**.

Z

Z Symbol for electric impedance (virtual resistance).

Zander, Jonas Gustav Wilhelm Swedish physician (1835–1920), who in 1865 established his Mechanico-Therapeutic Institution in Stockholm.

• **Zander apparatus.** Any of the numerous apparatuses or machines for exercise therapy, invented by Zander. Some of them are powered and impose passive movements upon the body; others impose a resistance to a given movement. Characteristically, they allow motion in only one plane.

• **Zander exercise.** Mechanotherapy with any of the apparatuses devised by Zander. The exercises may be of passive, active, or resistive type.

zero (0)

1. A grade in manual muscle testing, denoting absence of any visible or palpable contraction.
2. A grade in range-of-motion testing, denoting the zero position.

• **absolute zero.** See under **kelvin**.

zero cerebral muscle (0 c muscle) A muscle with loss of isolated voluntary motion, due to a cerebral lesion. It might still contract as part of a reflex. See also **confusion pattern**.

zero method See **neutral zero method**.

zero position See under **position**.

zone therapy Treatment that consists in the mechanical stimulation of an area located in the same longitudinal zone as the disorder. Called also Fitz Gerald method or treatment, after its proponent, William H. H. Fitz Gerald (1872–1939), American physician.

Zung Depression Scale An instrument commonly used to evaluate depression.

SECTION II

REHABILITATION ORGANIZATIONS

SELECTED NATIONAL AND INTERNATIONAL ASSOCIATIONS

AFTER Rehabilitation and Training Center for Limb Birth Deficiencies/Amputations
2559 Fairway Island Dr.
West Palm Beach, FL 33414
Phone: (407) 790-3589
May La Medica, Dir.

Founded: 1979. **Description**. Participants include social workers, physical and occupational therapists, psychologists, and parents of children with limb deficiencies caused by birth defects or amputations. Seeks to improve the self-image and independence of limb-deficient children; promotes public awareness of the needs of these children. Maintains support groups, conducts social activities, provides information, and offers referral services to their families. Operates Rehabilitation and Education Center, plans to maintain Sports and Education Center and provide psychological therapy on a sliding fee scale. **Formerly**: (1988) Amputees for Training, Education, and Rehabilitation.

American Academy of Physical Medicine and Rehabilitation (AAPMR)
122 South Michigan Ave., Ste. 1300
Chicago, IL 60603
Phone: (312) 922-9366
Fax: (312) 922-6754
Ronald A. Heinrichs, Exec. Dir.

Founded: 1938. **Members**: 3,200. **Description**: All members are certified as Diplomates of the American Board of Physical Medicine and Rehabilitation. Promotes the art and science of medicine and betterment of public health through an understanding and utilization of the functions and procedures of physical medicine and rehabilitation. Educational focus of the academy is on continuing education of physicians in physical medicine and rehabilitation. Sponsors continuing education courses. Bestows award. **Publications**: *American Academy of Physical Medicine and Rehabilitation Membership Directory, Archives of Physical Medicine and Rehabilitation, The Physiatrist.* **Formerly**: (1956) American Society of Physical Medicine and Rehabilitation.

American Association for Rehabilitation Therapy (AART)
P.O. Box 93
North Little Rock, AR 72115
Clarence English, Executive Officer

Founded: 1950. **Members**: 400. **Description**. Professional society of medical rehabilitation therapists and specialists and others interested in vocational rehabilitation of the mentally and physically disabled. Works to promote the use and advance the practice of curative technical and educational modalities within approved medical concepts of rehabilitation medicine; establish and advance standards of education and training of rehabilitation therapists and specialists; foster study and research; cooperate with other professional organizations with common objectives. **Publications**: *Newsletter, Rehabilitation Bulletin*.

American Board of Physical Medicine and Rehabilitation (ABPMR)
Northwest Center, Ste. 675
21 1st St., SW
Rochester, MN 55902
Phone: (507) 282-1776
Dr. Joachim L. Opitz, Exec. Dir.

Founded: 1947. **Description**: Certification board to establish qualifications, conduct examinations, and certify physicians whom the Board finds qualified to specialize in physical medicine and rehabilitation. **Publications**: Information booklet.

American Center for the Alexander Technique (ACAT)
129 W. 67th St.
New York, NY 10023
Phone: (212) 799-0408
Kathryn M. Miranda, Exec. Dir.

Founded: 1904. **Members**: 80. **Description**: Promotes the Alexander Technique, an educational technique that enables individuals to use their bodies with ease, grace, and flexibility and freedom from strain in any physical activity. Formed to assure further development of the technique in this country and to maintain its standards. **Publications**: *ACAT News*, newsletter.

American Congress of Rehabilitation Medicine (ACRM)
5700 Old Orchard Rd., 1st Fl.
Skokie, IL 60077
Phone: (708) 966-0095
Fax: (708) 966-918
Irene A. Tesitor, Exec. Dir.

Founded: 1921. **Members**: 3,300. **Description**: Physicians, surgeons, and other allied health specialists active in and contributing to advancement in the field of rehabilitation medicine. **Publication**: *Archives of Physical Medicine and Rehabilitation, Membership Directory*.

American Horticultural Therapy Association (AHTA)
362A Christopher Ave.
Gaithersburg, MD 20079
Phone: (301) 948-3010
Steven Davis, Dir.

Founded: 1973. **Members**: 690. **Description**: Professional horticultural therapists and rehabilitation specialists; horticultural therapy students. Promotes and encourages the development of horticulture and related activities as a therapeutic and rehabilitative medium. Horticultural therapy is considered particularly useful in the field of geriatrics and with regard to the mentally handicapped. Coordinates efforts of professional and educational organizations and conducts professional consultations. Operates placement service; provides resource information. **Publications**: *American Horticultural Therapy Association Newsletter; Journal of Therapeutic Horticulture; Organizing a Horticultural Therapy Workshop*.

American Kinesiotherapy Association (AKA)
c/o Ed Reiling
P.O. Box 611, Wright Brothers Sta.
Dayton, OH 45409
Phone: 800-26-0266
David Ser, Exec. Dir.

Founded: 1946. **Members**: 1,000. **Description**: Professional society of kinesio- and exercise therapists and associate and student members with interest in physical and mental rehabilitation and adapted physical education. Promotes and sponsors medically prescribed rehabilitation program; advances standards of education and clinical training in this field; encourages research and publication of articles dealing with therapeutic exercise. **Publications**: *American Kinesiotherapy Journal, Newsletter, Career in Kinesiology*. **Formerly** (1968) Association for Physical and Mental Rehabilitation; (1987) American Corrective Therapy Association.

American Massage Therapy Association (AMTA)
1130 West North Shore Ave.

Chicago, IL 60626
Phone: (312) 761-2682
Fax: (312) 761-0009
Flint Greene, Pres.

Founded: 1943. **Members**: 14,000. **Description**: Massage therapists or technicians. Provides referrals to area therapists and certified schools. Conducts community outreach programs and research and educational projects. Accredits massage training programs and offers a national certification program for massage therapists. **Publications**: *Hands On, Massage Therapy Journal, Membership Registry*. **Formerly**: American Association of Masseurs and Masseuses; (1983) American Massage and Therapy Association.

American Occupational Therapy Association (AOTA)
1383 Piccard Dr.
P.O. Box 1725
Rockville, MD 20849
Phone: (301) 948-9626
Fax: (301) 948-5529
Jeanette Blair, Exec. Dir.

Founded: 1917. **Members**: 45,000. **Description**: Registered occupational therapists and certified occupational therapy assistants who provide services to people whose lives have been disrupted by physical injury or illness, developmental problems, the aging process or social or psychological difficulties. Occupational therapy focuses on the active involvement of the patient in specially designed therapeutic tasks and activities to improve function, performance capacity, and the ability to cope with demands of daily living. Conducts research program and compiles statistics. **Publications**: *American Journal of Occupational Therapy, Occupational Therapy Week*; also publishes a catalog with more than 100 single titles. **Formerly**: National Society for the Promotion of Occupational Therapy.

American Physical Therapy Association (APTA)
1111 N. Fairfax St.
Alexandria, VA 22314
Phone: (703) 684-2782
William D. Coughlan, CEO

Founded: 1921. **Members**: 53,456. **Description**: Professional organization of physical therapists and physical therapist assistants and students. Fosters the development and improvement of physical therapy service, education, and research; evaluates the organization and administration of curricula; directs the maintenance of standards and promotes scientific research. Acts as an accrediting body for educational programs in physical therapy and is responsible for establishing standards. **Publications**: *American Physical Therapy Association Progress Report, Clinical Management in Physical Therapy, PT Bulletin, Today's Student in PT*. **Formerly**: (1922) American Women's Physical Therapeutic Association; (1949) American Physiotherapy Association.

American Psychological Association (APA)
750 First St., NE
Washington, DC 20002-4242
Phone: (202) 336-5500
Raymond D. Fowler, Exec. Dir.

Founded: 1892. **Members**: 120,000. **Description**: Psychologists who are active in advancing psychology as a science, as a professional, and as a means of promoting human welfare. It attempts to accomplish these objectives by holding annual meetings, publishing psychological journals, and working towards improved standards for psychological training and service. **Publications**: The APA publishes 29 periodicals, a monthly newspaper, books and a membership directory.

American Rehabilitation Counseling Association (ARCA)
c/o American Counseling Association
5999 Stevenson Ave.
Alexandria, VA 22304
Phone: (703) 823-9000
Fax: (703) 823-0252
Dr. Theodore P. Romley, Jr., Exec. Dir.

Founded: 1958. **Members**: 3,000. **Description**: A division of the American Counseling Association. Rehabilitation counselors and interested professionals and students. Purpose is to improve the rehabilitation counseling profession and its service to individuals with disabilities. Promotes high standards in rehabilitation counseling, practice, research, and education. Encourages the exchange of information between rehabilitation professionals and consumer groups. Serves as liaison among members and public and private rehabilitation counselors across the country. **Publications**: *ARCA News, Rehabilitation Counseling Bulletin.*

American Therapeutic Recreation Association (ATRA)
P.O. Box 15215
Hattiesburg, MS 39404
Phone: 800-553-0304
Fax: (601) 264-3337
Lamar Evans, Adm. Dir.

Founded: 1984. **Members**: 2,500. **Description**. Therapeutic recreational professionals and students, interested others. Promotes the use of therapeutic recreation in hospitals, mental rehabilitation centers, physical rehabilitation centers, senior citizen treatment centers, and other public health facilities. Conducts discussions on certification and legislative and regulatory concerns that affect the industry. **Publications**: *Employment Update, Newsletter, The Therapeutic Recreation Journal.*

Association of Academic Physiatrists (AAP)
7100 Lakewood Bldg., Ste. 112
5987 E. 71st St.
Indianapolis, IN 46220
Phone: (317) 845-4200
Fax: (317) 845-4299
Carolyn L. Braddom, Ed.D., Exec. Dir.

Founded: 1967. **Members**: 1,000. **Description**: Academic physicians practicing physical medicine and rehabilitation and certified by the American Board of Physical Medicine and Rehabilitation. Objectives include advancement of teaching and research in physical medicine and rehabilitation, and exchanging information. **Publications**: *American Journal of Physical Medicine and Rehabilitation, Membership Directory, Newsletter, Residency Program Directory.*

Association of Medical Rehabilitation Administrators (AMRA)
Children's Hospital & Health Center
8001 Frost Ave.
San Diego, CA 92123

Founded: 1953. **Members**: 250. **Description**: People engaged in administering medical rehabilitation programs for federal, state, and nongovernmental hospitals and centers. Fosters the concept of total rehabilitation for all disabled persons through coordination of multimedical specialties and the integration of such treatment with other medical, social, and economic aspects of a patient's rehabilitation.

Maintains American Board for Certification of Medical Rehabilitation Administrators. **Publications**: *Journal of Medical Rehabilitation Administration, Membership Directory*. **Formerly**: (1989) Association of Medical Rehabilitation Directors and Coordinators.

Association of Play Therapy
c/o Kevin O'Connor
California School of Professional Psychology
1350 M St.
Fresno, CA 93721
Phone: (209) 486-0851
Fax: (209) 486-0734
Kevin O'Connor, Exec. Dir.

Founded: 1982. **Members**: 2,900. **Description**: Professionals and students involved in play therapy. Promotes interests of members. **Publications**: *Association for Play Therapy Newsletter, International Journal of Play Therapy*.

Commission on Accreditation of Rehabilitation Facilities (CARF)
101 N. Wilmot Rd., Ste. 500
Tucson, AZ 85711
Phone: (602) 748-1212
Alan H. Toppel, Exec. Dir.

Founded: 1966. **Description**: Sponsored by 31 rehabilitation/habilitation organizations. The commission is the standard setting and accrediting authority for organizations providing services to people with disabilities. Encourages development and improvement of uniformly high standards of performance for all organizations servicing individuals with developmental, physical, or emotional disabilities. Surveys and accredits rehabilitation/habilitation organizations; conducts research and educational activities related to standards for organizations offering programs in comprehensive inpatient rehabilitation, spinal cord injury, chronic pain management, brain injury, outpatient medical rehabilitation, work hardening, vocational evaluation, and work adjustment. **Publications**: *CARF Report, Standards Manual for Organizations Serving People with Disabilities*.

Council on Rehabilitation Education (CRE)
P.O. Box 1788
Champaign, IL 61824

Phone: (217) 333-6688
Fax: (217) 244-6784
Elmer Broadbent, Exec. Dir.

Founded: 1972. **Members**: 5. **Description**: American Rehabilitation Counseling Association, Council of State Administrators of Vocational Rehabilitation, National Association of Rehabilitation Facilities, National Council on Rehabilitation Education, and the National Rehabilitation Counseling Association. Promotes effective delivery of rehabilitation services to people with disabilities. Surveys, critiques, and works to improve rehabilitation educational programs at the postgraduate level. **Publications**: *CORE News.*

Council of State Administrators of Vocational Rehabilitation (CSAVR)
P.O. Box 3776
Washington, DC 20007
Joseph H. Owens, Exec. Dir.

Founded: 1940. **Members**: 83. **Description**: Administrators of state vocational rehabilitation agencies. To serve as an advisory body to federal agencies and the public in the development of policies affecting rehabilitation of handicapped persons; to act as a forum for discussion on the provision of quality rehabilitation services. **Publications**: *CSAVR Memorandum, Proceedings of Conferences, State Rehabilitation Directors.*

Delta Society (DS)
P.O. Box 1080
321 Burnett Ave., S.
Benton, WA 98057
Phone: (206) 226-7357
Fax: (206) 235-1076

Founded: 1977. **Members**: 2,600. **Description**: Doctors, nurses, veterinarians, therapists, nursing home personnel, animal trainers and breeders, pet owners; psychology, therapeutic recreation, and other health fields. Seeks to study human-animal interactions and examine the bond that exists between people and the living environment. Assesses the role of animal companions in society and studies the effect of human-animal bonds on the mental and physical well-being of people. Seeks to establish an interdisciplinary approach to studying human-animal interactions and to increase awareness of these interactions among health and social care professionals. **Publications**: *Alert, Anthrozoos: A Multidisciplinary Journal on the Interactions of People, Animals, and Nature, InterActions.*

International Association of Laryngectomees (IAL)
c/o American Cancer Society
1599 Clifton Rd., NE
Atlanta, GA 30329
Phone: (404) 320-3333

Founded: 1952. **Description**: Persons who have had their larynxes removed, physicians, surgeons, speech therapists, rehabilitation experts, nurses, and others interested in the rehabilitation of laryngectomees. Encourages exchange of ideas and methods for training and teaching of alaryngeal methods of communication. Fosters recognized standards for the rehabilitation of laryngectomees. Maintains the Voice Rehabilitation Institute for training teachers of esophageal voice and the Lost Chord Clubs. **Publications**: Director, *IAL News.*

International Federation of Physical Medicine and Rehabilitation
Department of Rehabilitation Medicine
Mt. Sinai Hospital
800 University Ave.
Toronto, ON, Canada M6G 1X5
Phone: (416) 586-5033
Fax: (416) 586-8771
Jose Jimenez, M.D., Sec.

Founded: 1950. **Members**: 30. **Description**: National societies of physical medicine and rehabilitation controlled by and composed of qualified physicians and surgeons and approved by the federation's Internal Committee of Physical Medicine and Rehabilitation. Seeks to link, on an international level, societies of physical medicine and rehabilitation. Collects and distributes data on rehabilitation. Promotes equivalent standards in education and training, the total rehabilitation process, the importance of physical medicine and rehabilitation, and the exchange of information between medical and nonmedical workers in the field of rehabilitation. **Publications**: *Regulations and List of Members, White Book on Education and Training.*

International Rehabilitation Medicine Association (IRMA)
Dept. of Physical Medicine

1333 Moursund Ave., Rm. A-221
Houston, TX 77030
Phone: (713) 799-6066
Fax: (713) 799-5058
Donna Jones, Exec. Dir.

Founded: 1966. **Members**: 2,000. **Description**: Physicians from all specialties of medicine and surgery interested in promoting improvement of health through understanding and utilization of rehabilitation medicine. Goal is to convince governments and society that rehabilitation medicine services should be provided to aged, chronically diseased, and disabled persons who need help in entering the vocational and social mainstream of their communities. Provides a forum for continuous graduate medical education; provides speakers on rehabilitation medicine. **Publications**: *Book of Abstracts, Directory News and Views, Scientific Monographs.*

Laughter Therapy (LT)
2360 Nichols Canyon Rd.
Los Angeles, CA 90040
Phone: (213) 851-3394
Allen A. Funt, Pres.

Founded: 1981. **Description**: To supply tapes of *Candid Camera* to patients, nursing homes, doctors, hospices, and clinics. (*Candid Camera* was a regular weekly comedy series on CBS that ran from 1960 to 1967 and was produced by Allen Funt. The program displayed people from all walks of life and their reactions to strange or unexpected occurrences or situations.)

Medical and Sports Music Institute of America (MSMIA)
P.O. Box 70601
Eugene, OH 97401
Phone: (503) 344-5323
Fax: (503) 344-2925
James Sundquist, Pres.

Founded: 1985. **Description**: Develops and manufactures audio and videocassettes for exercise, insomnia, and stress management. Seeks to improve and maintain fitness levels for cardiac, drug, and physical rehabilitation.

National Association of Rehabilitation Facilities (NARF)
P.O. Box 17675

Washington, DC 20041
Phone: (703) 648-9300
Fax: (703) 648-0346
James Studzinski, Dir.

Founded: 1969. **Members**: 812. **Description**: Rehabilitation facilities in the U.S. and Canada; agencies operating established medical residential and vocational rehabilitation facilities. Promotes expansion and improvement of rehabilitation services to disabled persons as provided in rehabilitation facilities. Represents the concerns of rehabilitation providers before Congress and government agencies, is concerned with quality operation of rehabilitation centers and facilities. Conducts research and development programs in national rehabilitation policy. Maintains collection of periodicals, publications, and reprints on rehabilitation center services. **Publications**: *Rehabilitation Review, Newsletter*. **Formerly**: (1975) International Association of Rehabilitation Facilities; (1980) Association of Rehabilitation Facilities.

National Association of Rehabilitation Instructors (NARI)
633 S. Washington
Alexandria, VA 22314
Phone: (703) 836-0850
Fax: (703) 836-0840
Mary Chandler, Pres.

Members: 325. **Description**: Objective is to promote rehabilitation of all persons with disabilities. Acts as a medium through which rehabilitation instructors can coordinate their efforts with other instructors, facilities, workshops, individuals, and organizations serving persons with disabilities. **Publications**: *Bulletin*.

National Association of Rehabilitation Professionals in the Private Sector (NARPPS)
P.O. Box 697
Brookline, MA 02146
Phone: (617) 556-4432
Fax: (617) 556-0180
Bonnie Shelton, Exec. Dir.

Founded: 1977. **Members**: 3,500. **Description**: Private rehabilitation companies, insurance companies, rehabilitation nurses, and rehabilitation professionals in the private sector. Seeks to promote the field of private rehabilitation and to provide for information exchange on rehabilitation issues and techniques. **Publications**: *NAPPS Journal and News, National Directory of Rehabilitation Professionals, Vocational/Medical Facilities.*

National Council on Rehabilitation Education (NCRE)
c/o Dr. Garth Eldredge
Utah State Univ.
Dept. of Special Education
Logan, UT 84322
Phone: (801) 750-3241
Fax: (801) 750-3572

Founded: 1961. **Members**: 540. **Description**: Academic institutions and organizations; professional educators, researchers, and students. Goals are to assist in the documentation of the effect of education in improving services to persons with disability; determine the skills and training necessary for effective rehabilitation services; develop role models, standards, and uniform licensure and certification requirements for rehabilitation personnel; interact with consumers and public and private sector policy-makers. **Publications**: *Membership Directory; Rehabilitation Education; NCRE Newsletter.*

National Rehabilitation Association (NRA)
633 S. Washington St.
Alexandria, VA 22314
Phone: (703) 836-0850
Fax: (703) 836-0848
Dr. Ann Tourigny, Exec. Dir.

Founded: 1925. **Members**: 17,000. **Description**: Physicians, counselors, therapists, disability examiners, vocational evaluators, and others interested in rehabilitation of persons with disabilities. **Publications**: *Journal of Rehabilitation; NRA Newsletter; Report of the May E. Switzer Memorial Seminar*, monograph series.

National Rehabilitation Counseling Association (NRCA)
1910 Association Dr., Ste. 206
Reston, VA 22081
Phone: (703) 620-4404
Robert Neuman, Pres.

Founded: 1950. **Members**: 4,500. **Description**: A division of the National Rehabilitation Association. Professional and student rehabilitation counselors. Works to expand the role of counselors in the rehabilitation process and seeks to advance members' professional development. **Publications**: *Journal of Applied Rehabilitation Counseling, Professional Report of the National Rehabilitation Counseling Association.*

National Rehabilitation Information Center (NARIC)
8455 Colesville Rd., Ste. 935
Silver Spring, MD 20910
Phone: (301) 588-9284
Fax: (301) 587-1967
Mark Odum, Dir.

Founded: 1977. **Description**: Purpose is to improve delivery of information to the rehabilitation community. Maintains library of research reports, conference proceedings, books, microfiche, audiovisual material, material on individuals with sensory, physical, mental, or psychiatric disabilities, over 300 journals on the rehabilitation of persons with physical and mental disabilities. Disseminates the findings of programs funded by National Institute on Disability and Rehabilitation Research. **Publications**: *Directory of Librarians and Information Specialists in Disability and Rehabilitation, Guide to Disability and Rehabilitation Periodicals, Rehabdata Thesaurus, NARIC Quarterly.*

National Therapeutic Recreation Society (NTRS)
2775 S. Quincy St., Ste. 300
Arlington, VA 22206
Phone: (703) 820-4940
Fax: (703) 671-6772
Rikki S. Epstein, Prog. Mgr.

Founded: 1966. **Members**: 3,200. **Description**: Professional personnel whose full-time employment is to provide therapeutic recreation services to persons with disabilities in clinical facilities and in the community. Offers technical services and consulting to agencies, institutions, and individuals on matters related to the field. Encourages professional growth through studies and workshops. **Publications**: *NTRS Newsletter, Recreation Access in the 90's, Therapeutic Recreation Journal.*

Neurodevelopmental Treatment Association (NDTA)
P.O. Box 70
Oak Park, IL 60303

Phone: (706) 366-2454
Carol Kinsey, Exec. Sec.

Founded: 1967. **Members**: 4,000. **Description**: Physical and occupational therapists, speech pathologists, special educators, physicians, parents, and others interested in neurodevelopmental treatment. (NDT is a form of therapy for individuals who suffer from central nervous system disorders resulting in abnormal movement. Treatment attempts to initiate or refine normal stages and processes in the development of movement.) **Publications**: *Membership Directory, NDTA Newsletter.*

Rehabilitation International (RI)
25 E. 21st St.
New York, NY 10010
Phone: (212) 420-1500
Fax: (212) 505-0871

Founded: 1922. **Members**: 145. **Description**: Organizations in 83 countries conducting programs for the rehabilitation of people with physical and mental disabilities. Disseminates information on every phase of disability prevention and rehabilitation. Assists experts in planning work or study programs outside their own countries. Aids in practical development of national rehabilitation programs. **Publications**: *Directory, International Journal of Rehabilitation Research, International Rehabilitation Review, Proceedings of World Congress, Rehabilitation* (in Spanish).

U.S. Physical Therapy Association (USPTA)
1803 Avon Ln.
Arlington Heights, IL 60004
James J. McCoy, Pres.

Founded: 1970. **Members**: 12,700. **Description**: Professional physical therapists and assistants. Maintains U.S. Physical Therapy Academy, which conducts continuing education programs for members; sponsors workshops to acquaint personnel from other medical fields with physical therapy; accredits hospital and nursing home physical therapy departments, universities, and colleges of physical therapy; certifies physical therapists through board examinations. **Publications**: *Journal.*

SELECTED RESEARCH CENTERS AND INSTITUTES

Auburn University
Center for Special Services

Library Tower, 9th Fl.
7300 University Dr.
Montgomery, AL 36117
Phone: (205) 244-3468
Nancy McDaniel, Ed.D., Dir.

Research Activities and Fields: Works with existing agencies and information sources in securing data and services to meet the needs of Alabama's citizens and students with disabilities. Activities include development and implementation of postsecondary intervention program related to disabilities.

Dallas Rehabilitation Institute
9713 Harry Hines Blvd.
Dallas, TX 75220
Phone: (214) 358-6000
Fax: (214) 358-8453

Research Activities and Fields: Provides treatment and assesses physical disabilities, including those associated with spinal cord injury, head injury, stroke, arthritis, amputations, spinal pain, and other orthopedic or neuromuscular problems. Conducts cooperative studies on a human performance measurement system designed to assess 500 aspects of human performance.

Georgia Institute of Technology
Center for Rehabilitation Technology
490 10th St.
Atlanta, GA 30332
Phone: (404) 894-4960
Fax: (404) 853-9320
James C. Toler, Dir.

Research Activities and Fields: Develops equipment and procedures that help persons with disabilities to function effectively in various environments. Maintains design and development laboratories and a national information center for the collection and dissemination of information on all aspects of rehabilitation.

Harvard University/Massachusetts Institute of Technology
Rehabilitation Engineering Research Center

Massachusetts Institute of Technology
77 Massachusetts Ave., Rm. 2-137
Cambridge, MA 02139
Phone: (617) 253-8112
Fax: (617) 258-5802
Prof. Robert W. Mann, Dir.

Research activities and Fields: Development of quantitative measures of functional performance of persons with disabilities and of the technology to ameliorate various disabilities, including computer-aided surgical stimulation, gait analysis and synovial joint function, upper and lower extremity amputation prostheses, tremor and spasticity diagnosis and treatment, and functional neuromuscular stimulation.

Institute for Rehabilitation and Research
1333 Moursund Ave.
Houston, TX 77030
Phone: (713) 799-5000
Fax: (713) 797-5289
Charles C. Beall, Pres.

Research Activities and Fields: Clinical neurophysiologic, neuroendocrinologic, psychologic, and exercise tolerance studies of patients with severe spinal injuries; development and assessment of mechanical and electronic assistive devices for neurologically impaired individuals.

International Center for the Disabled (ICD)
340 E. 24th St.
New York, NY 10010
Phone: (212) 679-0100
Herbert H. Krauss, Ph.D., Dir. of Rehabilitation Research

Research Activities and Fields: Conducts research on promising techniques designed to prevent, reduce, and control disabilities arising from persistent physical disorders. Studies focus on the control of deterioration and disability associated with recurring ear infections in children, symptom magnification in those with disabling conditions, and factors associated with gainful employment.

Irene Walter Johnson Institute of Rehabilitation
509 S. Euclid Ave.

Box 8062
St. Louis, MO 63110
Dr. Thomas Thatch, Dir.

Research Activities and Fields: Conducts research into chronic diseases, neuromuscular function, biochemical basis for increases in muscle work-capacity with endurance exercise, rehabilitation procedure, and development of new methods of treatment of those diseases.

Kennedy Krieger Institute
707 N. Broadway
Baltimore, MD 21205
Phone: (410) 550-9483
Fax: (410) 550-9344
Gary W. Goldstein, M.D., Pres.

Research Activities and Fields: Pediatric rehabilitation evaluation, treatment and research including interdisciplinary studies in genetics, biochemistry, toxicology, neurochemistry, metabolic diseases, speech and hearing, and special education. Major emphasis is placed on physical rehabilitation, effectiveness of drug support, behavior modification, and developing and testing training techniques.

New York University
Medical Center Head Trauma Program
345 E. 24th St., Rm. 818
New York, NY 10010
Phone: (212) 263-6806
Fax: (212) 263-6807
Yehuda Ben-Yishay, Co-Director

Research Activities and Fields: Young adults suffering from head injuries. Conducts systematic remedial training in attention and concentration, various aspects of perception, perceptual-motor integration, and logical reasoning and interpersonal skills.

New York University
Medical Rehabilitation Research and Training Center
400 E. 34th St.
New York, NY 10016
Mathew Lee, M.D., Acting Chm.

Research Activities and Fields: Rehabilitation for brain trauma and stroke victims and comprehensive management of neuromuscular disease. Seeks to identify and validate specific treatment modalities applied to persons disabled by neuromuscular disorders, develop and improve new and existing treatment modalities, and quantify and standardize methods of evaluating disease activity and remission.

Northwestern University
Research and Training Center for Prevention and Treatment of Secondary Complications of Spinal Cord Injury
Rehabilitation Institute of Chicago
345 S. Superior St., 15th Fl.
Chicago, IL 60611
Phone: (312) 908-6207
Fax: (312) 908-2208
Zev Rymer, M.D., Ph.D., Dir.

Research Activities and Fields: Prevention of pressure sores, assessment and prevention of chemical dependence following a spinal cord injury, prevention of secondary complications through the use of electrical stimulation, prevention of thromboembolism in spinal cord injury, managing urinary tract infections, and managing the neurogenic bowel.

Packard Children's Hospital at Stanford
Rehabilitation Engineering Center
725 Welch Rd.
Palo Alto, CA 94304
Phone: (415) 497-8192
Fax: (415) 497-8154
Maurice LeBlanc, Dir. of Research

Research Activities and Fields: Rehabilitation technology, emphasizing speech aids, prosthetics, orthotics, and seating and mobility for people with disabilities.

Rancho Rehabilitation Engineering Program
Los Amigos Research and Education Institute
Bonita Hall
7503 Bonita St.
Downey, CA 90242
Phone: (310) 940-7994
Fax: (310) 803-6117
Don McNeal, Ph.D., Dir.

Research Activities and Fields: Application of functional electrical stimulation to improve methods of gait training and upper extremity rehabilitation, activate muscles in lower extremities with multichannel implants, and examine the effects of stimulus wave form and electrodes on comfort during controlled motor contractions.

Rehabilitation Institute of Chicago
345 E. Superior
Chicago, IL 60611
Phone: (312) 908-3381
Fax: (312) 908-2208
Dr. W. Zev Rymer, Dir. of Research

Research Activities and Fields: Rehabilitation medicine, brain trauma, stroke, atherosclerosis, neuromuscular diseases, applied neurophysiology, deep venous thrombosis, and communicative disorders.

Rehabilitation Institute of Michigan
261 Mack Blvd.
Detroit, MI 48201
Phone: (313) 745-9731
Fax: (313) 745-9863
Dr. Marcel Dijkers, Dir. of Research

Research Activities and Fields: Physical medicine and rehabilitation medicine, including electromyography, rehabilitation robotics, engineering, measures of rehabilitation outcome, and methods of evaluation and treatment of patients with closed head injuries, spinal cord injuries, cerebrovascular accidents, and other diagnoses.

Rehabilitation Research and Planning Center
Casa Colina Hospital for Rehabilitation Medicine
225 E. Bonita Ave.
Pomona, CA 91767
Phone: (714) 593-7521
Fax: (714) 593-0153
Robert Allen Keith, Ph.D., Dir.

Research Activities and Fields: Clinical research on physical medicine populations; organizational analysis of rehabilitation hospitals; program evaluation and design research studies conducted with hospital staff on head injury, stroke, spinal cord injury, and other conditions.

Research and Training Center in Vocational Rehabilitation
P.O. Box 1358

Hot Springs, AR 71902
Dr. Roy C. Farley, Dir.

Research Activities and Fields: Vocational rehabilitation for individuals with disabilities, including assessment, placement strategies, and skills for employment.

Sister Kenny Institute
800 E. 28th St. at Chicago Ave.
Minneapolis, MN 55407
Phone: (612) 863-4367
Fax: (616) 863-4507
Kent Canine, Dir. Research and Education

Research Activities and Fields: Physical medicine and rehabilitation. Aims at improving the quality and efficiency of rehabilitation patient care. Conducts research in spasticity management in post-polio and cardiovascular conditions; investigates the applications of functional electrical stimulation cycling for spinal cord–injured persons.

Southern Illinois University of Carbondale
Rehabilitation Institute
Rehn Hall, Rm. 317
Carbondale, IL 62901
Phone: (618) 536-7704
Fax: (618) 453-1646
Dr. Gary Austin, Dir.

Research Activities and Fields: Rehabilitation, including studies on the blind, developmentally and physically disabled adults and juvenile offenders, and economically disadvantaged. Conducts counseling process and outcome studies, counseling of special populations, and behavior therapy with diverse populations, including programs in alcoholism, substance abuse, and aging.

Syracuse University
Special Education Program
805 S. Crouse Ave.
Syracuse, NY 13244
Phone: (315) 443-9651
Fax: (315) 443-3289
Dr. Luanna Meyer, Chmn.

Research Activities and Fields: Applied studies focusing on special education and inclusive schooling. Projects include work on statewide educational systems change, facilitated communication, effect of special education program models, public policy affecting persons with disabilities, and attitudes toward people with disabilities.

Thomas Jefferson University
Regional Spinal Cord Injury Center of Delaware Valley
324 Main Bldg.
132 S. 10th St.
Philadelphia, PA 19107
Phone: (215) 955-6579
John F. Ditunno, Jr., M.D. Proj. Dir.

Research Activities and Fields: Acute care and rehabilitation for individuals disabled by spinal cord injury. Projects focus on evaluating therapeutic intervention such as surgery, traction, electrical stimulation, and biofeedback.

Tufts University
Medical Rehabilitation Research and Training Center
750 Washington St.
Box 75K/R
Boston, MA 02111
Phone: (617) 956-5622

Research Activities and Fields: Impact of rehabilitation on children with traumatic injury. Projects include maintenance of the National Pediatric Trauma Registry, development of clinical instrumentation to assess the physical affects of childhood injury, and a longitudinal follow-up study of the motor and functional outcomes of traumatic injuries in children.

University of Alabama at Birmingham
Medical Rehabilitation Research/Training for Prevention/Treatment of Secondary Complications of Spinal Cord Injury
UAB Sta.
Birmingham, AL 35294
Phone: (205) 934-3334
J. Scott Richard, Ph.D., Research Dir.

Research Activities and Fields: Prevention and treatment of secondary complications of spinal cord injury, including urologic, skin, and pulmonary complications, infertility and sexuality, spasticity, the role of nutrition in preventing secondary complications, psychosocial complications, and the effects of aging on persons with SCI.

University of Alabama at Birmingham
Spinal Cord Injury Care System
UAB Sta.
Birmingham, AL 35294
Phone: (205) 934-3330
Samuel L. Stover, M.D., Project Dir.

Research Activities and Fields: Rehabilitation needs of those with spinal cord injury, including urologic studies.

University of Arizona
Rehabilitation Center
College of Education
Tucson, AZ 85721
Phone: (602) 621-7022
Fax: (602) 621-9271
Dr. Amos Sales, Dir.

Research Activities and Fields: Psychological, social, medical, and vocational problems of rehabilitation, including interdisciplinary studies on various aspects of disability (with particular emphasis on relation of disability to everyday life), community organization for rehabilitation, and attitudes of educable high-school-age mental retardates.

University of Hawaii at Manoa
Rehabilitation and Training Center
Rehabilitation Hospital of the Pacific
226 N. Kuakini St., Rm 233
Honolulu, HI 96817
Phone: (808) 537-5906
Fax: (808) 537-8691
Daniel D. Anderson, Ed.D., Dir.

Research Activities and Fields: Medical rehabilitation, vocational rehabilitation, and special education in the Pacific area, including multicultural aspects of providing rehabilitation services in the developing Pacific areas, needs and follow-up training, referral systems and assessment methods, and transition study of community living.

University of Wisconsin–Madison
Rehabilitation Research Institute
Dept. of Rehabilitation and Psychology

432 N. Murray St.
Madison, WI 53706
Phone: (608) 262-5971
Fax: (608) 262-8108
George N. Wright, Ph.D., Dir.

Research Activities and Fields: Rehabilitation, including the role and professional function of vocational rehabilitation counselors and improvement of their effectiveness in coping with problems of the physically and mentally handicapped.

Virginia Commonwealth University
Rehabilitation Research and Training Center on Severe Traumatic Brain Injury
Box 677, MCV Sta.
Richmond, VA 23298
Phone: (804) 786-0213
Dr. David X. Cifu, M.D., Dir.

Research Activities and Fields: Severe brain injury. Specific projects, including studying changes in the circulation of brain fluid after an injury to develop treatments that minimize intellectual problems, investigating academic and emotional problems resulting from traumatic injury in children, and studying brain activity during coma.

SECTION III

HEALTH CARE ABBREVIATIONS AND SYMBOLS

Timothy J. Meline, Ph.D.
The University of Texas
Pan American
Edinburg, Texas

ABBREVIATIONS

Å	(a) Ångström units(s); (b) angstrom(s)
A	assessment; assistance; after
ā	(a) before ([L.] *ante*); (b) artery [L.] *arteria*)
(A)	axillary
A/A	auto accident
A.A.	Alcoholics Anonymous
āā	(a) the same quantity of each; (b) arteries ([L.] *arteriae*)
A.A.A.	American Academy of Audiology
AAC	augmentative and alternative communication
AADT	adaptive assistive devices team
A.A.H.A.	American Association of Homes for the Aging
A & O	alert and oriented
A.A.O.	American Association of Orthodontics
A.A.O.M.S.	American Association of Oral- Maxillofacial Surgeons
A.A.P.M.R.	American Academy of Physical Medicine and Rehabilitation
A.A.R.C.	American Association for Respiratory Care
AARF	acute alveolar respiratory failure
A/A ROM	active assistive range of motion
A.A.R.P.	American Association of Retired Persons
A.A.R.T.	American Association for Rehabilitation Therapy
A.A.S.W.	American Academy of Social Workers
AB	arm bike
Ab	antibody
ab	(a) abortion; (b) from ([L.] *ab*)
ABA	Apraxia Battery for Adults (Dabul)
ABCD	Arizona Battery for Communication Disorders
abd	abdomen
abdom	(a) abdomen; (b) abdominal
Abd. Hyst.	abdominal hysterectomy
abdu	abduction

ABE	acute bacterial endocarditis
ABI	atherosclerotic brain infarction
A.B.M.S.	American Board of Medical Specialties
abn	abnormal
ABP	arterial blood pressure
ABR	(a) absolute bed rest; (b) auditory brainstem response
ABS	acute brain syndrome
abs	absolute
abs. feb.	In the absence of fever (febrile)
aby	antibody
A/C	associated with
AC	(a) air conduction; (b) Activity Coordinator
Ac; ac	(a) alternating current; (b) air conditioning
a.c.	before meals ([L.] *ante cibum*)
ACA	anterior cerebral artery
ACC	anodal closing contraction
acc	(a) accuracy; (b) agenesis (of the) corpus collosum
accom	accommodation
ACD	assistive communication device
ACE	Award for Continuing Education
ACh	acetylcholine
AChE	acetylcholinesterase
ACL	Allen Cognitive Level (Scale)
ACLF	Adult Congregate Living Facility
A.C.P.A.	American Cleft Palate Association
ACR	acute respiratory failure
A.C.R.	American College of Radiology
act	activity
ACTH	adrenocorticotropic hormone
ACU	acute care unit
Ad	(a) adnexa; (b) to, up to
AD	(a) right ear ([L.] *auris dextra*); (b) Alzheimer's disease
A.D.A.	(a) American Dental Association; (b) American Diabetes Association
A.D.A. diet	American Diabetic Association diet
add	adduction
ADE	acute disseminated encephalitis
adenoca	adenocarcinoma
ADH	antidiuretic hormone
ADHD	attention-deficit hyperactivity disorder
ADL	activities of daily living
ADLT	activities of daily living test

ad lib	as desired ([L.] *ad libitum*)
adm	admission
admin	administer
adol	adolescent
ADON	Assistant Director of Nursing
ADP	adenosine diphosphate
ADR	adverse drug reaction
ADS	alternative delivery system
ADT	(a) admission, discharge, and transfer; (b) adenosine triphosphate
AE	above elbow
AED	antiepileptic drug
AEG	air encephalogram
AF	atrial fibrillation
Af	atrial flutter
A.fib	atrial fibrillation
AFO	ankle foot orthosis
AG	attached gingiva
AGA	acute gonococcal arthritis
A.G.A.	American Geriatrics Association
agglut	agglutination
agit	shake, stir ([L.] *agita*)
AGS	adrenogenital syndrome
A.G.S.	American Geriatrics Society
A.H.A.	American Hospital Association
A.H.C.A.	American Health Care Association
AI	(a) aortic insufficiency; (b) Allergy and Immunology
AIDS	acquired immunodeficiency syndrome
AIP	acute intermittent porphyria
AIT	administrator in training
AJ	ankle jerk
AJA	*American Journal of Audiology: A Journal of Clinical Practice*
AJOT	*American Journal of Occupational Therapy*
AJR	*American Journal of Roentgenology*
AJSLP	*American Journal of Speech-Language Pathology: A Journal of Clinical Practice*
AK	above knee
AKA	above the knee amputation
A.L.A.	American Laryngological Association
alb	albumin
ALD	(a) assistive listening device; (b) adrenoleukodystrophy

A.L.F.A.A.	Assisted Living Facilities Association of America
ALJ	administrative law judge
alk	alkaline
ALL	(a) acute lymphocytic leukemia; (b) Analysis of the Language of Learning: The Practical Test of Metalinguistics (Blodgett & Cooper)
ALOS	average length of stay
ALPS	Aphasia Language Performance Scales
A.L.R.O.S.	American Laryngological, Rhinological, and Otological Society
ALS	amyotrophic lateral sclerosis
A.L.S.A.	Amyotrophic Lateral Sclerosis Association
alt	alternate
ALTE	apparent life threatening event
alv	alveolar
A.M.	before noon ([L.] *ante meridiem*)
AMA	against medical advice
A.M.A.	American Medical Association
AMAP	as much as possible
amb	ambulate (ambulatory)
AMI	acute myocardial infarction
amorph	amorphous
amp; ampu	(a) amputation; (b) amplification; (c) ampule
amphet	amphetamine
amt	amount
an	aneurysm
A.N.A.	American Nurses' Association
ANE	active neck exercise
anes	anesthesia
angio	angiogram
ANI	acute neurological impairment
aniso	anisocytosis
ANS	(a) automatic nervous system; (b) anterior nasal spine
ANSI	American National Standards Institute
ant	anterior
ANUG	acute necrotizing ulcerative gingivitis
A & O	alert and oriented
A.O.A.	(a) American Orthopedic Association; (b) American Optometric Association
AOB	alcohol on breath
AOC	anodal opening contraction
AOD	arterial occlusive disease

AOL	acroosteolysis
AOM	acute otitis media
AOMD	adult onset diabetes mellitus
A.O.P.A.	American Orthotics and Prosthetics Association
aort. regurg.	aortic regurgitation
aort. sten.	aortic stenosis
A.O.S.	American Otological Association
A.O.T.A.	American Occupational Therapy Association
A.O.T.C.B.	American Occupational Therapy Certification Board
AP	anteroposterior
A-P	abdominal perineal
A & P	auscultation and percussion
A.P.A.	American Psychological Association
APC tabs	aspirin, phenacetin, and caffeine tablets
A-PD	anteroposterior diameter
APF	apically positioned flap
A.Ph.A.	American Pharmaceutical Association
A.P.H.A.	American Public Health Association
A.P.I.C.	Association for Practitioners in Infection Control
A-P & Lat	anterior-posterior and lateral
APOE	apolipoprotein
approx	approximately
appt	appointment
A-P rep	anterior-posterior repair
APRL	Army Prosthetics Research Laboratory
A.P.T.A.	American Physical Therapy Association
aq	aqueous (water)
aq. dist.	distilled water
AR	aural rehabilitation
A/R	apical/radial
A.R.A.	American Rheumatism Association
ARC	AIDS-related complex
ARD	acute respiratory disease
ARDS	acute respiratory distress syndrome
ARF	acute renal failure
A.R.F.	Association of Rehabilitation Facilities
ARM	age-related maculopathy
A.R.N.	Association of Rehabilitation Nurses
AROM	active range of motion
A.R.P.T.	American Registry of Physical Therapists
A/R ROM	active resistive range of motion
A.R.R.T.	American Registry of Radiologic Technicians

AS	(a) aortic stenosis; (b) arteriosclerosis
As	astigmatism
a.s.	left ear ([L.] *auris sinistra*)
ASA	acetylsalicylic acid (aspirin)
ASAP	as soon as possible
A-S attack	Adams-stokes attack
ASC	ambulatory-surgery center
ASCVD	arteriosclerotic cardiovascular disease
ASD	atrial septal defect
ASH	asymmetrical septal hypertrophy
A.S.H.A.	American Speech-Language-Hearing Association
ASHD	arteriosclerotic heart disease
A.S.H.T.	American Society of Hand Therapists
ASL	American Sign Language
ASLO titer	antistreptolysin-O titer
A.S.M.T.	American Society for Medical Technology
ASO	arteriosclerosis obliterans
ASO titer	antistreptolysis-O titer
assn	association
assoc	associated
A.S.R.T.	American Society of Radiologic Technologists
assist	assistance
as tol	as tolerated
ASYMP	asymptomatic
AT	ataxia telangiectasia
at. fib.	atrial fibrillation
ATG	antithymocyte globulin
ATN	acute tubular necrosis
ATNR	asymmetrical tonic neck reflex
ATP	adenosine triphosphate
ATR	registered art therapist
AU	(a) both ears ([L.] *auris unitus*); (b) each ear ([L.] *auris uterque*)
AUD	audiologist
aud	auditory
AV	atrioventricular
A-V	arteriovenous
AVG	ambulatory visit group
AVM	arteriovenous malformation
AVN	atrioventricular node
AVR	aortic valve replacement
AVS	arteriovenous shunt

A & W	alive and well
AWR	average weight range
Ax	axillary
ax	axis
AZT	azidothymidine
B	(a) both; (b) Black; (c) before
b	(a) born; (b) buccal
Ba	barium
bact	bacteria
Ba.E	barium enema
BaFPE	Bay Area Functional Performance Evaluation
BAL	blood alcohol level
bal	balance
bands	banded neutrophilis
barb	barbiturate
baso	basophils
Ba. swallow	barium swallow
BB	bile bag
B/B	bowel and bladder
BBA	born before arrival
BBT	basal body temperature
B. Bx	breast biopsy
BC	(a) bone conduction; (b) blood culture
BC/BS	Blue Cross and Blue Shield
BCC	basal cell carcinoma
BCG	ballistocardiogram
BCG Live	Bacillus Calmette Guerin Live
BCLP	bilateral cleft lip and palate
BCN	bilateral cortical necrosis
BCP	birth control pills
BCS	bilateral chest sounds
b.d.	twice a day ([L.] *bis die*)
BDAE	Boston Diagnostic Aphasia Examination
BDI	Beck Depression Inventory
BE	(a) below elbow; (b) barium enema
BEAM	brain electrical activity map
BEI	butanol-extractable iodine (test)
BF	Black female
BFO	balanced forearm orthosis
BG	blood glucose
BHS	beta-hemolytic streptococcus
BI	(a) brain injured; (b) Barthel index; (c) burn index

bib	drink ([L.] *bibe*)
b.i.d.	twice a day ([L.] *bis in die*)
BIH	benign intracranial hypertension
bil; bilat	bilateral
bili	bilirubin
b.i.n.	twice a night ([L.] *bis in noctus*)
BJM	bones, joints, muscles
BK	below knee
BKA; BK amp	below knee amputation
bkfst; bkt	breakfast
bl. cult.	blood culture
BLE	bilateral lower extremities
bl. obs.	bladder observation
Bl. T	blood type
bl. time	bleeding time
bl. x	bleeding time
BM	bowel movement
BMET	biomedical electronics technician
BMR	basal metabolic rate
BMT	bilateral myringotomy with tubes
B.N.D.D.	Bureau of Narcotics and Dangerous Drugs
BNO	bladder neck obstruction
BNT	Boston Naming Test
BO	behavioral objective
B & O	belladonna and opium
bol	bolus
BOM	bilateral otitis media
BOR	branchio-oto-renal (syndrome)
BOTMP	Bruininks-Oseretsky Test of Motor Proficiency
BoTox	botulinum toxin
BP	blood pressure
BPD	bronchopulmonary dyplasia
BPH	benign prostatic hypertrophy
BPM	beats per minute
BPRS	brief psychiatric rating scale
B.P.S.	Board of Pharmaceutical Specialists
BPVS	British Picture Vocabulary Scale
BQ	billing questionnaire
BR	(a) bed rest; (b) bathroom; (c) barium
BRATT	banana, rice, apple, tea, toast (diet)
BRB	bright red blood

B.R.C.	blind rehabilitation center
BRBPR	bright red bleeding per rectum
BRP	bathroom privileges
br. sounds	breath sounds
BS	(a) blood sugar; (b) body surface; (c) bowel sounds
BSB	body surface burned
BSD	bedside drainage
B.S.W.	Bachelor of Science in Social Work
BT	(a) bedtime; (b) brain tumor
BTB	breakthrough bleeding
BTE	behind the ear
BTWE	behind-the-wheel evaluation
BUE	bilateral upper extremities
BUN	blood urea nitrogen
BUS	Bartholin urethral skene
BVH	biventricular hypertrophy
BW	body weight
Bx	biopsy
C	(a) cervical; (b) cardiac arrest; (c) centigrade; (d) correct; (e) Celsius; (f) electrical capacitance
c	with ([L.] *cum*)
-¼c	one hundred ([L.] *centum*)
C_1 C_2	cervical vertebrae 1, 2, . . .
ca	about ([L.] *circa*)
Ca	calcium
CA	(a) carcinoma; (b) cancer; (c) chronological age
CABG	coronary artery bypass graft
CAD	coronary artery disease
CADL	communicative abilities in daily living
CAEPs	cortical auditory evoked potentials
CAFET	Computer-Aided Fluency Establishment Trainer
CAH	chronic active hepatitis
CAI	computer-aided instruction
cal	calorie
CALD	chronic active liver disease
canc	cancel
cap	(a) capsule; (b) capacity; (c) central auditory processing; (d) let him take ([L.] *capiat*)
CAPD	continuous ambulatory peritoneal dialysis
CAPP	Child Amputee Prosthetics Project
caps	capsules
cardiol	cardiology

CARF	Commission on Accreditation of Rehabilitation Facilities
CAS	carotid artery system
CAT	computerized axial tomography
Cath	Catholic
cath	catheter
caut	cauterize
C & B	chair and bed
CBC	complete blood count
CBD	chronic behavior disorder
CBR	complete bed rest
CBS	chronic brain syndrome
CBT	computed body tomography
CC	chief complaint
C/C	care and comfort
cc	cubic centimeter
c.c.	with correction
CCA	common carotid artery
CCC	cathodal closing contraction
CCC-A	Certificate of Clinical Competence in Audiology
CCC-SLP	Certificate of Clinical Competence in Speech-Language Pathology
CCCVC	consonant-consonant-consonant- vowel-consonant (words)
CCE	clubbing, cyanosis, or edema
CCF	compound comminuted fracture
CCM	congestive cardiomyopathy
CCMSU	clean catch midstream urine
CCP	complete cleft palate
CCPD	continuous cycler peritoneal dialysis
CCRC	continuing-care retirement community
CCSPEA	Classroom Communication Screening Procedure for Early Adolescents (Simon)
CCT	(a) certified corrective therapist; (b) crude coal tar
CCV	consonant-consonant-vowel (words)
CCVC	consonant-consonant-vowel- consonant (words)
CCW	counterclockwise
CCU	coronary care unit
C.D.	communicable disease
C/d	cigarettes per day
C & D	(a) cystoscopy and dilation; (b) cool and dry

CDC (a) Centers for Disease Control; (b) career development center
CDE chlordiazepoxide
CDH congenital dislocation of hip
CDR Clinical Dementia Rating
CE continuing education
CEBVD chronic Epstein-Barr viral disease
CED Clinical Evaluation of (Examination for) Dysphagia
CERT certification
CES continuous electric stimulation
CES-D Center for Epidemiological Studies Depression Scale
CEU continuing education unit
CF (a) cardiac failure; (b) cystic fibrosis
cf compare ([L.] *confer*)
CFP chronic false positive
CFR Code of Federal Regulations
CFS chronic fatigue syndrome
CFY Clinical Fellowship Year
cg centigram
CGD chronic granulomatous disease
CGL chronic granulocytic leukemia
cgm centrigram
CGN chronic glomerulonephritis
CGTT cortisone glucose tolerance test
ch chest
CHAMPUS Civilian Health and Medical Program of the Uniformed Services
CHB complete heart block
CHC community health centers
CHD (a) congenital heart disease; (b) coronary heart disease
CHF congestive heart failure
chg change
CHL conductive hearing loss
CHE cholinesterase
CHI closed head injury
CH-I child-initiated
CHO carbohydrate
chol cholesterol
chr chronic

chrg	charge
CHT	congenital hypothyroidism
CHTZ	chlorothiazide
Ci	Curie
CI	(a) cardiac infarction; (b) cerebral infarction
cib	food, meal ([L.] *cibus*)
CICU	cardiac intensive care unit
CID	cytomegalic inclusion disease
CIDS	cellular immunity deficiency syndrome
circ	circulation
circum	circumduction
ck	check
cl	(a) clear; (b) centiliter
Cl	chloride
CL	(a) clinic; (b) cleared
CLD	chronic liver disease
cldy	cloudy
CLIP	Clinical Language Intervention Program
CLL	chronic lymphocytic leukemia
cl. liq.	clear liquid
CLP	cleft lip (and) palate
CLQ	combined language quotient
CLS	Clinical Laboratory Scientist
CLT	clot-lysis time
clysis	hypodermocylsis
CM	costal margin
c.m.	tomorrow morning ([L.] *cras meridiem*)
cm	centimeter
CMA	certified medical assistant
CME	continuing medical education
CMG	cystometrogram
CMI	chronic mental illness
c/min	cycles per minute
CMO	cardiac minute output
CMP	competitive medical plan
CMS	circulation, motion, sensation
CMV	cytomegalovirus
CN	charge nurse
cn	(a) cranial nerve; (b) tomorrow night ([L.] *cras nocte*)
CNA	certified nurse assistant
CNE	chronic nervous exhaustion

CNH community nursing home
CNO chief nursing officer
CNS central nervous system
CNSLD chronic nonspecific lung disease
CNT could not test
CnX cranial nerve 10
CO (a) cervical orthosis; (b) certified orthotist; (c) carbon monoxide
c/o complains of
CO_2 carbon dioxide
COAD chronic obstructive airway disease
coag coagulation
COBRA Continued Omnibus Budget Reconciliation Act
COBS chronic organic brain syndrome
COC cathodal opening contraction
COD cause of death
COG (a) closed angle glaucoma; (b) cognitive
COHB carboxyhemoglobin
COLD chronic obstructive lung disease
CON certificate of need
conc concentration
cong congestion
cont continued
contr contracture
COPD chronic obstructive pulmonary disease
COPE chronic obstructive pulmonary disease
CORF Comprehensive Outpatient Rehabilitation Facility
COTA Certified Occupational Therapy Assistant
commun communicable
comp complication
conv convalescent
cort cortical
CP (a) cerebral palsy; (b) chronic pain; (c) cricopharyngeal
CPA cardiopulmonary arrest
CPAP continuous positive airway pressure
CPB cardiopulmonary bypass
CPC clinicpathologic conference
cpd compound
CpdE cortisone
CpdF hydrocortisone

CPE	chronic pulmonary emphysema
C Ped	certified pedorthist
CPF	coronally positioned flap
CPHI	Communication Profile for the Hearing Impaired
CPI	congenital/palatopharyngeal incompetence
CPK	creatinine phosphokinase
CPM	continuous passive motion
c.p.m.	cycles per minute
CPN	chronic pyelonephritis
CPO	certified prosthetist and orthotist
CPPB	continuous positive pressure breathing
CPPV	continuous positive pressure ventilation
CPR	cardiopulmonary resuscitation
cps	cycles per second
CPT	(a) current procedural terminology; (b) chest physiotherapy
CPZ	chlorpromazine (Thorazine)
CQI	continuous quality improvement
CR	(a) cardiac rehabilitation; (b) cardiorespiratory; (c) colon and rectal (surgery) (d) closed reduction
CRA	central retinal artery
cran	cranial
CRC	certified rehabilitation counselor
CRD	chronic renal disease
CRF	chronic renal failure
CRT	community readjustment training
crit	hematocrit
CRST synd	calcinosis, Raynaud's phenomenon, sclerodactyly, and telangiectasia syndrome
CRT	cardiac resuscitation team
crt	hematocrit
CRV	central retinal vein
crys	crystalline
C & S	culture and sensitivity
CSF	cerebrospinal fluid
CSH	chronic subdural hematoma
CSHEP	constriction, sclerosis, hemorrhage, exudate, papilledema
CSP	carotid sinus pressure
C-spine	cervical spine
CST	convulsive shock therapy
CSW	certified social worker

CT	(a) computed tomography; (b) corrective therapy; (c) corrective therapist
ct	count
cta	catamenia
CTB	ceased to breathe
CTD	carpal tunnel decompression
CTLO	cervicothoracolumbar orthosis
CTLS	cervical, thoracic, lumbosacral spine
CTLSO	cervicothoracolumbosacral orthosis
CTM	connective tissue massage
CTO	cervicothoracic orthosis
CT ratio	cardiothoracic ratio
CTRS	certified therapeutic recreation specialist
CTSP	called to see patient
CU	(a) copper; (b) cued
CUC	chronic ulcerative colitis
CUG	cystourethrogram
cu mm	cubic millimeter
CV	(a) cardiovascular; (b) consonant-vowel (words)
CVA	cerebrovascular accident
CVB	chorionic villus biopsy
CVC	consonant-vowel-consonant (words)
CVCC	consonant-vowel-consonant- consonant (words)
CVD	cardiovascular disease
cvd	curved
CVE	cerebrovascular episode
CVG	coronary vein graft
CVI	cerebrovascular insufficiency
CVP	central venous pressure
CVR	cardiovascular-respiratory
CVRD	cardiovascular renal disease
CVS	cardiovascular system
CWI	cardiac work index
CWT	compensated work therapy
CX	chest x-ray
Cysto	cystoscopy
D	(a) divorced; (b) distortion; (c) during; (d) dermatology; (e) dose; (f) dictated
D_1, D_2	dorsal vertebrae 1, 2, . . .
DAF	delayed auditory feedback
DAH	disordered action of the heart
DAS	developmental apraxia of speech

DAT	diet as tolerated
DB	date born
D/B	drain bag
db; dB	decibel
DBM	diabetic management
DBP	diastolic blood pressure
DC; D/C	(a) discontinue; (b) discharge; (c) direct current
D & C	dilation and curettage
DCA	desoxycorticosterone acetate
DCP	direct care provider
DC/POT	discharge plan of treatment
DD	developmental disability (delay)
DDD	degenerative disc disease
DDS	Disability Determination Service
DDST	Denver Developmental Screening Test
DDx	differential diagnosis
dec	decrease
dec'd	deceased
decr	decreased
decub	decubitus (ulcer)
def	definition
deform	deformity
degen	degeneration
delt	deltoid (muscle)
Dem	Demerol
dent	dental
depend	dependent
depr	depression
DER	dual energy radiography
Derm	dermatology
DES	diffuse esophageal spasm
Det	let it be given ([L.] *detur*)
determin	determination
dev	deviation
devel	development
df	dorsiflexion
D5 R/1	dextrose 5% in Ringer's lactate
DG	(a) dysphagiagram; (b) diastolic gallop
dgm	decigram
DHR	delayed hypersensitivity reaction
DHS	duration of hospital stay
DI	diabetes insipidus

DIA	(shortwave) diathermy
diab	diabetic
diag	(a) diagnosis; (b) diagnostic
diam	diameter
diath	diathermy
DIC	disseminated intravascular coagulation
dieb tert	every third day ([L.] *diebus tertiis*)
diff	differential
diff bc	differential blood count
diff diag	differential diagnosis
dig	digitalis
Dil	Dilantin
dil	(a) dilute; (b) dilate
dilat	dilation
DILD	diffuse infiltrative lung disease
diln	dilution
dim	(a) diminished; (b) one half
DIP	distal interphalangeal (joint)
diph	diphtheria
diph/tet	diphtheria-tetanus
diph tox	diphtheria toxoid
diph tox AP	diphtheria toxoid-alum precipitated
DIPJ	distal interphalangeal joint
Dip. O.T.	Diploma in Occupational Therapy
Dip. T. P.	diploma teacher of physiotherapy
dir	direct
dis	disease
disc	discontinued
disch	discharge
disloc	dislocation
dism	dismissed
disp	dispense
dissd	dissolved
dissem	disseminated
dist	(a) distance; (b) distilled
div	divide
DJD	degenerative joint disease
DJS	Dubin-Johnson syndrome
dk	dark
DKA	diabetic ketoacidosis
DL	(a) danger list; (b) direct laryngoscopy

dl	deciliter
DLE	discoid lupus erythematosus
DM	diabetes mellitus
DMD	Duchenne's muscular dystrophy
DME	durable medical equipment
DMS	dermatomyositis
DMSO	dimethyl sulfoxide
DN	(a) dicrotic notch; (b) depth of nasopharynx
DND	died a natural death
DNK	did not keep
DNR	do not resuscitate
DNS	did not show
DNT	did not test
DO	(a) Doctor of Osteopathy; (b) date of onset
DOA	(a) date of assessment; (b) dead on arrival; (c) date of admission
DOB	date of birth
DOE	(a) date of evaluation; (b) dyspnea on exertion
DOI	date of injury
DOL	Department of Labor
DON	determination of need
DOO	date of onset
DOT	(a) Doppler ophthalmic test; (b) Dictionary of Occupational Therapy
DP	(a) dorsalis pedis (pulse); (b) Discharge Planner
DPD	diffuse pulmonary disease
DPH	diphenylhydantoin
D. Phys. Med.	Doctor of Physical Medicine
DPM	Doctor of Podiatric Medicine
DPNMS	deep pharyngeal neuromuscular stimulation
DPOT	discharge plan of treatment
DPS	dysesthetic pain syndrome
DPT	diphtheria, pertussis, tetanus
DQ	developmental quotient
DQT	Denver Quick Test
DR	dressing removal
D.R.	dining room
Dr.	doctor
dr	dram
DRE	digital rectal examination
DRG	diagnosis related group

D.Rm.	dining room
DR Scale	(Rappaport) Disability Rating Scale
drsg	dressing
DS	dry swallow
D/S	dextrose and saline
DSD	dry sterile dressing
dsg	dressing
DSM	*Diagnostic and Statistical Manual (of Mental Disorders)*
D-spine	dorsal spine
D.S.W.	Doctor of Social Work
DT	double tachycardia
DTLA	Detroit Test of Learning Aptitude
DTN	dystonia
DTP	diphtheria, tetanus, pertussis
DTR	deep tendon reflex
DTs	delirium tremens
DTV	due to void
DTx	diagnostic therapy
DVA	Department of Veterans Affairs
DVT	deep vein thrombosis
DWR	desired weight range
Dx	diagnosis
E	(a) eye; (b) extremity
EA	Examining for Aphasia (Eisenson)
ea	each
E.A.A.	Educational Audiology Association
EAC	external auditory canal
EAI	equal-appearing interval (scale)
EAM	external auditory meatus
EB	epidermolysis bullosa
EBD	epidermolysis bullosa dystrophica
EBV	Epstein-Barr virus
ECC	Evaluating Communicative Competence (Simon)
ECF	(a) extended care facility; (b) extracellular fluid
ECG	electrocardiogram
ECHO	echocardiogram
ECO	ecological communication
ECS	environmental control system
ECT	electroconvulsive therapy
ECU	environmental control unit
EDC	expected date of confinement

EDF	elongation, derotation, and (lateral) flexion
EDx; El Dx	electrodiagnosis
EEC	electrodactyly-ectodermal dysplasia- cleft (syndrome)
EEE	Eastern equine encephalitis
EEG	electroencephalogram
EENT	eyes, ears, nose and throat
EG	esophagogastrectomy
e.g.	for example ([L.] *exempli gratia*)
EGG	(a) electroglottography; (b) electrogastrogram
EGJ	esophagogastric juncture
EGL	eosinophilic granuloma of the lung
EHO	extrahepatic obstruction
EHS	employee health service(s)
EI	early intervention
EIA	enzyme immunoassay
EIB	exercise-induced bronchospasm
EIP	extensor indicis proprium
EJB	extopic junctional beat
EKG	electrocardiogram
EKY	electrokymogram
ELA	expressive language age
elb	elbow
El Dx	electrodiagnosis
ELISA	enzyme-linked immunosorbent assay
elix	elixir
ELM	Early Language Milestone (Scale)
ELQ	expressive language quotient
elv	elevate
EM	Emergency Medicine
EMC	(a) electronic mail claims; (b) encephalomyocarditis
EMF	electromotive force
EMG	electromyogram
EMR	(a) emergency medical receiving; (b) educable mentally retarded
EMT	Emergency Medical Technician
emul	emulsion
EN	erythema modosum
endocrin	endocrinology
ENG	electronystagmogram
ENS	electric nerve stimulation

ENT	ears, nose and throat
EO	(a) elbow orthosis; (b) eyes open
eo	eosinophil
EOA	(a) examination, opinion and advice; (b) early-onset Alzheimer's (disease)
EOB	(a) emergency observation bed; (b) edge of bed
e.o.d.	every other day
EOG	(a) electro-oculogram; (b) electro-olfactogram
EOM	extraocular movements
eos	eosinophils
EP	evoked potential
EPA	Environmental Protection Agency
EPC	epilepsy
Epi	epinephrine
epith	epithelial
EPOT	evaluation plan of treatment
EPS	electrical programmed stimulation
EPSD	early and periodic screening, diagnosis, (and treatment program)
EPSF	early postsurgical fitting
eq	equivalent
ER	emergency room
ERA	evoked response audiometry
ERV	expiratory reserve volume
ES	electrical stimulation
ESM	ejection systolic murmur
esoph	esophagus
ess	essential
ess. neg.	essentially negative
est	estimated
EST	electroshock therapy
E-stim	electrical stimulation
ET	(a) eustachian tube; (b) educational therapist (therapy)
et al.	and others ([L.] *et alii*)
etiol	etiology
ETM	erythromycin
ETOH	ethyl alcohol
ETR	(a) enhancement of tissue repair; (b) exercise training range
ETT	(a) endotracheal tube; (b) exercise tolerance test
EUA	examination under anesthetic

EV extravascular
eval evaluate (evaluation)
EWB estrogen withdrawal bleeding
EWHO elbow wrist hand orthosis
ex (a) example; (b) exercise
exam examination
exp expressive
expir expiratory
exp lap exploratory laparotomy
expt expectorant
ext (a) extremity; (b) extract; (c) extension
ext rot external rotation
F (a) female; (b) fair; (c) Fahrenheit; (d) farad; (e) free
F_1, F_2 formant 1, 2, . . .
f frequency
facil facilitation
FAI functional aerobic impairment
fam. doc. family doctor
fam. phys. family physician
FAOTA Fellow of the American Occupational Therapy Association
FB foreign body
FBP femoral blood pressure
FBS fasting blood sugar
FC (a) finger counting; (b) functional capacity; (c) facilitated communication
F. cath Foley catheter
FCP Functional Communication Profile
FCT functional communication treatment
FDA (a) Food and Drug Administration; (b) Frenchay Dysarthria Test
FDG flurodeoxyglucose
FDS for duration of stay
Fe Iron
feb. dur. febrile duration (while the fever lasts)
Fe def iron deficient anemia
FEES fiberoptic endoscopic examination of swallowing
FEESS fiberoptic endoscopic examination of swallowing safety
FEF forced expiratory flow
FEGG fetal electrocardiogram

fem	femoral
FES	(a) functional electrical stimulation; (b) forced expiratory spirogram
FEV	forced expiratory volume
ff	force fluids
FF diet	fat-free diet
FH; F. Hx	family history
fib	fibrillation
FIG	fluency initiating gesture
filt	filter
FIM	Functional Independence Measure
fist	fistula
FL	fluoride
fl	fluid
FLB	funny-looking beat
fld	fluid
flex	flexion
fl oz	fluid ounce
FLS	Functional Life Scale (Sarno)
fluor	fluoroscopy
fl. up	follow up
fm	fine motor
FME	full mouth extraction
FMX	full mouth radiograph
FNP	family nurse practitioner
FO	(a) foot orthosis; (b) functional outcome
FOD	free of disease
FOH	fair oral hygiene
for. body	foreign body
FOW	fenestration oval window
FP	Family Practice
FR	French (catheter gauge)
fract	fracture
FRC	functional residual capacity
freq	(a) frequent; (b) frequency
frict	friction
FROM	full range of motion
Frx	fracture
FS	full and soft
FSH	follicle stimulating hormone
ft	foot (feet)
FTC	Federal Trade Commission

FTE	full-time equivalent
FTR	failed to report
FUO	fever of undetermined origin
f/u	follow up
FV	fluid volume
FVC	(a) false vocal cord; (b) forced vital capacity
FVU	first voided urine
FWB	full weight bearing
FW reaction	Felix-Weil reaction
Fx	fracture
Fx BB	fracture of both bones
FY	fiscal year
FYI	for your information
G	(a) good; (b) gastrostomy
g	(a) gravity; (b) gram
g.a.	ginger ale
GA	gestational age
ga	gauge
GABA	gamma-aminobutyric acid
gal	gallon
garg	gargle
GARS	Global Assessment of Recent Stress (Linn)
GAS	general adaption syndrome
GB	gallbladder
GBI	gingival bleeding index
GBS	gallbladder series
GC	gonococcus (gonorrhea)
g-cal	gram-calorie
GCS	Glasgow Coma Scale
gd	good
GDH	gonadotropic hormone
GE	(a) gravity eliminated; (b) gastroesophageal
GEA	general anesthesia
gen	general
Ger	geriatrics
GER	gastroesophageal reflux
GERD	gastroesophageal reflux disorder
GFTA	Goldman-Fristoe Test of Articulation
GGE	generalized glandular enlargement
GH	growth hormone
GHD	growth hormone deficiency

GI	gastrointestinal
GIK	glucose, insulin, (and) potassium
GIT	gastrointestinal tract
gl	gland
GLC	gas-liquid chromatography
glob	globulin
GLPP	glucose, postprandial
gluc	glucose
gm	gram
GM seizure	grand mal seizure
G/NS	glucose in normal saline
GOH	good oral hygiene
GP	general practitioner
GPB	glossopharyngeal breathing
GPO	Government Printing Office
gr	grain
GR	gastric resection
gran	granular
gran. o	no pregnancies
grd	ground
GRID	Gay Related Immune Deficiency
GRS	graphic representational system
GS	(a) general surgery; (b) gross substitution
G/S	glucose and saline
GSC	gas-solid chromatography
GSR	galvanic skin response
GSW	gunshot wound
gt	(a) gait; (b) g-(gastrostomy) tube
GTI	genital tract infection
GTT	glucose tolerance test
gtt	drops ([L.] *guttae*)
GU	genitourinary
GUS	genitourinary system
GVD	granulovacuolar degeneration
GVHD	graft-versus-host disease
G/W	glucose in water
GWE	glycerine and water enema
GXT	graded exercise testing
Gyn	gynecology
h	hour
H	(a) hold; (b) hypodermic (injection); (c) height; (d) hyperopia

(H)	hypodermic
Ha	absolute hypermetropia
HA	(a) headache; (b) hearing aid
H/A	height/age
hams	hamstrings
HAV	hepatitis A virus
HB	heart block
Hb	hemoglobin
HB/BW	hold breakfast for blood work
HBF	hepatic blow flow
HBHC	hospital-based home care
HBP	high blood pressure
HBS	hyperkinetic behavior syndrome
HBV	hepatitis B virus
HC	high caloric
HCC	health care center
HCFA	Health Care Financing Administration
HCP	(a) hearing conservation program; (b) health care provider
HCPCS	HCFA Common Procedure Coding System
hct	hematocrit
HCVD	hypertensive cardiovascular disease
HCW	health care worker
HD	(a) Huntington's disease; (b) hearing distance
h.d.	at the hour of bedtime ([L.] *hora decubitus*)
HD-h	Huntington's disease-hyperkinetic
HDL	high-density lipoproteins
HD-rb	Huntington's disease-rigid bradykinetic
HDW	hearing distance with watch
HEENT	head, ear, eye, nose, and throat
Hematol	hematology
hemi	hemiplegia
HEV	human enteric virus
HFHL	high-frequency hearing loss
HFRS	hemorrhagic fever with renal syndrome
Hg	mercury
Hgb	hemoglobin
HGG	human gamma globulin
HH	hiatal hernia
H & H	hemoglobin and hematocrit
HHA	(a) Home Health Agencies; (b) home health aide
HHC	Home Health Care

HHD	hypertensive heart disease
HHE	hemiconvulsions, hemiplegia, epilepsy
HI	head injury
HICN; HIC NO.	health insurance claim number
HIS	Hospital Information Systems
HIV	human immunodeficiency virus
H-K	heal to knee
HKAFO	hip-knee-ankle-foot orthosis
HKAO	hip-knee-ankle orthosis
HKO	hip-knee orthosis
HL	hearing level
H & L	heart and lungs
HLD	herniated lumbar disk
HLV	herpes-like virus
HMO	Health Maintenance Organization
HMP	hot moist packs
HN	head nurse
H & N	head and neck
HNV	has not voided
HO	(a) hand orthosis; (b) hip orthosis
H/O	history of
H_2O	water
H_2O_2	hydrogen peroxide
HOB	head of bed
HOCM	hypertrophic obstructive cardiomyopathy
HOH	hard of hearing
horz	horizontal
hosp	hospital
Hp	(a) hemiplegia; (b) hot pack
H & P	history and physical
HPE	history and physical examination
HPI	history of present illness
HPN	hypertension
HPV	human papilloma virus
HR	heart rate
hr	hour
H & R	hysterectomy and radiation
HRS	hepatorenal syndrome
h.s.	at bedtime ([L.] *hora somni*)
HSG	hysterosalpingogram
HSV	herpes simplex virus

HT	(a) hydrotherapy; (b) hypertension; (c) head trauma; (d) Hubbard task
Ht	total hyperopia
ht	height
HTE	hypertensive encephalopathy
HTN	hypertension
HTV	herpes-type virus
HUS	hemolytic uremic syndrome
husb	husband
HV	herpes virus
H & V	hemigastrectomy and vagotomy
HVD	hypertensive vascular disease
HVPC	high-voltage pulsed current
HW	housewife
Hx	history
hy	(a) hypermetropia; (b) hypropia
hypo	hypodermic
hys	hysteria
Hz	Hertz
IA	intra-arterial
IAC	internal auditory canal
IADL	instrumental activities of daily living
IAM	internal auditory meatus
IBD	inflammatory bowel disease
IBI	intermittent bladder irrigation
IBS	irritable bowel syndrome
IBW	initial body weight
IBQ	insurance billing questionnaire
IC	inspiratory capacity
ICC	intensive coronary care
ICCM	idiopathic congestive cardiomyopathy
ICCU	intensive coronary care unit
ICD	(a) International Classification of Diseases; (b) ideopathic cerebral dysfunction
ICD-9-CM	International Classification of Diseases, Ninth Revision, Clinical Modification
ICF	intermediate care facility
ICH	intracerebral hemorrhage
ICM	intercostal margin
ICN	Insurance Consultant Network
ICP	(a) intracranial pressure; (b) infection control program; (c) incomplete cleft palate

ICPS	Initial Communication Processes Scale (Schery & Glover)
ICS	intercostal space
ICT	inflammation of connective tissue
ict; ICT	(a) icterus; (b) intermittent cervical traction
ict ind	icterus index
ICU	intensive care unit
ICW	intracellular water
ID	(a) infectious disease; (b) identification; (c) initial dose
id	the same ([L.] *idem*)
I/D	intensity/duration
I & D	incision and drainage
IDA	iron deficiency anemia
IDB	interdental brush
IDD	insulin-dependent diabetes
IDU	injecting drug user
IDVC	indwelling venous catheter
IE	infective endocarditis
IEP	individualized education program
IFA	immunofluorescent assay
Ig	immunoglobulin
IH	infectious hepatitis
IHBT	incompatible hemolytic blood transaction
IHC	ideopathic hemachromatosis
IHD	ischemic heart disease
IHO	idiopathic hypertrophic osteoarthropathy
IHR	intrinsic heart rate
IL	independent living
I.L.A.	International Listening Association
ILDT	Interactive Language Development Teaching (Lee)
IM	(a) intramuscular; (b) internal medicine
IMH	idiopathic myocardial hypertrophy
immun	immunology
imp	impression
IMR	institution for the mentally retarded
IMV	intermittent mandatory ventilation
IN	intranasal
In	insulin
in	inch
inac	inactive

incl	include
incont	incontinent
incr	increased
ind	induction
indep	independent
inf	inferior
infec. dis.	infectious disease
inf. MI	inferior wall myocardial infarction
info	information
ing	inguinal
inh	inhalation
inj	(a) injury; (b) injection
inoc	inoculate
ins	insurance
INS	idiopathic nephrotic syndrome
inspir	inspiration
instr	instructed
in	internal
Int. Med.	internal medicine
Int CP	intermittent (in and out) catheter program
Intell	intelligibility
int rot	internal rotation
I & O	intake and output
IOFB	intraocular foreign body
IOM	Institute of Medicine
IOP	intraocular pressure
IP	(a) inpatient; (b) interphalangeal
IPA	independent practice association
IPAT	Iowa Pressure Articulation Test
IPD	intermittent peritoneal dialysis
IPF	idiopathic pulmonary fibrosis
IPG	impedance plethysmography
IPH	idiopathic pulmonary hemosiderosis
IPP & A	inspection, percussion, palpation, and auscultation
IPPB	intermittent positive-pressure breathing
IPOT	intervention plan of treatment
IPSF	immediate postsurgical fitting
IPT	intermittent pelvic traction
IPU	inpatient unit
IQ	intelligence quotient
IR	infrared

IRDS	idiopathic respiratory distress syndrome
irr	irradiation
irrig	irrigation
IRV	inspiratory reserve volume
IS	(a) intercostal space; (b) incentive spirometer
ISAAC	International Society for Augmentative and Alternative Communication
ISG	immune serum globulin
ISH	icteric serum hepatitis
ISW	interstitial water
IT	inhalation therapy
ITD	ideopathic torsion dystonia
ITE	in the ear
ith	intrathecal
ITP	idiopathic thrombocytopenic purpura
ITT	insulin tolerance test
IV	intravenous
IVD	intervertebral disk
IVF	intravascular fluid
IVGTT	intravenous glucose tolerance test
IVH	intraventricular hemorrhage
IVP	intravenous pyelogram
IVPB	intravenous piggyback
IVSD	intraventricular septal defect
IVT	intravenous transfusion
IVU	intravenous urography
IWMI	inferior wall myocardial infarction
IWRP	individualized written rehabilitation plan
J	Joule(s)
jaund	jaundice
jc	juice
J.C.A.H.O.	Joint Commission on Accreditation of Health Organizations
JCD	*Journal of Communication Disorders*
jct	junction
JD	juvenile dermatomyositis
JDM	juvenile diabetes mellitus
JEVS	Philadelphia Jewish Employment and Vocational Work Services Battery
JHFT	Jebson Hand Function Test
JJ	jaw jerk
JND	just noticeable difference

JODM;	
JOD	juvenile-onset diabetes
JPA	*Journal of Psychoeducational Assessment*
JRA	juvenile rheumatoid arthritis
JSHD	*Journal of Speech and Hearing Disorders*
JSHR	*Journal of Speech and Hearing Research*
jt	joint
juve	juvenile
JV	jugular vein
JVP	jugular venous pulse
K	(a) potassium; (b) kelvin; (c) kilo-
k	constant
KAFO	knee-ankle-foot orthosis
Kcal	kilocalorie
KCC	kathodal (cathodal) closing contraction
KCF	key clinical finding
KCG	kinetocardiogram
KCI	potassium chloride
KD	(a) knee disarticulation; (b) Korsakoff's disease
KELS	Kohlman Evaluation (of) Living Skills
kg	kilogram
kg-cal	kilocalorie(s)
kHz	kilohertz
KJ	(a) knee jerk; (b) knee joint
KK	knee kick
KLPA	Khan-Lewis Phonological Analysis
KLS	kidney, liver, spleen
km	kilometer
K-mod	K-module (heat therapy)
kn	knee
KO	knee orthosis
K/O	keep open
KOC	kathodal (cathodal) opening contraction
KOH	potassium hydroxide
KP	keratitis punctata
KS	Karposi sarcoma
KT	kinesiotherapist
KTA	Kitchen Task Assessment
K-therm	K-thermia (body temperature therapy)
KUB	kidney, ureter, bladder
KVO	keep vein open
L	(a) left; (b) liquid

l	(a) long; (b) length
L_1, L_2	lumbar vertebrae 1, 2, . . .
LA	(a) language age; (b) left atrium
lab	laboratory
lac	laceration
LAE	left atrial enlargement
LAM	late ambulatory monitoring
lang	language
LAO	left anterior oblique
LAP	left atrial pressure
lap	laparotomy
LARSP	Language Assessment, Remediation and Training Procedure (Crystal)
Laryng	laryngology
LAS	(a) local adaption syndrome; (b) Language Assessment Scales
LASER	light amplification by stimulated emission of radiation
lat	lateral
LAT	left anterior thigh
lat decub	lateral decubis
lax	laxative
LB	(a) large bowel; (b) leg bike
lb	pound ([L.] *libra*)
LBD	left brain damaged
LBP	low back pain
LCA	left coronary artery
LCL	hymphocytic lymphosarcoma
LCM	left costal margin
LCVA	left cerebrovascular accident
LD	learning disabled
L.D.A.	Learning Disabilities Association (of America)
LDD	lumbar disk disease
LDL	low density lipoproteins
L-dopa	levodopa
LDRP	labor and delivery/recovery and postpartum
LE	(a) lower extremity; (b) lupus erythematosus
LEA	lower extremity arterial
LED	lupus erythematosus disseminatus
LEP	limited English proficiency
LES	lower esophageal sphincter
leuko	leukocytes

LFx	left (arytenoid) fixation
lg	large
LGA	large for gestational age
LGB	Landry-Guillain-Barré
LH	left hemisphere
LHF	left heart failure
LHL	left hepatic lobe
Li	lithium
LIDC	low-intensity direct current
lig	ligament
LIH	left inguinal hernia
ling	linguistic
liq	(a) liquid; (b) liquor
lith	lithium
LK	left kidney
LKS	liver, kidney, spleen
LLB	long leg brace
LLC	long leg cast
LLL	(a) left lower lobe (of lungs); (b) left lower limb
LLLB	left lower leg brace
LLQ	left lower quadrant
LLT	left lateral thigh
LLWC	long leg walking cast
LM	lower motor
LMCA	left main coronary artery
L/min	liters per minute
LMN	lower motor neuron
LMNL	lower motor neuron lesion
LMP	last menstrual period
LMTA	Language Modalities Test for Aphasia
LN	lymph node
LOA	level of awareness
LOC	(a) loss of consciousness; (b) laxative of choice
LOM	left otitis media
LOS	length of service
lot	lotion
LP	lumbar puncture
LPA	left pulmonary artery
LPM	liters per minute
LPO	light perception only
LPT	(a) Language Proficiency Test; (b) licensed physical therapist

LPTA	licensed physical therapist assistant
LPV	left pulmonary veins
LPWM	lateral pharyngeal wall movement
lrln	left recurrent laryngeal nerve
LRQ	lower right quadrant
LRS	lactated Ringer's solution
LRT	lower respiratory tract
LS	lumbosacral
LSB	left sternal border
LSIO	lumbosacroiliac orthosis
LSK	liver, spleen, kidneys
LSLB	left short leg brace
LSM	late systolic murmur
LSO	lumbosacral orthosis
L-spine	lumbar spine
LSW	left-sided weakness
lt	left
LTCF	long-term care facility
LTG	long-term goal
lt. lat.	left lateral
LTM	long-term memory
LU	left upper
L & U	lower and upper
LUE	left upper extremity
LUL	(a) left upper limb; (b) left upper lobe (of lung)
LUQ	left upper quadrant
LV	left ventricle
LVDP	left ventricular diastolic pressure
LVE	(a) laryngeal video endostroboscopy; (b) left ventricular enlargement
LVF	left ventricular failure
LVH	left ventricular hypertrophy
LVN	licensed vocational nurse
lvs	laryngovideostroboscopy
LVSV	left ventricular stroke volume
LVSW	left ventricular stroke work
LW	left wrist
L & W	living and well
lymphs	lymphocytes
lytes	electrolytes
M	(a) male; (b) mega-
m	(a) meter; (b) minimum; (c) myopia; (d) muscle

Mμ	millimicron(s)
μm	micrometers
μV	millivolt(s)
M_1	mitral first heart sound
M_2	mitral second heart sound
MA	mental age
ma	milliampere
MAC	monomine oxidase inhibitors
MAE	(a) moving all extremities; (b) Multilingual Aphasia Examination
MAE-S	Examen de Afasia Multilingue (Spanish)
mag	large
malig	malignant
M + AM	(compound) myopic astigmatism
mand	mandible
manifest	manifestation
manip	manipulation
M.A.O.T.	Master of Arts in Occupational Therapy
MAP	modular assembly prosthesis
MAS	mobile arm support
masc	masculine
MAT	manual arts therapist
max	maximum
MBD	minimal brain dysfunction
MBS	modified barium swallow
MBSS	Modified Barium Swallow Study
MC	(a) millicurie; (b) maintenance candidate; (c) megacycle
M & C	morphine and cocaine
MCA	medial cerebral artery
mcg	microgram
MCL	midclavicular line
MCM	manual communication module
MCP	metacarpal phalangeal (joint)
MCPS	Missouri Children's Self Concept Scale
MCU	maximum care unit
MD	(a) medical doctor; (b) muscular dystrophy
MDD	mean daily dose
MDM	mid-diastolic murmur
MDR	minimum daily requirement
MDS	Minimum Data Set
MDT	motion-dependent torques

MDUO	myocardial disease of unknown origin
MDY	month, day, year
meas	measure
mech	mechanical
med	medicine
MED	minimal erythema dose
meds	medications
memb	membrane
MENS	muscular electrical nerve stimulation
ment	mental
met	metastatic
metab	metabolism
metas	metastatic
M & F	mother and father
MFS	mitral first sound
MG	myasthenia gravis
mg	milligram
mgtts	microdrops
MH	moist hat
mHz	megahertz
MI	(a) myocardial infarction; (b) mentally impaired
micro	microscopic
MICU	medical intensive care unit
MID	multi-infarct dementia
mid	middle
mid sag	midsagittal
millisec	millisecond
min	(a) minute; (b) minimum
MIS	management information system
misc	miscellaneous
MIT	Melodic Intonation Therapy
mixt	mixture
mj	millijoule
ML	midline
ml	milliliter
MLU	mean length of utterance
mm	(a) muscles; (b) millimeter
MM	mucus membrane
MMC	migrating motor activity
MMCPC	Multidimensional Measure of Children's Perception of Control
MMDDYY	month-day-year (numeric)

MMPI Minnesota Multiphasic Personality Inventory
MMR measles, mumps, (and) rubella
MMT manual muscle test
M/N midnight
M & N morning and night
MNCV motor nerve conduction velocity
mo month
mod moderate
MOM milk of magnesia
Mono infectious monoculeosis
morph morphology
mort mortality
mos months
MPO months postonset
MPS mucopolysaccharidosis
MPTP 1-methyl-4-phenyl-1, 23, 3, 6- tetrahydropyridine
MR (a) medical review; (b) medical records
M & R measure and record
M.R. × 1, × 2may repeat one time, two times, . . .
MRA medical record administrator
MRF mitral regurgitant flow
MRI magnetic resonance imaging
MRSA methicillin resistant staphylococcus aureus
MS (a) multiple sclerosis; (b) mechanical soft
ms; msec millisecond
M/S mother states
MSAFP maternal serum alpha-fetoprotein
MSDS material safety data sheet
msec millisecond
MSQ mental status questionnaire
M.S.S.W. Master of Science in Social Work
MST mean survival time
MSW Master of Social Work
MT (a) medical technologist; (b) maintenance therapy
MTDDA Minnesota Test for Differential Diagnosis of Aphasia (Schuell)
MTM method of time measurement
MTP metatarsophalangeal (joint)
MUAP motor unit action potential
mur murmur
musc muscles

muscle re-ed	muscle reeducation
MV	mitral valve
MVA	motor vehicle accident
MVP	mitral valve prolapse
MVR	mitral valve replacement
mvt	movement
MVV	maximum voluntary ventilation
my	myopia
mz	monozygotic
n	(a) nasal; (b) nerve ([L.] *nervus*); (c) normal
N	(a) nitrogen; (b) (licensed) nursing; (c) neurology
Na	sodium
NA	not applicable
N.A.	nursing assistant
N.A.A.	National Aphasia Association
NAB	National Association of Boards (of Examiners for Nursing Home Administration)
NaCl	sodium chloride
NAD	(a) no acute distress; (b) no appreciable disease
NAMB	non-A non-B (hepatitis) virus
narc	narcotic
NARIC	National Rehabilitation Information Center
NAS	no added salt
nas	nasal
nat	natural
N.B.A.S.L.H.	National Black Association for Speech, Language and Hearing
NBM	(a) nothing by mouth; (b) no bowel movement
NBN	narrow band noise
NBQC	narrow bone quad cane
NBS	no bacteria seen
NC	(a) noncontributory; (b) no change
N/C	no complaints
N.C.A.M.L.P.	National Certification Agency for Medical Laboratory Personnel
NCCEA	Neurosensory Center Comprehensive Examination for Aphasia
NCP	(a) no cleft palate; (b) nursing care plan
NCV	nerve conduction velocity
N/D	no defects

NDT	(a) neurodevelopment treatment (Bobath); (b) neuromuscular development technology
N.D.T.A.	Neurodevelopmental Treatment Association
nebul	nebulizer
NEC	necrotizing entercolitis
NED	no evidence of disease
neg	negative
NEMD	nonspecific esophageal motor disorder
NEP	non-English proficiency
nerv	nervous
NET	net torque
neuro	neurology
Neuro-Surg	neurosurgery
NF	nursing facility
NFT	neurofibrillary tangles
ng	(a) nasogastric; (b) nanogram
N/G	no good
NGO	nitroglycerin ointment
NGU	nongonococcal urethritis
NH	nursing home
NH_3	ammonia
NH_4CI	ammonium chloride
NHP	nursing home placement
NIA	no information available
NIC	nosocomial infection control
NICU	neonatal intensive care unit
NID	not in distress
NIDR	National Institute of Dental Research
NIHL	noise-induced hearing loss
nil	none
NIR	nosocomial infection rate
nitro	nitroglycerin
n/k	not known
NKA	no known allergies
NKFA	no known food allergies
n/l	normal limits
N.L.N.	National League for Nursing
N.L.R.B.	National Labor Relations Board
NM	(a) nuclear medicine; (b) non monitored
nm	nanometer
NMES	neuromuscular electrical stimulation
NMF	neuromuscular facilitative techniques

NMI	no middle initial
NMN	no middle name
NMR	nuclear magnetic resonance
NMSC	nerve and muscle stimulating current
nn	nerves ([L.] *nervi*)
no.	number
n/o	not obtained
noc	night ([L.] *nocte*)
noct	nocturnal (at night)
non rep	(a) no refill; (b) don't repeat ([L.] *non repetatur*)
norm	normal
NOS	not otherwise specified
noxt	at night
NP	(a) neuropsychiatric; (b) no potential; (c) neuropsychology
NPD	Neimann-Pick disease
NPH	normal pressure hydrocephalus
NPF	National Parkinson Foundation
NPI	no present illness
NPO	nothing by mouth ([L.] *non per os*)
nr	near
N/R	not remarkable
N.R.A.	National Rehabilitation Association
NRD	next review date
NRI	nerve root irritation
NS	(a) not significant; (b) no service; (c) normal saline; (d) neurologic surgery
NSA	no serious abnormality
N.S.D.A.	National Spasmodic Dysphonia Association
nsg	nursing
NS/NP	no service/no potential
NSQ	not sufficient quantity
NSR	normal sinus rhythm
NSS	normal saline solution
NSST	Northwestern Syntax Screening Test (Lee)
NSU	nonspecific urethritis
NT	not tested
NTG	nitroglycerin
NTGO	nitroglycerin ointment
NTI	no treatment indicated
NTP	normal temperature and pulse
N & T	nose and throat

NTS	nasotracheal suctioning
nunc	now
NV	nausea and vomiting
NVA	near visual acuity
NVD	nausea, vomiting, diarrhea
NVS	neurological vital signs
NWB	non-weight bearing
NYD	not yet diagnosed
O	(a) omission; (b) eye ([L.] *oculus*); (c) oxygen; (d) zero in muscle and range of motion testing
O2	both eyes
O_2	oxygen
o	(a) none; (b) bone ([L.] *os*)
o-	ortho
OA	osteoarthritis
O & A	observation and assessment
OAD	obstructive airway disease
OAE	(a) otoacoustic emission; (b) Orzeck Aphasia Evaluation
OB	obstetrics
obl	oblique
OBRA	Omnibus Budget Reconciliation Act (of 1987)
OBS	organic brain syndrome
obs	observed
obst	obstructed
O & C	onset and course
occ	occasionally
occup	occupation
OCV	ordinary conversational voice
OD	(a) overdose; (b) Doctor of Optometry
od	right eye ([L.] *oculus dexter*)
OE	ostectomy
OFD	oral-facial-digital (syndrome)
OG	obstetrics (and) gynecology
OH	oral hygiene
OHD	organic heart disease
OHI	oral hygiene instructions
OHS	open heart surgery
oint	ointment
o.j.	orange juice
OJT	on-the-job training
OK	okay; approved

ol	(a) oil; (b) left eye ([L.] *oculus laevus*)
ol oliv	olive oil
OM	otitis media
OMB	Office of Management and Budget
OME	otitis media (with) effusion
OMPA	otitis media, purulent, acute
OMSA	otitis media, suppurative, acute
OMSC	otitis media, suppurative, chronic
OOB	out of bed
op	operation
OP	(a) outpatient; (b) osteoporosis; (c) ophthalmology
OPA	oropharyngeal airway
OPB	outpatient basis
OPD	(a) outpatient department; (b) oto-palatal-digital syndrome (Taybi)
oper	operation
Ophth	ophthalmology
opp	opposite
OPS	outpatient service
OPT	(a) outpatient treatment; (b) outpatient physical therapy
OR	(a) operating room; (b) open reduction
Oral S	oral surgery
org	organic
orient x 3	oriented to time, place, person
ORIF	open reduction internal fixation
orig	origin
ORL	otorhinolaryngology
Ortho	orthopedics
OS	(a) left eye ([L.] *oculus sinister*); (b) orthopedic surgery
OSERS	Office (of) Special Education (and) Rehabilitative Services
osm	osmotic
OSMCP	occult submucous cleft palate
OSP	outpatient speech pathology
oss	(a) osseous; (b) bones ([L.] *ossa*)
OT	(a) occupational therapy; (b) otolaryngology; (c) oral transit
OTC	over the counter
OTD	out the door (discharge)
OTL	licensed occupational therapist

Olo	(a) otology; (b) otolaryngology
OTR	registered occupational therapist
OTR/L	registered licensed occupational therapist
ou	both eyes ([L.] *oculus uterque*)
OV	office visit
O/W	oil in water
oz	ounce
P	(a) phosphorus; (b) poor; (c) puréed
P	pulse
p	after ([L.] *post*)
PA	(a) posterior-anterior; (b) physician assistant; (c) pernicious anemia; (d) pathology
PACE	Promoting Aphasics' Communicative Effectiveness
PACO	pivot ambulating crutchless orthosis
pal	palpation
palp	palpable
palpit	palpitations
PALS	patients with amyotrophic lateral sclerosis
panendo	panendoscopy
pap	Papanicolaou (smear)
para; parap	paraplegic
parox	paroxysmal
PASARR	preadmission screening and annual resident review
pass	passive
PAT	paroxysmal atrial tachycardia
Path	pathology
pat med	patent medicine
PA-VF	pulmonary arteriovenous fistula
pb	phenobarbital
pbc	placebo
p.c.	after meals ([L.] *post cibum*)
PCA	posterior cerebral artery
PCC	Patient Care Conference
PCE	physical capacities evaluation
PCN	penicillin
PCP	pneumocystis carinii pneumonia
PCP	pneumocystic pneumonia
PCU	progressive care unit
PD	(a) Parkinson's disease; (b) peritoneal dialysis
p/d	packs per day

PDD pervasive development disorder

PDE predriver evaluation

PDIL Prueba Del Desarrollo Inicial Del Lenguage

PDMS Peabody Developmental Motor Scales

PDR; pdr (a) *Physician's Desk Reference*; (b) powder

PE (a) physical examination; (b) pulmonary embolism; (c) pressure equalization (tubes)

P-E pharyngeal esophageal

PEC Perfil De Evaluacion Del Comportamiento

PECT positron emission computerized tomography

Ped: PEDS pediatrics

PEEP positive end-expiratory pressure

PEG percutaneous endoscopic gastrostomy

PEL present education level

Pen penicillin

pent pentothal

per by ([L.] *per*)

perf perforation

periap periapical

PERL pupils equal, react to light

perm permanent

pers personal

PET pressure equalization tube

PETT position emission transaxial tomography

PE tube plastic eustachian tube

PF plantar flexion

PFS phonatory function study

PFT premium float pool

PG; Pg (a) progress; (b) pregnant

PH; PHx past (prior) history

phar pharmacy

PHC primary hepatic carcinoma

Ph.D. Doctor of Philosophy

PHMD pseudohypertrophic muscular dystrophy

PHN Public Health Nurse

phos phosphate

PHR post heart rate

PHS Public Health Service

PHT (a) pulmonary hypertension; (b) passive hyperimmune therapy

PHx past history

PHYS physician

phys dis	physical disability
Phys Med	physical medicine
PI	(a) present illness; (b) phonologically impaired
PICA	(a) Porch Index of Communicative Ability; (b) posterior inferior cerebellar artery (syndrome)
PID	pelvic inflammatory disease
pil	pill(s)
PIN	personal identification number
PIP	proximal interphalageal (joint)
PIVD	protruded intervertebral disk
PIVR	pacemaker-induced ventricular rate
PK	pack
PKU	phenylketonuria
PL	(a) perception of light; (b) plastic (surgery)
pl	plasma
plat	platelets
PLM	product line management
pls	(wall) pulleys
plt	platelet
PLWA	person living with AIDS
P.M.	afternoon ([L.] *post meridiem*)
PM	postmortem
PMH	past medical history
PMR; PM & R	physical medicine and rehabilitation
PMRS	physical medicine and rehabilitation service
PMV	prolapsed mitral valve
PN	peripheral nerve
Pn	pneumonia
PNF	peripheral nerve function; proprioceptive neuromuscular facilitation
PNI	progressive neurological
PND	paroxysmal nocturnal dyspnea
pneumo	pneumothorax
PNF	proprioceptive neuromuscular facilitation
PNI	peripheral nerve injury
PNS	(a) peripheral nervous system; (b) posterior nasal spine
pnx	pneumothorax
PO	postoperative
P/O	phone order
p.o.	by mouth ([L.] *per os*)

PO_4	phosphate
POC	(a) plan of care; (b) postoperative care
POH	poor oral hygiene
polio	poliomyelitis
PONS	Profile of Non-Verbal Sensitivity
Pos	positive
poss	possible
post	posterior
postop	postoperative
POT	(a) plan of treatment; (b) postoperative treatment
pot	potassium
powd	powder
PP	postpartum
PPD	(a) phonological (processing or production) disturbance; (b) purified protein derivative (TB test)
PPG	photplethysmography
PPE	personal protective equipment
PPN	peripheral parenteral nutrition
PPS	prospective pricing system
ppt	precipitate
PPVT-R	Peabody Picture Vocabulary Test– Revised (Dunn & Dunn)
ppw	posterior pharyngeal wall
pr	(a) pair; (b) process; (c) presbyopia
p.r.	per rectum
prac	practice
pract	practical
PRE	progressive resistance exercise
pref	preference
preg	pregnant
prelim	preliminary
prep	prepare
press	pressure
prev	previous
princ	principal
priv	privilege
PRM	preventive medicine
p.r.n.	as required ([L.] *pro re nata*)
prnts	parents
pro	(a) protein; (b) pronation
PRO	Peer Review Organization
prob	(a) probable; (b) problem

proc	procedure
Proct	proctology
prod	(a) product; (b) productive
prof	profession
prog	prognosis
proj	project
PROM	passive range of motion
pron	pronation
proph	prophylactic
prophy	(oral) prophylaxis
prosth	prosthesis
prot	protein
Prot	Protestant
prox	proximal
PS	(a) psychiatric services; (b) prognostic statement
PSA	prostatic specific antigen (test)
PSD	Professional Services Department
PSG	polysomnography
Psy	psychiatry
Psych	psychology
PT	(a) physical therapy; (b) physical therapist; (c) pharyngeal transit
pt	(a) patient; (b) prothrombin time
PT Reg	Physical Therapist, Registered (Canada)
PTA	(a) physical therapy assistant; (b) prior to admission
PTB	patellar tendon bearing
PTCA	percutaneous transluminal coronary angioplasty
PTD	prior to discharge
Pth	pathology
PTIP	physical therapist (in) independent practice
PTR	patient to return
PTS	(a) patient treatment stress; (b) patellar tendon supracondylar; (c) permanent (hearing) threshold shift; (d) patellar tendon
PTSD	posttraumatic stress disorder
PTT	prothrombin time
PU	peptic ulcer
P/U	pickup
PUD	(a) peptic ulcer disease; (b) pyroxin of unknown origin
pulm	pulmonary

PVD	peripherovascular disease
PVS	persistent vegetative state
pvt	private
PW	posterior wall
PWA	person with AIDS
PWB	partial weight-bearing
PWC	physical work capacity
PX	physical examination
Px	prognosis
Q	quantity
q	every ([L.] *quaque*)
QA	quality assurance
q. a.m.; q AM	every morning ([L.] *quaque ante meridiem*
q. d.	every day ([L.] *quaque die*)
q. 2 d.	every second day
q. h.	every hour ([L.] *quaque hora*)
q. 2 h.	every two hours ([L.] *quaque secunda hora*)
q. 3 h.	every three hours ([L.] *quaque tertia hora*)
q. h. s.	at bedtime ([L.] *quaque hora somni*)
q. i. d.	four times a day ([L.] *quaque in die*)
q. l.	as much as is desired ([L.] *quantum libet*)
qns	quantity not sufficient
q. o. d.	every other day ([L.] *quaque o. die*)
q. o. h.	every other hour ([L.] *quaque o. hora*)
q. o. n.	every other night ([L.] *quaque o. n.*)
q. p.	as much as you please ([L.] *quantum placet*)
q. p. m.; q PM	every afternoon ([L.] *quaque post meridiem*)
q. s.	a sufficient amount ([L.] *quantum sufficit*)
q.s. ad	to a sufficient quantity
QUAD	quadriceps exercise
quad	quadriplegic
quads	quadriceps (muscles)
qual	qualitative
quant	quantity
QUIL	Quick Incidental Learning
q.v.	as much as you wish ([L.] *quantum vis*)
R	(a) right; (b) resist; (c) recheck
(R)	rectal
r	(a) respiration; (b) rectal

RA	(a) rheumatoid arthritis; (b) rehabilitation aide; (c) restorative aide
Ra	radium
RACE	Rescue patients, sound the Alarm, Confine the fire, Extinguish (Evacuate) it
rad	radical
RAI	resident assessment instrument
RAIU	radioactive iodine uptake (test)
RAP	Resident Assessment Protocol
R & R	rest and relaxation
RAT	right anterior thigh
RB	right buttock
RBC	red blood count
RBD	right brain damaged
RBRVS	resource-based relative value scale
RC	(a) restorative candidate; (b) rehabilitative counseling (counselor)
RCBA	Reading Comprehension Battery for Aphasia
rCBF	regional cerebral blood flow
RCM	right costal margin
RCP	(a) resident care plan; (b) respiratory care practitioner
RCU	respiratory care unit
RCVA	right cerebrovascular accident
RD	reaction of degeneration
R.D.	registered dietitian
RDA	recommended dietary allowance
RDS	respiratory distress syndrome
RDT	regular dialysis treatment
RE; ref	referral
rec	(a) record; (b) recommendation
rect	rectum
recur	recurrent
Red	reduction
REEL	Receptive-Expressive Emergent Language Scale (Bzoch & League)
ref	refer
ref. doc.	referring doctor
ref. phys.	referring physician
reg	regular
regen	regenerate
rehab	rehabilitation

rel	relative
R-ELA	receptive minus expressive language age
rem	remove
rep	repeat
req	requested
RES	Rehabilitation Evaluation System
resp	respiratory
RESR	real ear saturation response
retro	retrograde
rev	review
RF	rheumatic fever
RFA	right femoral artery
RFX	right (arytenoid) fixation
RG	remedial gymnast
RGO	reciprocating gait orthosis
RH; Rh	(a) right hemisphere; (b) blood factor (Rhesus)
RHC	rural health clinic
RHD	rheumatic heart disease
RHF	right heart failure
RHR	resting heart rate
RIA	radioimmunoassay
RICE	Rehabilitation Institute of Chicago Evaluation (of Communication Problems in Right Hemisphere Dysfunction)
RICU	respiratory intensive care unit
RIH	right inguinal ligament
RIND	reversible ischemic neurologic defect
RIP	respiratory inductive plethysmography
RIPA	Ross Information Processing Assessment
RK	(a) right kidney; (b) radial keratotomy
RKT	registered kinesiotherapist
RL	right leg
RLA	(a) Rancho Los Amigos (scale); (b) receptive language age
RLE	right lower extremity
RLL	(a) right lower limb; (b) right lower lobe (of lung)
RLLB	right long leg brace
RLN	recurrent laryngeal nerve
RLQ	(a) right lower quadrant; (b) receptive language quotient
RLS	Ringer's lactate solution
RLT	right lateral thigh

rm	room
RM	repetition maximum
RN	registered nurse
RN-CS	registered nurse–clinical specialist
RN-NP	registered nurse–nurse practitioner
RND	radical neck dissection
RO	(a) routine order; (b) reality-oriented
R/O	rule out
ROM	(a) range of motion; (b) right otitis media
ROMT	range-of-motion test
ROS	review of systems
rot	rotate
rout	routine
row	rowers
RP	pulmonary resistance
RPA	right pulmonary artery
RPCH	rural primary care hospital
RPR	rapid plasma reagent (test)
RPT	registered physical therapist
RQ	response to a question
R & R	rate and rhythms
RR	recovery room
r r	respiratory rate
rrln	right recurrent laryngeal nerve
RRR	regular rate and rhythm
RRS	registered rehabilitation specialist
RRT	registered recreational therapist; registered rehabilitation therapist; registered respiratory therapist
RS	response to a statement
RSLB	right short leg brace
RSR	regular sinus rhythm
RSW	right-sided weakness
rt	(a) right; (b) reaction time; (c) return
RT	(a) registered technician; (b) respiratory therapy (therapist); (c) radiation therapy; (d) recreational therapist; (e) resuscitation therapist; (f) rehabilitation therapist
RTC	return to clinic
RTI	Routine Task Inventory
rt lat	right lateral
RTT	Revised Token Test

RUE	right upper extremity
RUL	right upper limb; right upper lobe (of lung)
rupt	rupture
RUTI	recurrent urinary tract infection
RV	residual volume
RVS	relative value scale
RW	right wrist
℞	prescription ([L.] *recipe*)
S	(a) single; (b) solid; (c) surgery; (d) sacral; (e) supper
-¼s	(a) without ([L.] *sine*); (b) sign ([L.] *signa*)
SA	sinoatrial
SAAT	Selective Auditory Attention Test
SAC	short arm cast
S & D	stomach and duodenum
SAD	seasonal affective disorder
SAI	School Activity Index
Sal	salmonella
SAQ	short arc quad
SAS	Sklar Aphasia Scale
sat	saturate
satis	satisfactory
Sb	strabismus
SBA	standby assist
SBD	senile brain disease
SBO	small bowel obstruction
SBR	strict bed rest
sc	subcutaneous
SCA	sex chromosomal abnormality
SCATBI	Scales of Cognitive Ability for Traumatic Brain Injury
SCC	squamous cell carcinoma
sched	schedule
schiz	schizophrenia
SCI	spinal cord injury
SCIC	self-clean intermittent catheterization
sclero	scleroderma
SD	(a) standard deviation; (b) speech discrimination; (c) septal defect; (d) spasmodic dysphonia; (e) skin dose
SDAT	senile dementia of the Alzheimer type
SDH	subdural hematoma

sds	sounds
SDT	speech detection threshold
sec	second
SECEL	Self-Evaluation (of) Communication Experience (after) Laryngectomy (Blood)
sect	section
Sed rate	sedimentation rate
SEIU	Service Employees International Union
SEO	shoulder-elbow orthosis
SEM	standard error (of) measurement
sep	separate
seq	sequence
seq luce	the following day ([L.] *sequenti luce*)
serv	service
SES	(a) socioeconomic status; (b) Self Esteem Scale (Rosenberg)
SEWHO	shoulder-elbow-wrist-hand orthosis
SEWO	shoulder-elbow-wrist orthosis
SF	standard form
SG	specific gravity
SGOT	serum glutamic-exalcacetic transaminase
SGPT	serum glutamic-pyruvic transaminase
Sh	shoulder
SH	social history
S & H	speech and hearing
S.H.E.A.	Society for Hospital Epidemiologists of America
SHFE	Smith Hand Function Evaluation
S.H.H.H.	Self Help for the Hard of Hearing
SI	(a) sacroiliac (joint); (b) International System of Units
sib	(a) sibling; (b) self-injurious behavior
SICD	Sequenced Inventory of Communicative Development
SIDA	sindrome de inmuno deficiencia adquirida
sig	(a) let it be labeled (write) ([L.] *signa*); (b) signature
SIO	sacroliac orthosis
SIPT	Sensory Information and Praxis Tests
SIS	(a) sensory information store; (b) shaken infant syndrome
SJP	static joint position
SJS	Stevens-Johnson Syndrome

SIW	self-inflicted wound
SKO	supracondylar knee orthosis
sl	slight
S.L.	sublingual
SLAP	Spanish Language Assessment Procedures
SLB	short leg brace
SLC	short leg cast
SLD	specific learning disability
SLE	systemic lupus erythematosus
SLN	superior laryngeal nerve
SLP	Speech-Language Pathologist
SLR	straight leg raises
SLST	symptom-limited stress test
sm	small
SMA	supplemental motor areas
SMCP	submucous cleft palate
SMI	sensory motor integration
S/N	signal to noise ratio
SN & SX	signs and symptoms
SNF	skilled nursing facility
SNHL	sensorineural hearing loss
SNS	sympathetic nervous system
SOAA	signed out against advice
SOAP	subjective data, objective data, assessment, plan
SOB	short of breath
SOC	start of care
soc sec	Social Security
sol	solution
SOMA	signed out against medical advice
SOMI	sternal occipital mandibular immobilizer
SOP	standard operating procedure
S.O.S.	one dose if necessary ([L.] *siopus sit*)
SP; sp	(a) speech pathologist; (b) senile plaques
S/P	status post
sp. cd.	spinal cord
spec	specimen
SPECT	single proton emission computed tomography
sp. fl.	spinal fluid
SPIN	Speech Perception in Noise (test)
spont	spontaneous
SQ	social quotient
sq	square

SR	(a) sinus rhythm; (b) suture removed
S/R	suture removal
SRE	schedule of recent experience
SROM	spontaneous rupture of membrane
SRT	speech reception threshold
SS	(a) Social Security; (b) stuttering severity (scale); (c) skilled service; (d) social services; (e) soap suds
S/S	signs and symptoms
ss	(a) simple substitution; (b) one-half ([L.] *semis*)
SSA	Social Security Administration
SS#	Social Security number
SSD	social service designee
SSDI	Social Security Disability Insurance
SSE	soapsuds enema
SS enema	saline solution enema
SSI	Supplemental Insurance Income
S & S	signs and symptoms
SSNB	supra scapular nerve block
S-spine	sacral spine
ST	(a) speech therapist; (b) speech therapy; (c) sinus tachycardia
stand.	standard
staph	staphylococcus
stat	immediately ([L.] *statim*)
STC	(a) sports training certificate; (b) single tip cane
STD	sexually transmitted diseases
std	standard
STF	special tube feeding
STG	short-term goal
stim	(a) stimulus; (b) stimulation
STM	short-term memory
STP	supracondylar tibial prosthesis
STT	skin temperature test
strab	strabismus
strep	streptococcus
struc	structure
subcut	subcutaneous
subling	sublingual
submand	submandibular
sub Q	subcutaneous
SUD	sudden unexpected (unexplained) death
suff	sufficient

sup	(a) superior; (b) supination
supp	suppository
suppos	suppository
Surg	surgery
susp	suspension
sut	suture
SVCS	superior vena cava syndrome
SVI	stroke volume index
SW	social worker
SWD	short wave diathermy
SWE	simulated work experience
SWI	stroke work index
Sx	symptom
sym	symmetry
symb	symbol
sympat	sympathetic
sympt	symptom
syn	syndrome
syph	syphilis
syr	syrup
sys	system
sz	seizure
T	(a) temperature; (b) tension; (c) trunk; (d) thoracic; (e) transcribed; (f) temporal; (g) Trace: muscle testing
T_1, T_2	thoracic vertebrae 1, 2, . . .
T & A	tonsillectomy and adenoidectomy
tab	tablet
tachy	tachycardia
talc	talcum powder
TAPS	Test of Auditory Perceptual Skills
TAWL	Teachers Applying Whole Language
TB	tuberculosis
T/B	tonic bite
tbc	tuberculosis
TBG	thyroxine-binding globulin
TBI	traumatic brain injury
tbsp	tablespoonful
TBW	total body weight
TC	throat culture
TCA	tricyclic antidepressant
TCN	tetracycline

TCNS	transcutaneous nerve stimulator
TD	tactile defensiveness
T/D	treatment discontinued
TE; T-E	tracheoesophageal
te	tetanus
T & E	trial and error
teasp	teaspoonful
tech	technician
TED	(a) thromboembolic (disease): (b) Test of Emotional Development
TEF	tracheoesophageal fistula
TEFRA	Tax Equity and Fiscal Responsibility Act
Temp	temperature
TEN	toxic epidermal necrolysis
TENS	transcutaneous electrical neuromuscular stimulation
TEP	tracheal esophageal puncture
term	terminate
tert	tertiary
TEW	tolerates exercise well
TF	tube feeding
TG	triglycerides
T/G	thermal gustatory
th	(a) therapist; (b) thoracic
ther	therapy
therm	thermal
THR	total hip replacement
TIA	transient ischemic attack
t.i.d.	three times a day ([L.]*ter in die*)
tinct	tincture
TJ	triceps jerk
TK	Through-knee
TKO	to keep open
TL	thick liquid
TLC	(a) total lung capacity; (b) tender loving care
TLSO	thoracolombosacral orthosis
TLV	total lung volume
TM	tympanic membrane
TMA	transcortical motor aphasia
TMJ	temporomandibular joint
TMR	trainable mentally retarded
TMP-SMX	trimethoprim-sulfamethoxazole

TMT	treadmill test
TNTC	too numerous to count
T-O	time out
T(O)	temperature (oral)
T/O	telephone order
TOA	task-oriented assessment
tol	tolerate
tomo	tomogram
top	(a) topical; (b) termination of pregnancy
TOPS	Test of Problem Solving
TOT	tip of the tongue
tox	toxic
TP	(a) total protein; (b) trigger point
TPN	total parenteral nutrition
TPR	temperature, pulse, respiration
TQM	total quality management
tr	(a) tincture; (b) trace
T(R)	temperature (rectal)
trach	tracheostomy
trach. asp.	tracheal aspiration
tract	traction
train	training
trans	transverse
transm	transmission
transpl	transplant
TRH	thyrotropin releasing hormone
trig	triglycerides
TRIP	Tennessee Test of Rhythm and Intonation Patterns (Koike & Asp)
trt	treatment
TS	(a) thoracic surgery; (b) test solution
TSA	transcortical sensory aphasia
TSH	thyroid stimulating hormone
tsp	teaspoon
T-spine	thoracic spine
TT	(a) Token Test; (b) tilt table
TTA	transtracheal aspiration
TTBL	tilt table
TTS	temporary threshold shift
TTWB	toe touch weight bearing
TTY	teletypewriter
T.U.	type undetermined

tuberc	tuberculosis
TUR	transurethral resection
tuss	cough ([L.] *tussis*)
TV	tidal volume
TVC	timed vital capacity
TVPS	Test of Visual Perceptual Skills
TWB	total weight bearing
TWE	tap water enema
TWF	Test of Word Finding (Gorman)
Tx	(a) treatment; (b) traction
tymp. mem.	tympanic membrane
tymps	tympanograms
typ	typical
U	urology
u	unit
UA	urinalysis
UCHD	usual childhood diseases
UCLP	unilateral cleft lip and palate
UCR	usual, customary, and reasonable
UE	upper extremity
UES	upper esophageal sphincter
UGI	upper gastrointestinal (tract)
UHF	ultrahigh frequency
U & L	upper and lower
UKN	unknown
ULQ	upper left quadrant
ULT	Utley Lipreading Test
UM	upper motor
UMN	upper motor neuron
UMNL	upper motor neuron lesion
uncomp	uncomplicated
uncon	unconscious
uncond	unconditioned
uncond. ref.	unconditioned reflex
uncorr	uncorrected
undet. orig.	undetermined origin
undiff	undifferentiated
ung	ointment ([L.] *unguentum*)
unilat	unilateral
UNIT	Universal Nonverbal Intelligence Test
univ	universal
unk	unknown

unsat	unsatisfactory
up ad lib	out of bed as desired
UPIN	unique physician identification number
UPPP	uvulopalatopharyngoplasty
ur	urine
UR	utilization review
URD	upper respiratory disease
ureth	urethra
URI	upper respiratory infection
uro-gen	urogenital
Urol	urology
URQ	upper right quadrant
US	(a) ultrasonic; (b) ultrasound
US/ES	ultrasound with electrical stimulation
USI	urinary stress incontinence
U.S.S.A.A.C.	United States Society for Augmentative and Alternative Communication
UT	urinary tract
Ut	diet as directed ([L.] *ut dictum*)
UTI	urinary tract infection
UV	ultraviolet
UVL	ultraviolet light
V	(a) vision; (b) velum
v	(a) vein; (b) volt
VA; V/A	visual acuity
VABS	Vineland Adaptive Behavior Scale
vac	vacuum
vacc	vaccinate
vag	vaginal
var	(a) variable; (b) variance
vasc	vascular
vas. dis.	vascular disease
VAT	Visual Action Therapy
VC	(a) vital capacity; (b) color vision; (c) vowel-consonant (words); (d) voluntary closing
VCC	vowel-consonant-consonant (words)
VCF	velocardiofacial syndrome
VCR	videocassette recorder
VD	venereal disease
Vd	voided
VDE	videodeglutition examination
VDG	venereal disease–gonorrhea

VDRL	Venereal Disease Research Laboratory (test)
VDS	venereal disease, syphilis
VEED	videoendoscopic evaluation of dysphagia
ventr	ventral
VEP	visual evoked potentials
VER	visual evoked response
vert	vertical
ves	vessel
VESS	videoendoscopic swallowing study
vest	vestibular
V.f.	visual field
VFs	vocal folds
VFSS	videofluoroscopic swallowing duty
VHD	valvular heart disease
VIB	volumetric interstitial brachytherapy
vib	vibration
vis	(a) vision; (b) visual; (c) visual improvement service
visc	visceral
Vit	vitamin
vit	vital
vit. cap.	vital capacity
viz	namely
VJ	ventriculojugular (shunt)
VLDL	very low density lipoproteins
VM	(a) vestibular membrane; (b) ventromedial
V.N.A.	Visiting Nurses Association
VO	voluntary opening
V/O	verbal order
VOD	vision right eye
vol	volume
VOS	vision left eye
VOT	voice onset time
VP	(a) venous pressure; (b) velopharyngeal; (c) visual perception
VPC	video positioning chair
VPI	velopharyngeal insufficiency
VPM	ventro-posteromedial
VPOH	very poor oral hygiene
v.p.s.	vibrations per second
VR	(a) vocal resonance; (b) virtual reality
VRT	vocational rehabilitation therapist (therapy)

vs, VS	(a) versus; (b) vital signs
V/S	vital signs
VSS	(a) vital signs stable; (b) visit
VT	ventricular tachycardia
vv	veins
VV	varicose veins
VW	vessel wall
W	(a) White; (b) walker; (c) watt(s)
WA	when awake
WAB	Western Aphasia Battery
WAIS	Wechsler Adult Intelligence Scale
Wass	Wasserman test (for syphilis)
WB	Western blot
WBC	white blood count
WBTT	weight bearing to tolerance
W/C	wheelchair
W & D	warm and dry
WD	well developed
wds	wounds
WF	(a) White female; (b) word fluency (measure)
WFL	within functional limits
wh	white
WHO	(a) World Health Organization; (b) wrist-hand orthosis
whpl	whirlpool
wk	(a) walker; (b) week
WKL	workload
wks	weeks
WL	waiting list
WM	White male
W/M	warm and moist
WMS	Wechsler Memory Scale
WN	well nourished
WNF	well-nourished female
WNL	within normal limits
WNM	well-nourished male
W/O	written orders
w/o	without
wp	(a) wet pack; (b) whirlpool
wr	wrist
WR	Wassermann reaction
wt	weight

w/u	workup
WV	whispered voice
x	(a) axis; (b) times
x3, x4	3 times, 4 times, . . .
x2d, x3d	for 2 days, for 3 days, . . .
XBX	ten basic exercises
XRT	external radiation therapy
yd	yard
yel	yellow
Y/O	years old
YOB	year of birth
yr	year
Z	zero
ZE syn	Zollinger-Ellison syndrome
ZIG	zoster immune globulin
ZN	zinc

SYMBOLS

/	extension
+	(a) positive; (b) plus; (c) excess
+/-	present on one side/absent on the other side
?	questionable
-	(a) negative; (b) minus; (c) deficiency
↑	increase
↓	decrease
✓	flexion
>	greater than
<	less than
≤	less than or equal to
≥	more than or equal to approximate
=	equals
Δ	change
μM	micrometers
μV	microvolt
Mμ	millimicrons
Ω	ohm
//	parallel bars
+	slight trace
+ +	trace
+ + +	moderate amount

+ + + +	large amount
+ reaction	acid reaction
− reaction	alkaline reaction
↑↑	extensor response (Babinske sign)
↓↓	plantar response (Babinske sign)
1x, 2x	one time; two times . . .
o	degree
1°, 2°	primary; secondary . . .
’	foot
″	inch
Δt	time interval
24°	24 hours
#	(a) number; (b) pound; (c) weight; (d) gauge
@	at
:	ratio
::	proportionate to
/	per
♂,□	male
♀,○	female
†	death
*	birth

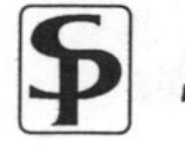

Springer Publishing Company

PERSONALITY AND ADVERSITY

Psychospiritual Aspects of Rehabilitation

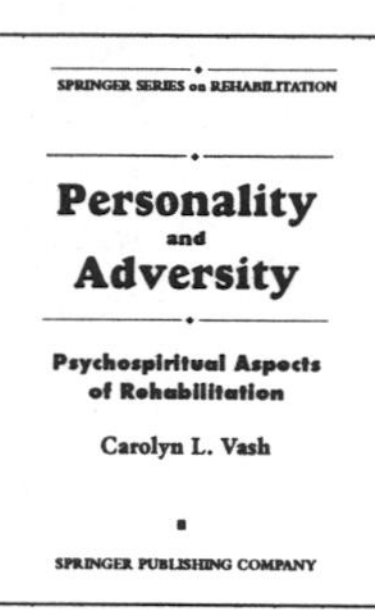

Carolyn L. Vash, PhD

The author of the acclaimed *Psychology of Disability* draws on her own experiences as a person with severe disabilities to bring us her newest textbook, *Personality and Adversity.* The main theme of this new work centers on adversity as a catalyst for pyschospiritual growth. Using her artistic creativity, the author incorporates ideas from philosophy, religion, and art to provide effective strategies for coping with disabilities.

Contents:

Springer Series on Rehabilitation
1994 304pp 0-8261-8040-X hardcover

536 Broadway, New York, NY 10012-3955 • (212) 431-4370 • Fax (212) 941-7842